"Richard Lathe has written a remarkable synthesis of the biomedical evidence relevant to understanding the causes of autism spectrum conditions. As an excellent scientist, he is concerned with achieving an objectivity in his review of a very large number of studies. He draws on evidence from the diverse fields of genetics, endocrinology, immunology, toxicology, virology, and neuroscience, to name just a few.

There are few individuals with his grasp of the basic science who could have pulled off such a masterly review. He balances his theory of environmental (heavy metal toxicity) factors with a recognition of genetic susceptibility factors. His book will be of great value to researchers, as well as to parents or people with an autism spectrum condition, who are interested in a serious summary of the science of autism."

– Simon Baron-Cohen
Professor of Developmental Psychopathology at Cambridge University
and Director of the Autism Research Centre, Cambridge

"This book should be required reading for any practitioner who is involved in treating children with autism spectrum disorders. It is exceptionally well written, logically organized and covers the topic from several interesting angles. If you knew nothing about autism spectrum disorders before you opened this book you would still be able to read it and understand the facts, hypotheses and concerns that are paramount in the recent concern about the cause, effects and possible treatments for these illnesses.

The author does an excellent job presenting the basic research observations from many areas and relevant clinical studies. He also ties these together in an impressive manner. The presentation of the limbic brain structure and dysfunction are very well done, as are the biochemical and physiological explanations. The book is informative, interesting, presents new ideas and is an excellent read."

– Boyd Haley
Professor and Chair, Department of Chemistry, University of Kentucky

Autism, Brain, and Environment

of related interest

Autism – The Search for Coherence
Edited by John Richer and Sheila Coates
ISBN 1 85302 888 6

Asperger's Syndrome
A Guide for Parents and Professionals
Tony Attwood
Foreword by Lorna Wing
ISBN 1 85302 577 1

Children, Youth and Adults with Asperger Syndrome
Integrating Multiple Perspectives
Edited by Kevin P. Stoddart
ISBN 1 84310 319 2

Diet Intervention and Autism
Implementing the Gluten Free and Casein Free Diet for Autistic
Children and Adults – A Practical Guide for Parents
Marilyn Le Breton
Foreword by Rosemary Kessick, Allergy Induced Autism
ISBN 1 85302 935 1

Autism, Brain, and Environment

Richard Lathe

Jessica Kingsley Publishers
London and Philadelphia

First published in 2006
by Jessica Kingsley Publishers
116 Pentonville Road
London N1 9JB, UK
and
400 Market Street, Suite 400
Philadelphia, PA 19106, USA

www.jkp.com

Copyright © Richard Lathe 2006

Library of Congress Cataloging in Publication Data
Lathe, Richard, 1952-
  Autism, brain, and environment / Richard Lathe.
    p. cm.
  Includes bibliographical references and index.
  ISBN-13: 978-1-84310-438-4 (hardback : alk. paper)
    ISBN-10: 1-84310-438-5 (hardback : alk. paper) 1. Autism--Pathophysiology. 2.
Autism--Environmental aspects. I. Title.
  RC553.A88 L38 2006
  616.85'882--dc22
                                2006005650

British Library Cataloguing in Publication Data
A CIP catalogue record for this book is available from the British Library

ISBN-13: 978 1 84310 438 4
ISBN-10: 1 84310 438 5

Printed and bound in the United States by Thomson-Shore, Inc.

For our children

*In remembrance of Jeffrey Gray,
who pointed the way forward*

To L, who taught what it is to be autistic

Contents

List of figures and tables

Preface

This analysis is offered in the hope that it may help to place a new and oddly shaped piece, autism, at its proper place within a much bigger jigsaw puzzle – and one whose ramifications may be far wider than autism spectrum disorders.

The book, originally intended for professionals, has been broadened to make the material accessible to non-specialists – families, medical practitioners, teachers, support workers, psychologists, political/environmental lobbies, and to autistic individuals themselves. Serving these different audiences in a single work is not an easy undertaking, and the assistance of informed readers in this task has been very helpful.

My first encounter with autism, in the child of a close acquaintance, was a surprise and an enigma. A surprise because autism was entirely new to me; my mother taught special needs children for many years but autism was scarcely in evidence. And it was an enigma too – I was intrigued by the striking resemblance between autistic behavior and cases of injury to a specific brain region: the hippocampus and its anatomical extension, the amygdala. Over more than a decade earlier my researches focused on brain genes and biochemistry, dwelling on the hippocampus, this unusual structure toward the center of the brain. Many odd features of autism – the repetitive behavior and anxiety – conspicuously reiterated some common effects of hippocampal damage. The same oddities were seen again and again in other children with autism of varying severity. The question could not be avoided – is the hippocampus somehow involved in autism?

As the investigations advanced, more parallels and overlaps emerged. Epilepsy and even pain insensitivity gave further clues. Then a wealth of evidence emerged that the key brain regions are unusually and exquisitely sensitive to environmental toxicity. There was finally no avoiding the conclusion that the physiological problems seen in autism, including gastrointestinal inflammation with hormone excesses and deficiencies, might reflect damage to just these key brain regions, and could also contribute to such damage – and, if so, perhaps provide a primary focus for medical intervention.

Autism can be a debilitating disorder. Thorough understanding offers hope of remedial therapies that could have a real prospect of ameliorating the condition.

Richard Lathe
Edinburgh, December 2005

Acknowledgements

Sincerest gratitude is owed to John O. Bishop and Caroline Lathe who commented extensively on the majority of the text, and to Ken Aitken, David St. Clair, Anna Lathe, Steve Hillier, and Corinne Skorupka who visited sections of the manuscript with helpful suggestions. Bob Isaacson, Richard Mills, Mike Ludwig, Linda Mullins, John Mullins, Evelyn Tough, Gareth Leng, Steve Hillier, Boyd Haley, William J. Walsh, Jonathan Seckl, John Arthur, Ian Reid, Sofie Dow, John Dean, Robert DeLong, Corinne Skorupka, and Robert Nataf are thanked for their many comments on different aspects of this text, and Simon Baron-Cohen, Robert DeLong, and Dennis P. Hogan for as yet unpublished manuscripts.

The following are gratefully acknowledged for personal communications of new data and ideas: James Adams, Lisa A. Croen, Julia Drew, Dennis Hogan, Wendy Kates, Vlad Kustanovich, Anne McLaren, David St. Clair, Corinne Skorupka, and William J. Walsh. Noburu Komiyama and Yuri Kotelevtsev gave invaluable assistance with translations. All those who granted permission to reproduce published figures and data are gratefully thanked. Staff at the Erskine Medical Library, the British Library, and the National Library of Scotland are thanked for their cheerful and efficient assistance.

Richard Morris is acknowledged for initiation into the world of the limbic brain, Marie-Paule Kieny for advice on vaccines, Mike Ashburner spelled out the importance of fruitflies, Pierre Chambon first pointed to direct hormone effects on the brain, while Richard Grantham introduced me to environmental issues.

Much of my research has been funded over the years by the Biotechnology and Biological Sciences Research Council (BBSRC), the Medical Research Council (MRC), the Wellcome Trust, the Department for Environment, Food and Rural Affairs (DEFRA), and the European Commission (EC-BIOTECH). I am very grateful for their support.

My children Anna, Mhairi, Clémence, James, and Constance have been a source of inspiration and assurance. Without M. McClenaghan and G.H. Lathe this book would not have seen light of day; I am too inarticulate to put it otherwise. True thanks are due to Jessica Kingsley, the publisher, whose perception and support brought this project to completion.

RL

Chapter 1

Introduction

Autism stands out from the crowd. The child seems aloof, a little anxious and withdrawn, preferring to engage in solitary activities rather than to mix in with children of the same age. Some, because of their inward focus and devotion, have extraordinary mastery of facts and figures. For these children, autism is not a disability, rather a different way of looking at the world.

But it is not always like that. A majority of those with autism and related disorders are more seriously affected. "At 12 months Austin began to box his ears at loud noises and cry for no apparent reason." Sometimes with "intermittent rhythmic, repetitive movements of the head and entire body."[1] At 18 months, Austin spoke only a few words (e.g. Mama, Daddy, juice), yet these few words soon disappeared from his speech. Austin's parents were frightened and concerned – his father observed, "I knew that something was different about him. My wife and I were very nervous about bringing him to the evaluation." This is how one autism expert recounts the story of a young subject.[1] The severe type of autism is, unfortunately, the most common.

Even so, the tendency to social withdrawal and self-absorption are features both of high-functioning autism and of this more severe type. This has led many to argue that these are part of a continuum, and the term autistic spectrum disorder[2,3] (or autism spectrum disorder) has entered common parlance.

The specific term "autistic" was introduced in the 1940s by Hans Asperger in Vienna[4,5] and Leo Kanner in Baltimore[6–8] who described the key features of autism for the first time. The use of the word "autism" reflects the unusual self-absorption (*autos* is Greek for self) to the exclusion of others. However, the term had been used earlier – "*Das autistische Denken*"[9] – and this description of a similar if not identical condition probably predated both Kanner and Asperger.[9,10]

Autism and autistic spectrum disorders (ASDs) are now defined by a triad of impairments – in social interaction, in communication including language, and in restricted or repetitive behaviors and activities (the following chapter discusses this in more detail). But the blandness of the "triad" conceals a wealth of paradoxical anomalies and deficits, best illustrated through description of specific children.

The following extracts are taken from a paper by Hauser, DeLong, and Rosman, published in 1975, which presents detailed descriptions of autistic children.[11] The extracts have been paraphrased to illustrate the scope and diversity of the disorder, while underlining a basic commonality. I am indebted to Robert DeLong for permission to reproduce these edited accounts.

> Child JS, 3½ years. Early developmental milestones were normal or advanced. He said "mama" and "bye bye" at 11 months but failed thereafter to develop more speech. Behavioral difficulties were first noted after age 2½ years. He became increasingly hyperactive with a notably short attention span. He came to occupy himself with purposeless and often repetitive activities such as turning a light switch on and off, and watching running water or spinning objects. By age 3½ years his vocabulary had increased to an estimated 75 words, but much of his speech remained unclear. The mother thought he had lost some words previously known but used infrequently. He appeared not to know the names of colors. No knowledge of numbers could be demonstrated. He could not count. He grasped a pencil crudely and scribbled busily, but was unable to copy a circle. There were several behavioral peculiarities: preoccupation with sameness; fascination with objects such as bright lights and rotating bicycle wheels.

> Child HFJ. 6 years old. The boy's behavior was always characterized by a marked lack of emotional or affective response and a paucity of social interaction. He was, in addition, hyperactive, self-mutilating, destructive, and ritualistic. He turned switches on and off and ate ravenously.

> Child NZ. At 4½ years she often sat alone, shaking her hands in front of her. She was hyperactive, hyper-exploratory, and hypersensitive to loud noises. She would line things up and was obsessed with wrist watches and with a particular old hat that she always wore. She had no recognizable speech, but rather uttered primitive sounds seemingly unrelated to words. She could copy a straight line but not a circle.

> Her first seizure was noted at age 2 years and 9 months. Three further seizures, each associated with fever and apparent bronchitis, occurred during the next six months. After a period in hospital, she had become almost uncontrollably hyperactive. In a world of her own, she made no social contacts and established no eye contact. She had no purposeful activity but would pick up objects randomly and put them in her mouth.

> Child PK, 5 years. Speech: age 15 months, "mama"; age 4, mute but good comprehension of language. He now identifies objects, colors, numbers. Affection-

ate, playful with family. When left alone turns violent, destructive, hits head; helps in house, watches television, dances to music, fascinated with water.

Child AP. At 2 years old, affectionate and responsive; but became unresponsive, lost eye contact, screamed when touched; now, at age 11, she recognizes people and gestures. Extremely obsessive, lines things up, preserves sameness in environment; pain-insensitive.

Child DC. A boy aged 3 years and 7 months. Ignores all people but does cry when mother leaves. Hyperactive, aimless, hyper-exploratory; temper tantrums, bangs head and screams, rocks head for hours; bizarre gait, walks on toes.

Child LB. At 2 years and 5 months, this girl wanders aimlessly, ignoring people and toys; flaps hands, bangs arms, makes clicking sound with mouth; insensitive to pain; will remain in awkward position without moving; constant writhing movements of fingers with loss of use of hands for all purposeful activity.

These cases, all quite severely affected, illustrate the diversity of impairments. The failure to acquire language, or loss of words already learned, is a key feature; others include the lack of interaction with peers and family and eye-contact avoidance. Regarding repetitive activities, Rapin[1] recounts that the most common stereotypy is flapping the hands, but rocking, pacing, jumping, twiddling the fingers, shaking a string, and many others are frequent.

Rapin[1] also notes other puzzling features of these children: "Squinting, looking out of the corner of the eyes, gaze aversion, staring at the shadows of waving fingers, smelling food and people, gagging on chocolate pudding, and craving pretzels are other paradoxical sensory responses." She observes: "It is not clear whether infants who stiffen and arch their backs when you want to cuddle them are demonstrating heightened tactile sensitivity or social aversion."[1]

These studies amply illustrate the enormously debilitating nature of severe childhood autism, both for the child and the family. The lifelong forecast for a child with such impairments, without appropriate treatment, is generally held to be poor.

There have been, nevertheless, many suggestions that marked improvement is possible. Boy JS described above, at 3½ years of age, was severely impaired: he produced only a few utterances, mostly unintelligible single words. He named a "kitty-kat" from a picture book but did not name a dog, a car, a wagon. He had a greater interest in objects than in people; total lack of play with other children, coupled with a tendency to hit or strike them unpredictably; and poor attention span.[11] But, by 7½ years, there had been dramatic improvement in the area of interpersonal contacts. He was now quite sociable and initiated conversation. By age 8½ years his speech was improved. When last seen at age 11 years, his language had improved further. "He spoke openly of his concerns regarding his difficulties."[11]

Austin, the child first discussed here, by 8 years has also improved. "He enjoys riding his bicycle, bowling with his father, and playing with his mother. His parents wonder if there are any new effective medications for symptoms of autism and if there will ever be a cure."[1]

Kaufman provides a description of another boy who, by all accounts, was markedly impaired in childhood. By adulthood he had fully recovered functionality in all areas,[12] and was able to lecture on his experience. Unfortunately, such cases of full recovery are the exception. Most individuals with autism, especially those most seriously affected, will depend on lifetime care from family and community.

Jarbrink and Knapp[13] estimate the average lifetime cost (2001) for a person with autism at £2.4 million (4.1 million US dollars), primarily reflecting the need for full-time care, medical assistance, and speech and education therapists. The figures are generally accepted to be underestimates.[14]

The total per year cost to the UK was put at one billion pounds, based on a prevalence of just 5 per 10,000. Rates now are ten-fold above that, pushing the UK cost to £10 billion (17 billion US dollars). When extrapolated to the USA with a population of just over 290 million, in comparison to the UK's figure of nearly 60 million inhabitants, the yearly cost to the USA rises to 84 billion dollars, much the same as for hurricane Katrina, and every year.

Other major disorders, including cancer, diabetes, and hypertension, differ from autism in that onset is much later in life. Many with these conditions are able to lead productive lives despite their ongoing medical problem, and can look after themselves. Only Alzheimer disease and senile dementia come close to autism in their dependence on constant help from others, and these are diseases of the elderly. Autism is unusual in that onset is in the earliest years of life, and lifelong dependence is often the result. Therefore, autism is clearly among the most worrying of all conditions, particularly because the rates in children appear to be rising steadily.

Therapeutic intervention in severe autism is essential, and to this end an understanding of the condition and its causes is required. This book looks critically at the different features of autism and autistic spectrum disorders, focusing on diagnostic criteria, the genetic contribution, and the rise in prevalence. It then moves to a detailed treatment of the brain regions involved, and whether early brain damage can explain the deficits seen in autism.

The second half of the book dwells on the likely contribution of the environment, and emphasizes the fact that subjects with autism have a diverse set of physiological impairments in addition to their psychological and cognitive difficulties. Many practitioners treating autism over the last 30 years resist the view that there is any significant physiological dysregulation, but recent evidence now contradicts that position. It is argued here that environmental toxicity in concert with this physiological dysregulation combine to exacerbate damage to key brain regions.

A further objective of this book is to dispel the view, perhaps still too prevalent, that psychological/psychiatric disorders are somehow separate, distinct, and immune from the physiological dysregulation(s) they can both produce and be exacerbated by.

The final thrust is to argue that therapy of autism and related disorders should focus on biomedical rectification of environmental toxicity and physiological problems. Though focused on ASD in the first instance, there are important ramifications for other brain disorders including anxiety, attention deficit, cerebral palsy, epilepsy, Alzheimer, and schizophrenia. Only with thorough understanding of the specific biochemical and physiological deficits, rather than focusing on purely behavioral abnormalities, can one hope to prevent, ameliorate, or even cure the behavioral deficiencies that cause such distress to affected children and their families.

Chapter 2

Autism and Autism Spectrum Disorders: An Introduction to the Problem of Recognition and Diagnosis

Autism is difficult to describe, though trained clinicians say it is as distinctive as a sunset or a symphony. Some disorders are easily defined by markers, such as the extra chromosome found in Down syndrome. Others can be ascertained by numerical values: for example, of blood pressure in the assessment of hypertension, or of blood sugar in diabetes. No essential markers have yet been identified in autism, and none may exist. Instead the criteria for autism are now widely accepted to involve anomalies in three central categories, known as the triad of impairments, as set out by Wing and Gould:[1]

- deficits or marked abnormalities in social interaction
- deficits or marked abnormalities in communication including language
- restricted and often repetitive behavioral repertoires, interests, and activities.

Of course, many childhood problems meet one or more of these criteria, and the experienced physician relies on other clues to venture a precise diagnosis of autism rather than another disorder. For instance, an unusual enjoyment of spinning objects, flapping movements of the hands, an intriguing fixation on the sense of smell – with newcomers being greeted with a sniff rather than a "hello" – are all seen in autism. But these features are difficult to quantify. And, though described and discussed, such as in the work of Gillberg and Coleman,[2] only a proportion of children labeled as being autistic show such specific behaviors. The borderline between autism and the "normal" range of behaviors is blurred, particularly in less severely affected children.

Pervasive developmental disorders

The term autism is now associated with a range of conditions collectively known as pervasive developmental disorders, or PDDs. "Pervasive" indicates that many different areas of development are involved, not merely speech or communication. As defined (see below), PDDs include autism proper (often termed autistic disorder or autistic syndrome to distinguish it from the larger grouping) and Asperger syndrome, as well as PDD-NOS (not otherwise specified), Rett syndrome, and childhood disintegrative disorder (CDD). Autistic disorder (autism proper) and PDD-NOS are the most common, Asperger represents a small fraction of cases, while Rett and CDD are very rare (see Figure 2.1). The

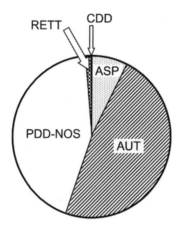

Figure 2.1 Pervasive developmental disorders. Approximate proportions of different diagnostic groups within the DSM-IV diagnostic grouping. The fractions presented are the averages given in two different recent studies[4,5] and do not address temporal changes in diagnosis or prevalence rates. AUT, autistic disorder; PDD-NOS, pervasive developmental disorder, not otherwise specified; RETT, Rett disorder; CDD, childhood disintegrative disorder; ASP, Asperger disorder. The latter review (Tidmarsh and Volkmar[4]) is based on data collated by Fombonne[6,7] and recently revised,[8] building on several larger prior studies such as that of Baird et al.[9] These reports concur that rates of autistic disorder and PDD-NOS are not dissimilar (but with perhaps a slight excess of PDD-NOS), Asperger represents a small fraction of all cases, while CDD and Rett are very rare indeed. Despite subtle differences in diagnostic criteria, the relative proportions according to DSM-IV and ICD-10 are comparable.

inclusion of quasi-similar conditions – ranging from severe impairment to specific performance elevation – has led to the introduction of the term "autism spectrum disorder" (ASD) to reflect this diversity.[2,3] ASD and PDD are seen as synonyms in much of the autism literature.

Rigorous definition of these disorders is provided by two authorities. The World Health Organization publishes an International Classification of Diseases, the most recent issue being ICD-10,[10] while the American Psychiatric Association provides a Diagnostic and Statistical Manual of Mental Disorders, the current edition being DSM-IV.[11] These are not exactly identical; parallels and differences are shown in Table 2.1.

Both DSM-IV and ICD-10 recognize a disorder similar to autism but which fails to meet the precise diagnostic criteria for autistic disorder. This variant autism is termed "Pervasive developmental disorder – not otherwise specified" by the DSM-IV. This equates to the condition "atypical autism" in ICD-10. Both systems recognize the late age of onset in this atypical autism, but whereas DSM-IV speaks of atypical or sub-threshold (mild) symptoms, ICD-10 states that it may be characterized by severe retardation and language impairment.

A further difference is the inclusion in ICD-10 of some rarer conditions including overactive disorder with mental retardation and stereotyped movements.

A large number of disorders are superficially similar to autism and ASDs but are not included in the definition of PDDs. For completeness many of these are summarized in Table 2.2 (ICD-10), noting the inclusion of attention deficit disorder (F90.0 ADD) and attention deficit with hyperactivity (F98.8 ADHD) whose definitions overlap with an ASD condition (F84.4 overactive disorder with mental retardation, also characterized by hyperactivity and inattention).

PDDs including autism are generally far more common in males than in females (see Chapters 3 and 4), but some have questioned whether girls with the same underlying disorder might present with a subtly different clinical picture. The exact male-to-female ratio depends on severity, as discussed later, with more boys than girls displaying a milder form of the disorder. It is possible that girls with "mild autism" are not recognized as having any impairment, or indeed have an impairment that fails the specific criteria for autism.[12]

In modern diagnostic manuals autism is grouped alongside Asperger, a far less debilitating condition with superior abilities in some individuals. Even so, it has been argued that Asperger's may be wholly distinct from autism and should not be considered to be a mild form of autism.[13] Others suggest that Asperger syndrome is really not a separate entity and most Asperger patients are in fact autistic.[14] The debate continues.

Table 2.1 DSM-IV and ICD-10 criteria for pervasive developmental disorders, otherwise known as autism spectrum disorders (Gillberg and Coleman;[2] Wing[3]). All characteristics and definitions have been abridged. * Indicates a significant discrepancy between the two systems of classification. ICD-10 specific criteria are not specified where they are similar to DSM-IV

DSM-IV criteria, pervasive developmental disorders	*ICD-10 pervasive developmental disorders*
Characterized by severe and pervasive impairment in several areas of development: reciprocal social interaction skills, communication skills, or the presence of stereotyped behavior, interests, and activities. The qualitative impairments that define these conditions are distinctively deviant relative to the individual's developmental level or mental age.	Defined by abnormalities in reciprocal social interactions, patterns of communication, and by a restricted, stereotyped, repetitive repertoire of interests and activities. These are a pervasive feature of the individual's functioning.
299.00 Autistic disorder	**F84.0 Childhood autism**
Impaired social interaction	· impaired non-verbal behaviors (eye gaze, expression, postures, and gestures) · peer relationships impaired · failure to initiate social contact, lack of social or emotional reciprocity	Impairment of reciprocal social interaction
Impairments in communication	· impaired spoken language and communication · impaired initiation/ maintenance of conversation · stereotyped/repetitive language · deficit in symbolic or imaginative play/social play	Impairments of communication
Repetitive/ stereotyped activities	· preoccupation with restricted interest · adherence to routines or rituals · stereotyped/repetitive actions	Restricted, stereotyped, repetitive behavior

Continued on next page

Table 2.1 cont.

DSM-IV criteria, pervasive developmental disorders		ICD-10 pervasive developmental disorders	
299.00 Autistic disorder		**F84.0 Childhood autism**	
Onset prior to age 3 years*		Impaired development before the age of 2 years*	
		Other common features:	• phobias, sleeping and eating disturbances, temper tantrums, and (self-directed) aggression
299.80 Pervasive developmental disorder – not otherwise specified (PDD-NOS)		**F84.1 Atypical autism**	
Any of the specified impairments:	• reciprocal social interaction • or communication skills • or stereotyped activities	Impairments as specified	
But do not meet the criteria for autistic disorder in view of:	• late age of onset, or • atypical symptomatology, or • subthreshold symptomatology*	But late age of onset or do not fulfill all diagnostic criteria	• e.g. impairments only after age 3 years, or • failing to fulfill all three diagnostic criteria • most often with severe retardation and language impairment*
299.80 Asperger disorder		**F84.5 Asperger syndrome**	
Impairment in social interaction	• use of non-verbal behaviors, e.g. eye-to-eye gaze, facial expression, posture, and gestures • impaired peer relationships • lack of spontaneous social sharing • lack of social or emotional reciprocity	Social interaction impairment as in autism	

Restricted, repetitive, activities	• preoccupation with stereotyped/restricted patterns of interest • adherence to non-functional routines or rituals • stereotyped/repetitive motor mannerisms • preoccupation with parts of objects	Restricted, stereotyped, repetitive interests and activities

299.80 Asperger disorder

Significant impairment in social/occupational etc. function

Differs from autism:	• no delay in language • no delay in cognitive development other than in social interaction	

F84.5 Asperger syndrome

Differs from autism:	• no general delay or retardation in language or in cognitive development • often marked clumsiness

299.80 Rett disorder

Normal early development	
Regression:	• deceleration of head growth between ages 5 and 48 months • loss of hand skills at 5–30 months • development of stereotyped hand movements

Early loss of social engagement

Poorly coordinated gait or trunk movements

Impaired expressive and receptive language development

Psychomotor retardation

F84.2 Rett syndrome

Normal early development	
Followed by loss of:	• only in girls; onset usually between 7 and 24 months of age • speech, locomotion skills, hand use, deceleration in head growth • hand-wringing stereotypies and hyperventilation are characteristic • mental retardation commonly follows

Continued on next page

Table 2.1 cont.

DSM-IV criteria, pervasive developmental disorders	ICD-10 pervasive developmental disorders
299.10 Childhood disintegrative disorder	**F84.3 Other childhood disintegrative disorder**
Normal development for 2 years	Normal early development
Loss of previously acquired skills before age 10 in some of the following: · expressive or receptive language · social skills or adaptive behavior · bowel or bladder control · play · motor skills	Loss of previously acquired skills
Subsequently: · impaired social interaction · impairments in communication (e.g. language delay, impairment in initiation/maintenance of conversation) · repetitive/stereotyped activities including motor stereotypies	Typically with: · loss of interest in the environment · stereotyped, repetitive motor mannerisms · autistic-like abnormalities in social interaction and communication
	F84.4 Overactive disorder associated with mental retardation and stereotyped movements · children with severe mental retardation (IQ below 35) · hyperactivity and inattention · stereotyped behaviors
	F84.8 Other pervasive developmental disorders
	F84.9 Pervasive developmental disorder, unspecified

Table 2.2 Other disorders (ICD-10) potentially overlapping with ASD

I. Mental and behavioral disorders (F00–F99)

F70–79. Mental retardation

Poor mental development, impaired skills manifested during the developmental period, skills contributing to cognitive, language, motor, and social abilities

F90–F98. Behavioral and emotional disorders with onset usually occurring in childhood and adolescence

F90. Hyperkinetic disorders	• Early onset (usually in the first five years of life); lack of persistence; tendency to move from one activity to another; disorganized and excessive activity
	• Often reckless, impulsive, disciplinary issues trouble because of unthinking breaches of rules (rather than deliberate defiance); socially disinhibited
	• Common impairment of cognitive functions; frequent delays in motor and language development
F90.0 Disturbance of activity and attention	• Attention deficit disorder with hyperactivity
F90.1 Hyperkinetic conduct disorder	• Hyperkinetic disorder associated with conduct disorder
F91. Conduct disorders	• Repetitive, persistent, dissocial, aggressive, or defiant conduct
F91.1 Unsocialized conduct disorder	• Persistent dissocial or aggressive behavior
	• Pervasive abnormalities in relationships with peers
F91.2 Socialized conduct disorder	• Disorder involving persistent dissocial or aggressive behavior
F91.3 Oppositional defiant disorder	• Usually occurring in younger children
	• Defiant, disobedient, disruptive behavior
	• Does not include delinquent acts

Continued on next page

Table 2.2 cont.

F92 Mixed disorders of conduct and emotions	• Aggressive, dissocial, or defiant behavior with depression, anxiety, or other emotional upsets
F92.0 Depressive conduct disorder	• Conduct disorder (F91) with depression of mood (F32)
F92.8 Other mixed disorders of conduct and emotions	• Conduct disorder (F91) with emotional symptoms, e.g. anxiety, obsessions or compulsions, depersonalization or derealization, phobias, or hypochondriasis
F93 Emotional disorders with onset specific to childhood	• Exaggerations of normal developmental trends; the key diagnostic feature regards developmental appropriateness
F93.2 Social anxiety disorder of childhood	• Apprehension or anxiety in new or socially threatening situations. Used only where such fears arise during the early years
F94. Disorders of social functioning with onset specific to childhood and adolescence	• Abnormalities in social functioning with onset during the developmental period, but which (unlike PDD) are without social incapacity or pervasive deficit. Environmental distortions may play a role in etiology
F94.0 Elective mutism	• Selectively in speaking: language competence in some situations but failure to speak in other (definable) situations • Usually associated with social anxiety, withdrawal, sensitivity, or resistance
F94.1 Reactive attachment disorder of childhood	• Onset in first five years • Anomalous social relationships associated with emotional disturbance • Reactive to environmental circumstances (e.g. fearfulness and hypervigilance, poor social interaction with peers, aggression towards self and others, misery, and growth failure in some cases)
F94.2 Disinhibited attachment disorder of childhood	• Onset in first five years • Anomalous social functioning • Non-selectively focused attachment behavior • Attention-seeking • Indiscriminately friendly behavior • Poorly modulated peer interactions

F95 Tic disorders	• Syndromes in which the predominant manifestation is some form of tic (involuntary, rapid, recurrent, non-rhythmic motor movement or vocal production of sudden onset and without apparent purpose). Exacerbated by stress; disappear during sleep
	
	Examples: • Repetitive gestures, facial grimacing
	               • Vocal tics
	               • Complex: hitting oneself, jumping, and hopping

F98 Other behavioral and emotional disorders with onset usually occurring in childhood and adolescence	• With childhood onset, differ from other conditions and often associated with psychosocial problems
F98.4 Stereotyped movement disorders	• Repetitive, stereotyped, non-functional movements • Non self-injurious: body-rocking, head-rocking, hair-plucking, hair-twisting, finger-flicking mannerisms, and hand-flapping • Self-injurious: banging, face-slapping, eye-poking, and biting of hands, lips, or other body parts • Most frequently in association with mental retardation
F98.8 Other specified behavioral and emotional disorders with onset usually occurring in childhood and adolescence	• Attention deficit disorder without hyperactivity

F00–F09. Organic, including symptomatic, mental disorders

F06.7 Mild cognitive disorder	• Impairment of memory, learning difficulties, and reduced ability to concentrate on a task for more than brief periods. Often a feeling of mental fatigue • Only recognized in association with a specified physical disorder. May precede, accompany, or follow a wide variety of infections and physical disorders, both cerebral and systemic • Restricted range of generally mild symptoms, usually shorter duration

Continued on next page

Table 2.2 cont.

F50–F59 Behavioral syndromes associated with physiological disturbances and physical factors

F54 Psychological and behavioral factors associated with disorders or diseases classified elsewhere	• Psychological or behavioral influences playing a major part in the etiology of physical disorders. Usually mild mental disturbances, often prolonged (e.g. worry, emotional conflict, apprehension) • Psychological factors affecting physical conditions
	Examples of the use of this category are: • Asthma F54 and J45 • Dermatitis F54 and L23–L25 • Gastric ulcer F54 and K25 • Mucous colitis F54 and K58 • Ulcerative colitis F54 and K51 • Urticaria F54 and L50

F80–F89. Disorders of psychological development

	(a) Onset invariably during infancy or childhood; (b) delayed development/maturation of the central nervous system; (c) a steady course without remissions and relapses. In most cases, the functions affected include language, visuo-spatial skills, and motor coordination. Usually, impairment present from earliest ages, may diminish progressively with age
F84. Pervasive developmental disorders	See Table 2.1
F80 Specific developmental disorders of speech and language	• Disturbed language acquisition from the early stages of development. Not directly attributable to neurological or speech mechanism abnormalities, sensory impairments, mental retardation, or environmental factors. Often followed by difficulties in reading and spelling, abnormalities in interpersonal relationships, emotional and behavioral disorders
F80.0 Specific speech articulation disorder	• Use of speech sounds below mental age, but in which there is a normal level of language skills
	Examples: • Phonological disorder • Speech articulation disorder • Dyslalia • Functional speech articulation disorder • See also aphasia NOS (R47.0) and apraxia (R48.2)

F80.1 Expressive language disorder	· Use of expressive language below mental age; language comprehension within normal limits. Sometimes with abnormalities in articulation
F80.2 Receptive language disorder	· Understanding of language below mental age. Expressive language is usually affected, abnormalities in word-sound production are common
F80.3 Acquired aphasia with epilepsy [Landau-Kleffner]	· Onset usually between the ages of 3 and 7 years. Loss of receptive and expressive language skills after a period of normal language development, general intelligence retained. Onset accompanied by paroxysmal EEG abnormalities, also with epileptic seizures in a majority. May be due to an inflammatory encephalitic process. About two-thirds of patients are left with a receptive language deficit

II. Symptoms and signs involving speech and voice (R47–R49)

R47 Speech disturbances, not elsewhere classified

R47.0 Dysphasia and aphasia

R47.8 Other and unspecified speech disturbances

R48 Dyslexia and other symbolic dysfunctions, not elsewhere classified

R48.0 Dyslexia and alexia

R48.1 Agnosia

R48.2 Apraxia

In a careful follow-up, Hippler and Klicpera[15] analyzed the original records of Hans Asperger[16] in Vienna and reported that, according to modern (DSM-IV) criteria, the majority of his subjects would have been categorized as having Asperger syndrome and only 25% as having autism proper. However, the authors of this work stated that "current ICD-10 and DSM-IV criteria for Asperger's do not quite capture the individuals originally described by Asperger and his team," and continue: "they appear to differentiate Asperger's from autism solely based on the onset criteria, regardless of the patient's social impairment later in life."[15]

Specifically they note that Hans Asperger's study group was selected from upper strata of Viennese society, with almost one-third of the fathers and a quarter of the mothers having a university degree, a rather unrepresentative selection of the population.

In contrast, the children studied by Kanner[17–19] in Baltimore at the same time seem to be more typical of severe autism (autistic disorder). Kanner noted at the time that the condition he was observing was something new and distinct from previously described disorders.

A diagnosis of ASD is not exclusive, and autism and ASDs are commonly seen in association with other disorders.[20] These include mental retardation – a majority of children with classic autism have marked impairment of intellectual performance, with IQ ratings under 70. Other disturbances include anxiety, sensory (sight, hearing, pain) disturbances (with increased or diminished sensitivity), and psychological depression. Epilepsy is very common, affecting one-quarter to one-third of subjects, and other physiological disturbances including gastrointestinal problems are often encountered. Therefore, further assessment is warranted even when a primary diagnosis has been provided.

Gillberg and Coleman[2] state that many individuals with autism meet fully the diagnostic criteria for attention deficit hyperactivity disorder (ADHD), but are at pains to note that "associated problems – not the core diagnostic symptoms – can be those that cause the most suffering."

There is also a diagnostic dilemma when ASD arises in later life. Both DSM-IV and ICD-10 restrict the diagnosis of autism proper to cases where onset is early (at or before age 2–3 years) and refer to PDD-NOS or atypical autism when onset is later on. When previously acquired skills are lost both systems refer to childhood disintegrative disorder (CDD) – typically the symptoms are of autism, but involve loss of social skills and language taking place before age 10 under DSM-IV (see Table 2.1).

Case reports describe onset of typical autism at 11 or 14 years of age following herpes simplex encephalitis.[21,22] A further report was of a previously healthy man who contracted herpes encephalitis at the age of 31 years: over the following months he developed all the symptoms considered diagnostic of autism.[23] The diagnostic criteria would seem to exclude these subjects, even though the impairments are, as far as one can tell, identical. Nevertheless, these reports do underscore the conclusion that specific brain damage can underlie autistic behavior.

Early diagnosis

Concerns regarding proper development are most commonly expressed by parents and carers at the age of 2–3 years, but there are many earlier signs. In children later becoming autistic, behavioral signs are already seen in the first year of life. Because intervention is likely to be of most benefit if implemented at the earliest possible opportunity, researchers have sought to produce easily applied methods for use in the youngest children.

Baird, Cass, and Slonims[24] give a useful breakdown of the earliest key features, noting lack of "babble," or pointing, or other gestures, and lack of imitation or spontaneous showing and sharing of toys with others. Filipek et al.[25] recommend intensive evaluation if the child fails to meet any one of several developmental milestones – babbling (12 months), gesturing (12 months), single spoken words (16 months), two-word phrases (24 months), or loss of language or social skills at any age.

The Checklist for Autism in Toddlers, or CHAT, devised by Baron-Cohen and colleagues[9] in the UK, puts to the parent a number of key questions such as "Does your child ever use his/her index finger to point, to *ask* for something?" or "Does your child ever bring objects over to you (parent) to *show* you something?" For the physician there are further simple questions: "Point across the room at an interesting object and say: 'Oh look, there's a [name of toy]' – watch the child's face. Does the child look across to see what you are pointing at?"

This very useful test has, with modifications and updates devised by researchers across the world, been very successful in identifying children with autism and related disorders. Baron-Cohen and colleagues point out, however, that many children who fail the test on first trial are cleared on retesting.

Sixteen thousand children aged 18 months were screened with CHAT, and then retested with more conventional methods at between 3 and 5 years of age. The original CHAT screen identified 19 cases of autism, but follow-up revealed a total of 50 cases of childhood autism.[9] Thus the sensitivity of the CHAT was less than 50%, though the specificity was good – 98% of children scoring positive were confirmed to be autistic.

Like CHAT itself, the modified checklist "M-CHAT" (devised by Robins and colleagues[26] in the USA) has been shown to be powerful. In a follow-up study[27] 4200 children earmarked by primary care services as being at risk were screened, revealing 236 as "positives" on the M-CHAT. These were followed up with intensive evaluation with other accepted tests including DSM-IV. Of the 236 children, 165 were found to have an autism spectrum disorder, 67 had a developmental impairment that was ruled to be distinct from autism, and only four were found to be false positives, and were in fact developing normally.[27] This puts the accuracy of the test for all developmental disorders at better than 95%, and of these a majority were ASD. It was felt that few children with neurodevelopmental problems went undiagnosed.

More intensive and accurate diagnostic instruments are available for the slightly older child. These include the Autism Diagnostic Interview – Revised (ADI-R) and the Autism Diagnostic Observation Schedule – Generic (ADOS-G).

ADI-R[28] is based on DSM-IV and ICD-10, focuses on the triad of impairments, and relies on responses to a questionnaire from parents and carers. Reliability as assessed by repeat rating by an independent evaluator was over 90%. ADOS-G[29] is a structured evaluation of social interaction, communication, and play – consisting of several modules, each of which is attuned to different levels of development and language use, and is therefore applicable to both language-impaired infants and adults with fluency. Specificity and sensitivity, distinguishing autistic disorder and PDD-NOS from non-ASD conditions, were excellent. Other common instruments include the somewhat older CARS (Childhood Autism Rating Scale)[30] that also can distinguish between autism and PDD-NOS.[31]

Autism, a preferred diagnosis?

A later chapter discusses evidence for a rise in the rates of autism and ASDs, but one major complicating factor is that autism might be preferred by clinicians and families over other diagnoses. With the success of the film *Rain Man*, depicting a high-performing and talented individual with a disorder on the autistic spectrum, the term autism does not share the unfortunate and unwarranted negative connotations of terms such as mental retardation.

It does seem that there may be a preference for autism as a diagnosis. A population-based survey of California birth cohorts recorded an increase in the rates of autism diagnosis at the same time as the rate of mental retardation declined by approximately the same amount.[32] Nevertheless, as will be debated, this is not the whole story; indeed another study across the USA found no concomitant decrease in the separate categories of mental retardation or speech and language impairment,[33] while ASD continued to rise.

The broader phenotype

Many observers, going back to Hans Asperger, have noted that close relatives of autistic subjects often have mild behavioral anomalies surprisingly reminiscent of autism.[15] Other disorders of brain and behavior, dubbed the "broader phenotype,"[34] are somewhat more frequent in family members of ASD subjects.[35-38] While this has important implications when we come to consider the genetic contribution to autism and ASDs (Chapter 3), it does also emphasize that autism is not a precisely defined condition with a specific cut-off point. Practitioners may disagree about the diagnosis of many subjects, and the deficits of many will not be sufficiently pronounced to warrant any diagnosis, even though some subtle behavioral idiosyncrasies are apparent. At the other end of the spectrum, the severest forms of autism may be categorized as non-specific mental retardation or general brain impairment such as cerebral palsy, and not ASD, even though the underlying biochemical, genetic, and physiological causes could be the same.

Is there really such a thing as autism? Subtypes

Each individual is different. A major effort will be needed to subtype ASDs according to physiological rather than psychological parameters.[39-41] This provides a formidable obstacle to the analyst, particularly when intrusive methods of investigation are employed, such as blood sampling or brain scanning – techniques that require active cooperation. Many ASD children find it impossible to keep still for more than a moment; the idea of lying motionless in a brain scanner for ten minutes an anathema. For some, even a visit to a general practitioner for routine evaluation can be a logistic nightmare for the parents. This means, of course, that when we speak of hormone levels in ASD children, or brain measurements, we run the risk of looking at selective subsets, perhaps skewed toward the more mildly affected.

Despite efforts to adopt uniform diagnostic instruments and methods, there will be local variations – what one research team regards as atypical autism (and excluded from study) is included in other studies. Literature reports sometimes refer to autism, other times to the autistic spectrum, and these published studies may therefore not be strictly comparable. To give an example, one research paper (not cited) refers to autistic spectrum disorders in the title, but in the details of the methods it is revealed that the majority of the subjects were Asperger and a minority were high-functioning autism. Verbal IQ scores were above average and they were keen participants in demanding tests. The authors worried: "it is unclear how applicable these results are to lower-functioning autistic individuals."

Many reports do not explicitly recognize other conditions that go along with autism – frequently investigators present no data on whether their subjects have other difficulties such as epilepsy or gastrointestinal problems, both common in ASD children, and which potentially could complicate interpretation.

Nevertheless, a start must be made. There are, one hopes, sufficient common features between autism and related spectrum disorders to allow comparison and meaningful consolidation of the evidence. For simplicity, and to avoid chopping and changing, this book employs the term autistic spectrum disorder,[2,3] (ASD) to denote the group of related PDDs. Most subjects studied fall into the categories of autistic disorder (autism proper) or PDD-NOS, with Asperger disorder a further subgroup; specific rarer disorders (such as Rett) are only discussed where they are particularly informative.

There is something called autism, but what is it? As we will perhaps see later in this book, once one turns to brain and biochemistry, the classification and understanding of ASDs subtly begins to change, offering hope for new therapeutic interventions.

Key points

Autism and related disorders represent a spectrum of abilities; the term autism spectrum disorder (ASD) is often used to denote the grouping of pervasive developmental disorders (PDDs).

Autism spectrum disorders, or PDDs, are subdivided into autistic disorder, Asperger disorder, PDD-NOS (not otherwise specified), Rett, and childhood disintegrative disorder (CDD).

The majority of ASD cases are either autistic disorder or PDD-NOS. Asperger represents less than 10%, while Rett and CDD are very rare.

ASD is more common in boys than in girls.

Two diagnostic systems are used currently – ICD-10 (Europe) and DSM-IV (USA) – that are similar but not quite identical.

Many ASD subjects suffer from other disorders including anxiety, sensory disturbances, and epilepsy.

Behavioral signs are commonly seen in the first year of life; early diagnosis is important.

Chapter 3

Genetic Contribution to Autistic Spectrum Disorders: Diversity and Insufficiency

There is strong evidence that genes underpin autism and autistic spectrum disorders. In other words, ASD only develops in susceptible children – and the susceptibility is dictated by particular gene variants (alleles) or combinations of variants. One task for modern genetic research is to identify these genes, with the hope that they might possibly indicate therapies or even preventative measures. However, this area is fraught with difficulty, not least the conclusion that the data clearly distinguish ASD from single-gene conditions like cystic fibrosis or sickle-cell anemia, and point away from an "autism gene" that might underpin most ASD cases.

Genetic predisposition to ASD

The clearest line of evidence for a genetic predisposition comes from studying close relatives of subjects with ASD. Twins are particularly informative. Studies on identical (monozygotic, MZ) twins, where one is affected by ASD, show that most of the other co-twins have the same condition, i.e. are concordant. An early study put concordance at well over 60% in MZ twins, while there was no concordance (0%) between non-identical (dizygotic, DZ) twin pairs.[1] Generally, monozygotic concordance in ASD exceeds dizygotic concordance by a large margin,[1-4] as reviewed.[5]

The exact definition of ASD clearly plays a role. When a broader definition was adopted, monozygotic concordance was 92% versus 10% in non-identical pairs.[4]

Looking more widely, it has been reported that close relatives of subjects with autism have an elevated frequency of Asperger and schizo-affective and anxiety disorders.[6-9] Thus, the genetic risk factors for ASD may extend to other brain conditions that are diagnostically distinct. In Hans Asperger's original study group of "autistic" subjects (roughly one-quarter autistic disorder and the majority Asperger disorder) his notes record that in the majority of cases there was a resemblance between the subject and one or more family members – fathers (52%) were reported as having a similar (odd, aloof, or "nervous") personality with some deviant behaviors or low social competence.[10]

A second line of evidence comes from the finding that far more boys are affected than girls. Consistently across the published literature the incidence of autism is higher in males than in females. One study put the male to female ratio at 2.6 to 1,[11] another at 4.1 to 1.[12] A more recent estimate reports an average male–female ratio of 3.8:1.[13] The excess of males suggests that the sex chromosomes play a part in establishing the risk of ASD development.

Despite a bias toward males, when only severely affected subjects are considered the ratio changes markedly. One early study[14] found a *higher* proportion of females with an IQ below 34. The male–female ratio diminished in more severely affected children,[15] and declined to 2.1 to 1 when only markedly affected individuals were included.[11] This means, in effect, that for severe disablement the split is less in favor of males.

Given the overall excess of males, the data show that more boys than girls exhibit a mild version of the disease. Even so, it could be that mildly affected girls do not meet the traditional diagnostic criteria of autism or ASD. For instance, depression and anxiety were roughly twice as common in girls referred to Swedish child and adolescent psychiatric services.[16] It is an open question whether these conditions might reflect the same underlying genetic and/or biochemical disturbances as in mild ASD in boys.

Despite the undoubted role of gender in determining susceptibility to ASD, it could be argued that this is not a genetic phenomenon – but that instead something about the male brain makes it particularly susceptible to perturbation.

How important are genes in ASD? Heritability

If a disorder is entirely environmental, only exposed individuals will develop the condition. Conversely, if the condition is entirely genetic, only subjects with specific genes will have the disorder.

Most human disorders are a combination of environmental and genetic factors, and the term "heritability" is a mathematical measure of the degree of genetic contribution. Heritability can be calculated from the frequency at which identical twins develop an identical disorder, and also from the rate at which parents and children, or non-identical siblings, share the same condition. Heritability estimates are imprecise because they depend on how different practitioners assess subjects (diagnostic accuracy), but nevertheless it has proved very useful.

For major depression, heritability is about 40%,[17] for bipolar disorder around 60%, and somewhat over 80% for schizophrenia.[18] Autism proper (autistic disorder) has a calculated heritability of over 90%, making it one of the most highly gene-dependent of all disorders affecting the brain. It is to be noted that heritability and twin concordance are not the same – a heritability of over 90% is consistent with concordance rates in identical twins of only 50%. Both measurements point to environmental factors overlaid on a genetic predisposition.

The high heritability of ASD raises the question of what specific genes contribute to ASD. Overall, 10–15% of ASD cases in the last 20 years have been associated with *known* genetic abnormalities including chromosome rearrangements; 3% of subjects with mental retardation and/or autism of unknown cause had abnormal karyotypes[19] while discernible chromosome abnormalities were seen in 3–9%[20] or 2–5%[21] of autistic individuals. Large chromosome 7 deletions have been observed[22] while a chromosome 15 partial duplication[23] appears to be one of the more common anomalies.[21] In these cases a causal relationship with disease development has not been formally demonstrated.

The most common genetic association is Fragile X,[24] affecting 10% of autistic males in some earlier studies. The gene inactivated in Fragile X is FMR-1[25] (for Fragile-X mental retardation), encoding a novel RNA-binding protein implicated in the control of gene expression; inactivation is associated with expansion of a CGG trinucleotide repeat within the gene. Chromosome abnormalities in ASD have been reviewed.[26]

Known single gene deficits in ASD are extraordinarily diverse, including all types of metabolic and housekeeping functions.[5,27] The long list (not reviewed comprehensively here; see [28]) includes deficits in amino acid metabolism (histidinemia,[29] phenylketonuria,[30] and oxoprolinase deficiency[31]), or purine metabolism (hyperuricosuria,[32] adenylosuccinate lyase deficiency,[33] and xanthinuria[34]). Others affect sterol metabolism (Smith-Lemli-Opitz syndrome – SLOS[35]) or mitochondrial function[36,37] and oxidative metabolism (succinic semialdehyde dehydrogenase[38]). Non-enzymatic deficits include neuronal cell-adhesion molecule mutations (neuroligins[39]) and methyl DNA binding protein (MeCP2) deficiency,[40] this latter being most commonly encountered in Rett syndrome. Many very different gene defects can cause ASD.

Insufficiency of genetic predisposition

These specific genetic deficiencies are rare, and cannot explain more than a tiny proportion of ASD cases. But they do illustrate one important point – that the genetic risk factor is not itself sufficient to cause the development of ASD.

As with identical twins, where the development of ASD in one co-twin is often not accompanied by ASD in the other, in the known genetic conditions (at least where good data are available) the picture is of diverse impairments but with only a sub-fraction of subjects being affected.

For instance, Fragile X is a known risk factor, but only one in five boys with Fragile X are diagnosed with ASD.[41] Mutations in the tuberous sclerosis genes TSC1 and TSC2 underlie a further small proportion of ASD cases, but again there is no 1:1 link between TSC mutations and ASD development:[42,43] most children with TSC mutations do not develop ASD. Children and adolescents carrying the MeCP2 gene mutation range from severely impaired to essentially unaffected.[44,45]

In a family with histidinemia, only a son displayed ASD but other family members had the same elevated levels of histidine.[29]

Phenylketonuria is a case in point. This condition results from an inability to assimilate the amino acid phenylalanine, resulting in toxic excess, with damaging effects on the brain. If diagnosed early, however, children are put on a diet free of phenylalanine, and may suffer no long-term adverse effects. Though the link with ASD is well established, none of 62 patients with classic phenylketonuria diagnosed early met criteria for ASD; only 2 of 35 patients diagnosed late (i.e. after chronic dietary exposure to phenylalanine) fulfilled the diagnostic criteria.[30]

In adenylosuccinate lyase deficiency "striking variable expression" was reported.[46] For SLOS, only 9 of 17 subjects (53%) met the diagnostic criteria for ASD.[35]

Thus, in these cases, ASD is not the inevitable consequence of a particular genetic combination, and instead one must speak of risk factors – does a particular gene predispose to ASD and, if so, by how much?

The search for new genes

Other genetic factors, so far unknown, clearly contribute to autism,[8,41,47,48] and a major thrust of research is the identification of new autism genes. This is most generally attempted through association studies as follows.

Throughout the genome are thousands of small differences in chromosome sequences, termed polymorphisms. For the most part, they come in two versions –

for instance, the A version and the B – and the difference is generally thought to be without any obvious phenotypic consequence. The frequency of A versus B in the population ranges, depending on the site, from around 50% to extremely rare (less than 1%) – and researchers focus on polymorphisms that are fairly abundant (in the order of 10%).

Long lists of these polymorphisms such as the haplotype map (HapMap),[49] and how to detect them, have been prepared by genome researchers. These afford extremely useful markers to detect genes that might contribute to ASD.

The underlying assumption is that a new mutation arising in the human genome is inevitably adjacent to one or more polymorphisms on the same chromosome, with either the A or B form. As the population expands, despite much re-assortment through recombination processes at every generation, because of physical proximity the new mutation remains associated with the same polymorphic variant (but not with polymorphisms at a distance or on a different chromosome).

The basic approach is to perform association studies. Using molecular techniques a large number of these polymorphisms are typed (A or B) in hundreds of subjects. The simplest comparison is to compare ASD with control children for each polymorphism, though some studies have compared affected children with unaffected siblings. Other comparisons are possible.

The question is, for each polymorphism, does it associate with ASD? In other words – is it near to the gene or mutation that contributes to ASD? If it is, the original version (either A or B) will be significantly more abundant in ASD children, but not in controls, and the bias pinpoints the location of the ASD gene mutation.

The extent of the bias is measured by statistical methods, the most commonly employed measure being "log of the odds," or LOD score, that reflects the probability that the bias was not by chance. Using logarithmic scales reduces the numbers to manageable figures – a 100-to-1 score rates as LOD=2, while 1000-to-1 gives LOD=3.

LOD scores of at least 3 are generally needed to indicate a significant gene locus is nearby. This is for a simple reason – if a sufficient number of polymorphisms are studied there will always be one or two that, by chance, appear to associate with the condition under exploration. To illustrate: when throwing dice, the likelihood of casting 6 sixes in series is extremely low. But, if 10,000 dice are each thrown 6 times, it suddenly becomes possible, even likely, that purely by chance one or more will generate a series of 6 sixes. For this reason the statistical cut-off point needs to be set high, and a LOD score under 3.0 is generally regarded as inconclusive.

In multiple studies to date on ASD and control children, a number of markers have been found to be biased. However, LOD scores have been generally low, rarely exceeding 3.0. This is to be contrasted with, for example, the scores of markers near the gene causing cystic fibrosis, where LOD scores in excess of 60 were reported.[50] Spelled out, there is a 10 to the power 57 difference in the strength of the statistical association.

Potential ASD genes

Despite the weak statistical significances, some associations have been considered to be meaningful. Deviations in marker frequencies have been seen on chromosome 7 in the q31–35 region, on chromosome 15 (region q11–13), and on chromosome 16 (region p13.3),[8,51] as reviewed.[52] A recent study gave evidence for polymorphism linkage on chromosomes 17 (p11) and 19 (p13)[53] but in all cases LOD scores have been low (under 3.5). (See Figure 3.1.)

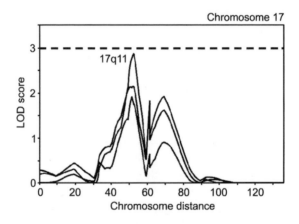

Figure 3.1 An example of genome-wide screening for ASD genes. The frequency of polymorphic marker bias (LOD) is plotted against position, revealing at least two peaks under which potential ASD genes might lie. The different curves represent different parametric models for contribution to ASD (e.g. dominant versus recessive alleles). Modified with permission of BioMed Central from Figures 2 and 3 of McCauley et al.[53]

Though the particular genes involved are not yet known, the prominent chromosome 15q locus (which encodes a GABA receptor subunit) is a potential candidate.[54] GABA (gamma-amino butyric acid) is the major inhibitory neurotransmitter in the brain – stimulation of the GABA receptor suppresses neuronal firing, and many anti-epileptic drugs operate by activating this receptor. Defective GABA receptor function could contribute to the epilepsy and EEG (electroencephalogram) abnormalities often seen in ASD (see Chapter 6).

Alarcón and colleagues[55] split their family groups according to specific criteria – including the age at which the children spoke their first word (the WORD group) and the age at which the first phrase of several words was spoken (the PHRASE group). Genome-wide analysis revealed a probability peak on chromosome 7q, with a LOD score of around 3, but only in the PHRASE group. Without ranking according to language trait, the region would not have been considered further. Molloy and co-workers used a different criterion – evidence of developmental regression.[56] This definition also highlighted a similar region on 7q, and a further locus on 21q, also with LOD scores around 3.

Shao and colleagues[57] also subtyped strictly defined autistic disorder into two categories – those characterized by repetitive behaviors (RB) and a second group with the common feature of experiencing particular difficulties if routine or environment were changed ("insistence on sameness"). When genetic linkage was now performed, focusing only on the RB subjects and their families, a peak probability value (LOD score) of as high as 4.7 was achieved for chromosome 15 (region q11–13) containing the GABA receptor type β3. Without such subdivision, the LOD score was only 1.45. No linkage was found with the second group. While highlighting the role of the GABA receptor, this study demonstrates that genetic susceptibility factors differ between individuals.

Recent genome-wide computer analysis of likely candidate ASD loci yielded 383 genes which could be involved. These were reduced, using a number of predictive techniques based on known associations, signaling pathways, and evidence for involvement in brain function, to 58 primary suspects. The final shortlist included genes encoding tumor necrosis factor (TNF), interleukins (ILs -6,-7,-8], and the serotonin transporter (SLC6A4/5HTT).[52]

An ongoing initiative sponsored by the National Alliance for Autism Research (NAAR, soon to be known as Autism Speaks Inc.) is using DNA chip technology to scan 6000 samples of DNA from 1500 multiplex families from the USA, Canada, and Europe, each consisting of two children with ASD and their parents.[58] Results will be awaited eagerly. A parallel scan is being undertaken by researchers at the Autism Genetic Resource Exchange (AGRE), who are typing 586 families using many thousands of polymorphic markers.[59] The results of this study are likely to be highly informative. Finally, a large new study is gearing up at Cold Spring Harbor Laboratory, New York, to scan the genomes of children with ASD, siblings, and other family members, to identify new disease genes in autism.[60]

Problems with the genome approach

The paucity of significant LOD scores need not be an insurmountable problem. A score of only 2.5 is compatible with a relative risk (in individuals carrying the gene or allele) of up to five-fold – even though such a low score would normally be put aside as inconclusive.

A complication (addressed by the NAAR study) is that the susceptibility allele need not be carried by the individual with ASD, but instead by his or her mother. This has been documented in one specific instance. Maternal anti-epileptic medication during gestation can cause ASD in children, and a specific enzyme (methylene tetrahydrofolate reductase, MTHFR) is implicated in the effect. There was a clear excess of particular MTHFR gene variants in the mothers of affected children, but no bias in the children themselves.[61]

Genes affecting ASD in males could also be different from those affecting females: evidence in support of this idea has been presented.[62]

It is quite possible that gene alleles contributing to ASD in one family or cohort will not contribute in another group. A model in which there are multiple interacting genes is widely accepted to underlie most cases of ASD, but the more genes that are involved the less likely it becomes that unique gene combinations will, across different populations, underlie the development of ASD.

Finally, chromosomes are not the only genetic material we inherit from our parents. Mitochondria are sub-cellular organelles with their own small genome, and are required for energy generation in the cell. Some cases of ASD are associated with defective mitochondrial genes – 14 of 69 children with ASD were found to have excess blood lactate (a marker of energy impoverishment), and of these roughly half were classified as having a mitochondrial disorder.[63] The authors suggested that this might be one of the most common genetic associations of autism (7% of cases). In a small study of subjects with ASD with a family history of mitochondrial defects, four provided evidence of a mitochondrial DNA mutation while more than two-thirds of mitochondria were lost from muscle tissue of the fifth.[37]

Overall, the diversity of the gene mutations identified in individuals with ASD suggests that there is no "autism gene." Instead, one is led to the conclusion that any one of a variety of metabolic insults, perhaps in combination with other toxic factors, can trigger a transition from sub-threshold disease to a disorder discernible by standard diagnostic criteria. Also, as in the case of Fragile X, ASD is not the inescapable consequence of a given genetic deficiency. Another triggering factor is required to precipitate clinical disease.

The patchwork genome

Further confounding analysis, and to the surprise of researchers, the human genome is not a defined and constant entity. In a chromosome sizing experiment on 98 normal individuals, significant size differences were seen, on average, in four chromosomes in every subject.[64] Large blocks of DNA are inverted in up to 48% of the population.[65] In a systematic survey, large duplications and deletions were found to be extremely common – among a group of 20 normal subjects, each individual differed from the others by, on average, 11 large-scale rearrangements.[66] The human genome is a patchwork:[67] each individual bears a unique combination of large changes. The extent to which such changes contribute to phenotypic diversity and disease has not yet been assessed.

Epigenetics and brain disorders

A final problem is that we do not only inherit genetic material from our parents. Specifically, we inherit characteristics, termed "epigenetic," that are independent of changes in gene sequences, but can have a major impact on how children develop.

This is because many sites in the human genome are modified through the addition of methyl groups to the DNA.[68,69] Such DNA methylation can dictate whether a particular gene will be expressed or not. For some (but not all) genes, the methylation pattern is conserved over many rounds of cell division and even during reproductive processes giving rise to eggs and sperm. The laying down of this heritable methylation pattern is termed "imprinting." On–off imprinting of specific gene expression can be inherited from one generation to the next, and children tend to resemble their parents (and even grandparents) more than just through the chromosomal DNA sequences they inherit.

Importantly, the inherited pattern of methylation (and gene expression) depends on the origin of the DNA – if an allele is inherited from the mother, versus the father, the expression may be different (sex-specific imprinting).

The importance of epigenetic inheritance has been highlighted in conditions like schizophrenia, where (as in ASD) heritability is very high, but where identical twin concordance is little better than 50%. In twins discordant for schizophrenia the phenotype correlates with DNA methylation levels.[70,71] In bipolar disorder, particular gene alleles account less for the disorder than the source of the allele – the risk depends more on whether the genes are inherited from the mother or the father,[71] and less on their identity, a classical case of epigenetic inheritance.

An epigenetic contribution to ASD is strongly suggested by the fact that Rett syndrome, one of the pervasive developmental disorders that include autism proper, is due to a mutation in the gene encoding the protein that recognizes and binds to DNA bearing methyl groups, known as MeCP2.[40] It is possible that imprinting errors make a specific contribution to the development of the ASD phenotype, though the specific genes involved are not known.

Generally, it is held that imprinting differences could contribute to twin discordance,[72–75] a major consideration in ASD which, like schizophrenia, has high heritability but where identical twin concordance is only around 50%.

Twinning is itself an additional risk factor for developmental disorders.[76] Phenotypic development of one embryo may influence the co-twin, a concept dubbed "mirror-imaging."[77] In the case of ASD, it is possible that developmental events taking place in one twin can bias events in the other, such that (of the two) only one develops ASD. Such influences may further complicate the unraveling of genes contributing to the disorder.

Genes and environment

The rising prevalence of ASD (see Chapter 4) points to an environmental factor involved in the development of the disorders. However, only a fraction of the population is affected, and it would seem that the environmental factor only damages individuals with a genetic predisposition. This means that there needs to be a combination of both genetic susceptibility, which could extend across several genes, and exposure to an environmental factor, perhaps during a window of susceptibility in the developing child. A combination of genetic liability with an additional risk factor (a "two-hit" mechanism) may be needed to take individuals from a milder and more diffuse phenotype to a seriously handicapping disorder.[78]

Key points

ASD has a major genetic component, demonstrated by the elevated frequency of autism in co-twins. The heritability of ASD may be as high as 90%.

The male to female ratio declines in markedly affected individuals – pointing to a large pool of boys with a milder version of ASD.

Some 10–15% of ASD have known genetic abnormalities such as Fragile X, but such abnormalities are extraordinarily diverse.

In no case is the genetic risk factor sufficient to produce ASD in all subjects with the gene anomaly.

Studies are underway to search for new genes contributing to ASD. Association is based on a probability score known as log of the odds (LOD), but LOD scores have consistently been low, pointing away from an "autism gene."

Subdividing subject or kindred groups (according to precise impairments) before gene typing has improved associations with specific genes, suggesting that gene variants linked to ASD differ between individuals.

Gene analysis may be complicated if maternal genes are a risk factor, by mitochondrial inheritance, and by non-genetic (epigenetic) effects.

A "two-hit" mechanism – a combination of diffuse genetic liability with an environmental risk factor – may be needed to produce ASD.

Chapter 4

New Phase Autism: Rising Prevalence

When autism was first described in the 1940s by Kanner and Asperger it was a rare condition. But now autism spectrum disorders (ASDs) appear to be reaching epidemic proportions. This argues against the possibility that genes alone might explain the rise – a change in the distribution of genes in the population requires dozens of generations, with strong selective pressures. There have certainly been many suggestions that the prevalence of ASD has steadily risen over the intervening years, with increasing skepticism that ASDs are primarily genetic disorders. But, unfortunately, the evidence has been patchy and there are many variables which cloud the issue. This chapter critically evaluates the evidence for a rise in autism.

The debate

Over the 1950s to 1970s there were no systematic surveys of the prevalence of ASD, and in the absence of a firm baseline it has been difficult to assess the possibility of a rise. Moreover, there has been a change in diagnostic criteria with successive updates of both US and international criteria, the most recent being DSM-IV[1] and ICD-10[2] as discussed in Chapter 2. Is it possible that changes in diagnostic criteria might explain some of the rise?

The ICD-10 forerunner, ICD-9, covered the period 1979 up to and through 1992. While the diagnostic categories are not identical to ICD-10, autism disorders were clearly delimited – with specific recognition of speech delay, social interaction impairment, eye-gaze avoidance, and resistance to change.

DSM-III was established in 1980, and followed by a revised edition (DSM-III-R, 1987), to be replaced by DSM-IV in 1994. Though there have been arguments that DSM-III-R broadened the diagnostic concept of autism,[3] the recommendations of III-R are largely reiterated in DSM-IV, and substantially parallel ICD-10.[4] Thus, for the most critical period under scrutiny (the early 1990s onwards), there has been no significant evolution of diagnostic criteria.

During this time period there has been increasing awareness of the conditions, both by professionals and by the public, illustrated by vocal protestations in the USA and UK regarding some childhood vaccinations. Nevertheless, it is possible that autism is now given as a diagnosis for conditions that were, formerly, labeled as something else.[5] In some cases, one suspects that autism could even have become a preferred diagnosis for some childhood disorders as it is seen as a less negative designation, without the unfortunate associations of mental retardation or childhood schizophrenia. Parents may also have sought a diagnosis of autism, in preference to other diagnoses, following formal recognition of the condition by government authorities dispensing welfare and support for affected families. Family migration to areas where the condition is well diagnosed and help provided could produce a seeming rise in prevalence where none such exists.

In 1996, the situation was summarized by an expert[6] as follows:

> Autism seems to be on the increase. This at least is the feeling of many professionals in the field of child development in Britain, who believe that in recent years they have been seeing more children with autistic spectrum disorders. [But]...there is no firm evidence for or against a general rise in the prevalence of "typical autism" or other autistic spectrum disorders. The impression that there is a rise could be due to a change in referral patterns, widening of diagnostic criteria for typical autism (which are difficult to apply with precision anyway), and increased awareness of the varied manifestations of disorders in the autistic spectrum (especially those associated with higher IQ). On the other hand, there might be real changes in prevalence, locally or nationally, due to temporary or permanent factors.

Ten years later the situation has not radically altered. A 2005 paper, also by an expert in the field, states: "Over recent decades there has been a major rise in the rate of diagnosed autism. The main explanation for this rise is to be found in better ascertainment and a broadening of the diagnostic concept. Nevertheless, some degree of true rise cannot be firmly excluded."[7]

Both experts urge the need for caution, but neither rules out the possibility that there may have been an increase in prevalence. It is therefore important to consider the primary data that might argue for, or against, the contention that ASDs are becoming steadily more common, and not as a consequence of greater awareness or other complicating factors.

Increasing prevalence

Until the 1990s ASD was diagnosed at no more than ~5 cases per 10,000. Examples of large studies include the UCLA-Utah study, giving a prevalence rate of 4 per 10,000 population.[8] A large survey of over 500,000 children in Denmark (1991–1998) gave a prevalence (8 years of age) of 7.7 per 10,000 for autism disorder and 22.2 per 10,000 for other ASDs.[9]

Rates in the UK and the USA are now higher. The diagnosis of ASD increased approximately four-fold in the period 1988–1993[10] and, by 2001, as many as 1 in 166 children under 8 (60 per 10,000) in the UK were affected.[11] Higher rates have been reported in UK schools (1 in 86[12]) while a recent audit in Scotland reported prevalence averaging at 1 in 200 (50/10,000) but as high as 1 in 44 in certain regions.[13] All contributors to the Scotland study acknowledged that the figures are underestimates.

In the USA, data from California point to a steady and substantial increase over the period 1987–2002,[14] a profile mirrored elsewhere in the USA.[15] (See Figure 4.1.) For children born after 1992, national data on special education rates has confirmed that prevalence has increased with each successive year.[16]

A review of data presented by the Danish Psychiatric Central Register concluded that the prevalence of childhood (age 5–9) autism has increased from less than 10 per 10,000 population range (1980–90) to over 70 (2000–02).[17] The rise in ASD rates in Denmark has been confirmed.[18]

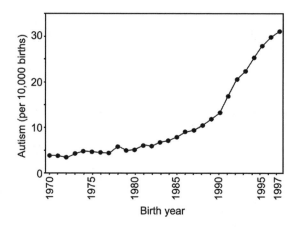

Figure 4.1 Birth year prevalence rates (1970 to 1997) for the 2002 population of persons with autism, defined as autistic disorder of DSM-IV or "infantile autism residual state" of DSM-III (1980). Other PDDs were not included. Data from the California Department of Developmental Services.[14]

Despite these indicators of a strong rise, and opinions that ASDs are much more common than previously thought,[19,20] the view has been that the available data do not provide an adequate test of changing incidence.[21,22] However, Blaxill,[23] in a review of over 50 studies, states: "A comparison of UK and US surveys, taking into consideration changing definitions, ascertainment bias, and case-finding methods, provides strong support for a conclusion of rising disease frequency," and continues: "Reported rates for ASDs in both countries have risen from the 5 to 10 per 10,000 range to the 50 to 80 per 10,000 range."

Why do different studies seem to give different rates?

Some studies have yielded exceptionally high rates, while others remain low. Williams et al.[24] comprehensively overviewed prevalence data on autism and autism spectrum disorders (ASD) published over the period 1966–2004 to explore what factors might underlie the different rates. Using model-fitting approaches, they systematically addressed the reasons for inter-study variability. Three separate factors were inferred to explain most (61%), but not all, of the variation.

The first factor, urban versus rural residence, reiterates the conclusions of several investigations showing that living in a town is a major risk factor for the development of autism and ASD,[25,26] providing strong evidence of an environmental component to the disorder. It also seems likely that over the last 40 years an increasing fraction of the population resides in urban areas. The second factor, age of the child, was also important. With increasingly young children, the Williams et al. study recognized a clear rise in the prevalence of the disorders with, according to their best-fit model, an approximately 10% increase per year as progressively younger children were studied. Factor three concerned the diagnostic criteria, either current (DSM-IV[1] or ICD-10[2]) versus alternatives including DSM-III and ICD-9. This factor therefore also includes a strong temporal feature, because ICD-9 was introduced in 1992, and DSM-IV in 1994.

It appears unlikely that the more recent diagnostic methods encompass a wider range of children, because all include the key features of autism disorders with specific recognition of speech delay, social interaction impairment, eye-gaze avoidance, and resistance to change.

Both the second and third factors therefore address temporal evolution of population rates, with factor one confirming an environmental contribution. This paper is worthy of serious study, and the prevalence data (Figures 1 and 2 of Williams et al.[24]) demonstrate an ongoing rise. For autistic disorder, mean rates have increased from approximately 2 per 10,000 (1980) to just under 30 per 10,000 (2004), while ASD overall increased from around 5 per 10,000 (1980) to around 70 per 10,000 (2004). Moreover, there is generally a delay of a year (or more) between data collection and publication. The data reviewed by Williams *et al.*[24] therefore demonstrate that current (2005) rates of autism and ASD are, on average, in the range of 35 per 10,000 and just over 90 per 10,000 respectively, and surely higher in urban areas and in younger children.

In the early 2000s, therefore, the prevalence of ASD has rapidly approached 1%. Rates in the 1980s to 1990s were no more than 0.1%. The combined evidence points to a ten-fold rise in prevalence in recent years that remains to be explained.

Potential confounding factors

Changes in the way autism is diagnosed could possibly account for part of the rise in prevalence. It has been reported[27] that as the rate of ASD increased there was a decline in the prevalence of mental retardation. Nevertheless, this analysis has been challenged[28] and the conclusion was subsequently withdrawn by the authors.[29] Another larger study ruled out a concomitant decline in the separate categories of either mental retardation or speech and language disability,[16] while ASD continued to rise.

Furthermore, in cases where investigators have retrospectively evaluated diagnostic criteria, or applied identical criteria to historic and current ASDs, no such bias was found.

When rates for all ASDs (pervasive developmental disorders according to DSM-IV) in the UK General Practice Research Database over the period 1988–2001 were analyzed, an increase was confirmed.[30] A significant feature of this analysis was that it retrospectively inspected diagnostic accuracy and found this to exceed 90% over the entire study period. This argues against the possibility that evolution of diagnostic criteria underlies the rise.

An increase (~ ten-fold) has also been described in the rates of diagnosis of autism in children in Olmsted County, Minnesota, over the period 1976–1997.[31] Though the rates (4.5 per 10,000 in 1995–1997) were lower than in other more recent studies, the analysis is distinguished because it applied identical diagnostic criteria (DSM-IV) to the early and late groups, eliminating the possibility that a change in criteria could underlie the observed rise. (See Figure 4.2.)

The extensive and authoritative study performed by Byrd and colleagues[32] at the MIND Institute in California addressed many of the issues raised (earlier age of diagnosis, broadening criteria, families migrating to access better services, increased diagnosis in specific ethnic groups) and concluded that the observed rise in ASD rates cannot be explained by a loosening in the criteria used to make the diagnosis, or any other factors, pointing to a real increase. As noted, there is little if any evidence that changes in survey methods can explain the apparent rise in autism.[23]

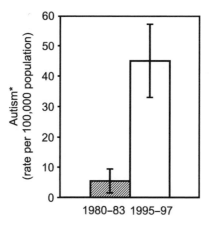

*Figure 4.2 Olmsted County ASD prevalences in two different timeframes. *Here, rates were assessed according to identical (DSM-IV) diagnostic criteria; error bars are 95% confidence intervals. Data from Barbaresi and co-workers.[31]*

Other evidence addressing a rise

Frequencies alone do not convincingly demonstrate a rise in prevalence or its absence. Therefore we must turn to other independent measures that could contradict or confirm the change in prevalence rates.

Younger age groups

If prevalence rates are increasing, for a condition with early onset, it is predicted that a greater number of ASD children will be found in younger age groups. This is confirmed by data from New Jersey, where there are five-fold more children aged 6 with a diagnosis of ASD than there are at age 16.[33] In Minnesota, the increase was confined to children born after 1987.[31] A similar bias to younger age groups is seen in Australia,[34] Denmark,[17] England,[12] Iceland,[35] Scotland,[13] and broadly across the USA.[16]

One possibility meriting serious consideration is that young children with ASD lose the distinguishing features of the disorder as they grow into adolescence and adulthood. Seltzer and co-workers[36] suggested that perhaps 40% of ASD children may lose some features of the disorder with time. However, a more detailed study on 48 children diagnosed with autism at age 2–4 years was less optimistic, with only two or four failing to meet diagnostic criteria in adolescence depending on diagnostic method[37] – though parents reported significant improvements with age. The lifetime evolution of ASD is therefore unable to explain the large (at least five-fold) reduction in prevalence rates among older children (see Figure 4.3).

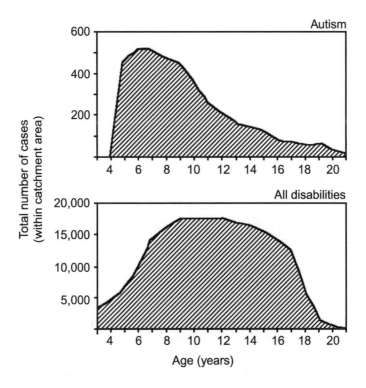

Figure 4.3 Rates of "autism" and all disabilities, according to age. The first age of diagnosis/ recognition determines the cut-off at the left (younger) end of the curves. Data from New Jersey, December 2001.[33]

Changing spectrum of impairments

It has been reported[14] that the cognitive ability of persons in California with ASD declined from 81% with moderate to profound retardation in 1987–88 to 45% in 2001–02. At the same time, the Byrd[32] study also in California reported that the proportion of ASD subjects with Asperger dropped from 15% to 2% (1983–85 versus 1992–95). If the frequency of Asperger has remained constant, this would point to a ~8-fold rise in non-Asperger PDD including autistic disorder. At the same time mental retardation (MR) fell from 55% to 25% while ASD subjects with a family history of MR simultaneously fell from 30% to 16%. In Australia, autism proper as a fraction of total ASD cases is also evolving – with rates of autistic disorder, as a percentage of the total, being highest in the younger age groups.[34]

These data suggest that the pattern of presentation of the disorder has altered over the 1980s through 2000s, with autistic disorder becoming more prevalent with respect to other conditions. The data are therefore consistent with a change in prevalence.

Evolution of twin concordance rates

Historically, autism was felt to be purely environmental, but the first studies on twins showed that when one twin has the disorder, the other identical co-twin often does too.[38] This would tend to suggest underlying genetic factors are the major determinant. However, concordance rates in twins are changing markedly, consistent with an increasing environmental contribution. Early studies reported a very high concordance, 60–100%, between identical or monozygotic (MZ) twin pairs, with no concordance (0%) between non-identical, i.e. dizygotic (DZ), twin pairs.[38,39]

Even when a broader definition of ASD was adopted, concordance in identical twins was 92% while only 10% of non-identical pairs shared the condition.[40] In this time period, the concordance shown by monozygotic twins far exceeded that seen in dizygotic twins, as reviewed.[41] It needs to be remembered, however, that identical twins are concordant in gender – both are either male or female – and therefore in a condition which shows a strong gender bias (with a marked excess of males) then one must always *expect* higher concordance in identical twins versus non-identical twins.

Analysis could also be complicated if it is found that ASD children are more common in twins versus singleton births.[42] This highlights the possibility that we may be dealing with non-genetic factors associated with twinning, including prematurity and increased risk of perinatal injury including hypoxic-ischemic damage. However, the suggestion has been refuted by a later study.[43]

Recent data do suggest that the rates of twin concordance are changing. Specifically, the excess of monozygotic versus dizygotic concordance appears to be diminishing. In one study (based on parent/practitioner accounts of zygosity), only 58% of identical twin pairs were concordant versus 36% of non-identical pairs (Croen, L.A., pers. comm.). In an extended twin group,[44] basing concordance and zygosity on parent accounts only, eight identical pairs were concordant, but the majority (21 identical pairs) were discordant; one pair was unclear. A small bias may have been introduced by the selection protocol, but this places identical twin concordance at only 26% (Kates, W., pers. comm.).

In a larger study, including triplets and some quadruplets, applying a strict definition of concordance (V. Kustanovich, Autism Genetic Resource Exchange, pers. comm.), 33 out of 41 (80%) identical twins were concordant but only 17 out of 46 (37%) non-identical twins; when a wider definition of concordance was applied 41 out of 41 (100%) monozygotic twins were concordant as against 29 out of 46 (63%) non-identical twins.

Together, these three studies suggest a trend that the nature of ASD is changing, away from concordance only in monozygotic twins, and toward surprisingly high concordance rates (e.g. 63%) in dizygotic twins. This increase in dizygotic concordance suggests evolution away from a purely genetic disorder to one determined centrally by environmental factors, though still with an important genetic susceptibility component.

Decline of a specific genetic contribution: Fragile X

If the population prevalence of ASD is evolving from a purely genetic disorder to one with a major environmental contribution, one prediction is that the relative rates of ASD associated with a known specific genetic cause *must* decline in a population where the causation, in most cases, is independent of the genetic risk factor. This is addressed through evaluation of Fragile X rates in ASD.

Many gene and chromosome abnormalities have been described in ASD, including Fragile X, tuberous sclerosis, and phenylketonuria.[41,45] Fragile X syndrome is associated with an anomaly on chromosome X (specifically at region q27.3), and a link between Fragile X and mental retardation has long been established. Although a proportion of subjects with this abnormal chromosome have no obvious impairment, the general phenotype includes subtle changes to facial features, mildly shortened stature, and characteristic behavior often resembling autism spectrum disorder.[46] A proportion of children with Fragile X present with autistic features.[47,48] Conversely, early work showed that as many as 10% of children diagnosed according to standard criteria for autism are subsequently found to have the Fragile X anomaly.[49]

The frequency of Fragile X in ASD is of interest as it can cast light on prevalence. The assumption is that the rate of Fragile X in the population (around 2–3 per 10,000) is fairly constant – if the prevalence of autism is rising, the proportion of individuals with ASD who harbor Fragile X must fall.

This is borne out by the literature. In a survey of published papers and reviews addressing the frequency of Fragile X in ASD subjects, principally males and more rarely females, there was a strong reduction in the proportion of ASD subjects with the Fragile X anomaly over the period 1985 through 2005 (see Figure 4.4). Recent figures confirm this low rate of Fragile X in present-day ASD.

Three pooled reports of children (n=266) under 10 years old diagnosed for autism revealed just two with Fragile X,[50–52] overall 0.7%.

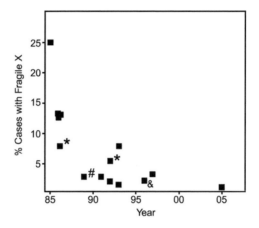

Figure 4.4 Frequency of Fragile X observed in subjects diagnosed with ASD plotted against date of publication (or date of survey where this was specified to be different) [47,53–65]. ∗ *: reviews, data points included were from* [47,62]. #: *time period 1980–98,* [62] *plotted at 1989.* &: *results from a survey carried out in 1996.* [61]

Possibly some centers might use Fragile X to exclude subjects from a diagnosis of "pure" autism, but this is not documented nor substantiated by either ICD or DSM guidelines. In all likelihood, children in this specific subset, prior to any chromosome analysis, are referred (along with other similarly behaviorally affected children) to specialist clinics for a diagnosis of autism – in which case the figures are probably reliable.

Fragile X prevalence in the population is assumed to be fairly constant, though improvements in diagnostic methods suggest that cases established by chromosome analysis rather than molecular technology may have overestimated[66] or underestimated[67] the true frequency.

Therefore, the reduction in the proportion of ASD children displaying Fragile X most likely reflects dilution. In other words, Fragile X children constitute a smaller proportion of total ASD children because, in recent years, the total number of ASD children has risen.

The data allow a tentative measure of current ASD prevalence. On the assumption that the frequency of the Fragile X anomaly in the population has not changed, the relative rates of ASD may be estimated. Comprehensive and authoritative review[68] provided an accurate figure, 2.3/10,000, for the prevalence of

Fragile X syndrome (males). The precise proportion of Fragile X subjects presenting with autism is not known, but the published figures (also for males) of 12.3%[47] and 50%[48] are plausible; mean 31%. For females, rates may be lower, to be balanced against the suspicion that the higher published figure[48] is the more reliable, and further diminished as a factor of concern because of the strong over-representation of males with both ASD and Fragile X syndrome.

Thus, one may estimate the total rate of ASD due to Fragile X is 0.71 per 10,000 population (i.e. $2.3/10,000 \times 31\%$). From this, if only 1% of current ASD children are found to have Fragile X, the overall prevalence of autism must be 71/10,000, or 1 in 142. This figure is consistent with recent (higher) estimates from population surveys of younger children, and confirms a rise in ASD prevalence.

Summary of observations

The combined evidence from several large recent surveys points to a real increase in the prevalence of autism and ASDs from the 1980s through 2000s. A broadening of diagnostic criteria does not afford a likely explanation, as these have not changed significantly since before 1990, and the steepest incline of the rise only commenced after this time (see Figure 4.1). Retrospective analyses do not support a change in criteria.

Four different independent criteria are consistent with increased prevalence – the over-representation of ASD in the younger age groups; the reduction in Asperger as a percentage of total; the marked increase in dizygotic concordance; and the decline in the frequency, among ASD subjects, of Fragile X.

Is there an epidemic of autism?

It is important to be cautious when considering these data. Fombonne[69] makes four points which need to be carefully thought through before reaching conclusions. First, many prevalence estimates provide numbers rather than frequencies. Regarding the California (Byrd[32]) study, the population in the younger age group has also increased; so any increase in ASD prevalence must allow for this change. However, the population increase over the study period (approximately 1.25-fold) is small in comparison to the documented increase. Second, changes in diagnostic criteria are a plausible concern, but recent analyses have confirmed a rise despite application of identical criteria. Third, earlier diagnosis would not alter population rates once all children have been assessed. Fourth, upward trends are also seen in some other disorders including cerebral palsy, attention deficit, and epilepsy. This specific point is readdressed in Chapter 11 regarding the likely environmental contribution to disorders that extend beyond ASD.

Conclusion. The rise may be real: new phase autism

It is hard to dispute the fact that there has been a real change in the prevalence of ASDs, as recent opinion has asserted.[23,30,70–72] All aspects of the disorder have changed in a direction consistent with an increasing environmental contribution. Specifically, an increase in ASD of only four-fold would indicate that 75% of new cases have a cause distinct from classical autism, and 90% if the prevalence has risen ten-fold, as the figures suggest.

There will be, even among specialists, concerns that the rise in rates is an artifact, due to some as yet unexplained quirk of assessment and recording procedures. Perhaps, one must concede, autism has always been with us, and is only now receiving the attention it deserves. The final word is left to an MD general practitioner of 30 years' experience, who observes: "I never encountered autism until my last year in practice, when a young lad, severely affected, came to my practice."[73]

The debate regarding a true increase, or an explanation in terms of recognition/diagnostic issues, may be to some extent academic. Issues not under discussion include the fact that the condition was largely unknown 50 years ago, but now among younger age groups, in recent years, perhaps 1% of children are affected. Debate apart, ASDs are of major concern, and demand an understanding.

Key points

Most studies confirm that there is an ongoing rise in ASD prevalence.

This could perhaps be due to changes in diagnostic criteria and/or increased awareness.

Retrospective studies addressing earlier diagnostic accuracy, or using identical criteria to compare historic and present-day rates, confirm an increase in prevalence.

The increase is supported by:

1. the excess of younger children

2. the decline in Asperger disorder as a percentage of ASD

3. the evolution of twin concordance rates (non-identical twins used to be almost always discordant – today there is a surprisingly high concordance rate)

4. the decline of Fragile X in ASD children (once this was found in over 10% of ASD – the rate is now less than 1%).

Overall, ASD prevalence can be calculated to now be between 90 and 100 per 10,000 (~1%), in excess of earlier estimates, pointing to a real increase – "new phase autism."

Chapter 5

Brain Abnormalities: Focus on the Limbic System

To understand a brain disorder it is first necessary to determine which brain areas are affected. Only then can one address whether these changes are consistent with the observed behavioral changes. This chapter considers structural and imaging studies on the autistic brain. For the most part, the neurological data reviewed here span the period of changes in prevalence, and caution is needed in extrapolating from historic ASD to the new phase of increasing prevalence.

Brain structure

The human brain is a large and exceptionally complicated organ, impossible to cover properly here. For structural details the interested reader is referred in the first instance to illustrative internet conceptualizations such as "Build a Brain,"[1] to databases including the "Digital Anatomist Information System"[2] and the Whole Brain Atlas,[3] and to a general comprehensive textbook.[4] However, in the context of autism and autistic spectrum disorders it will be important to distinguish the major regions of the brain (see Figure 5.1).

The cerebrum or cerebral cortex is the largest part of the human brain. The surface is highly convoluted with many deep fissures: dividing the mass of the brain on each side into four lobes – the frontal, parietal (the outer wall), occipital (the back), and temporal (within the temples). The cortex is the major information storage and processing region of the brain.

Behind and below the cortex is the cerebellum (little brain), known to participate in movement and motor coordination. The cerebellum attaches to the top of the brainstem, a region that controls automatic functions including respiration and heartrate.

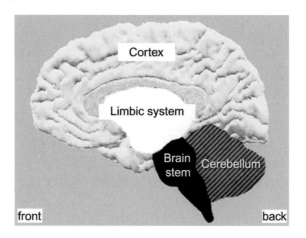

Figure 5.1 Major subregions of the human brain (simplified).

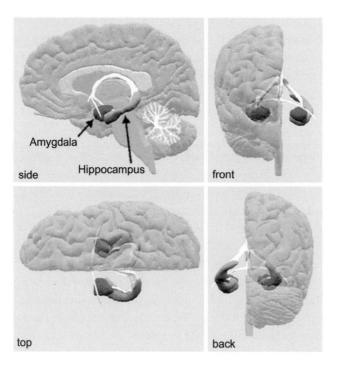

Figure 5.2 Hippocampus and amygdala viewed from different directions. Adapted from the Digital Anatomist Information System[2] with permission from the Structural Informatics Group, Digital Anatomist Project, University of Washington.

The limbic system is predominantly found within and underlying the temporal lobes, on the fringe (*limbus*, Latin) between the cerebrum/cortex and the brainstem. It is involved in emotion and memory and includes the hippocampus and adjoining amygdala (see Figure 5.2).

Most of the brain (with the exception of the brainstem and lower brain), and including the limbic system, is divided into two halves (hemispheres); these halves are connected by the corpus callosum which allows information to pass from one side to the other.

Limbic structure

The hippocampus is so termed because of its apparent resemblance in shape and in cross-section (see Figure 5.3) to the sea-horse (*Hippocampus* species); the amygdala is a short nut-shaped extension of the hippocampus (Latin, *amygdala*, almond). The limbic system extends beyond the hippocampus and amygdala to include other adjacent structures including the entorhinal cortex, the connecting fibers of the fornix and septum, with adjoining mammillary bodies and limbic nuclei of the thalamus. These will not be described in any detail here.

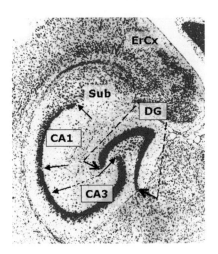

Figure 5.3 Hippocampal substructure. CA1, CA3, regions of the cornu ammonis; CA2 (not labeled) is the small area separating CA1 and CA3; DG, dentate gyrus; ErCx, entorhinal cortex; Sub, subiculum. Though the photograph is from mouse, the structure in primates including humans is very similar, although the alignment of neurons (stained dark) is a little more diffuse. From Lathe,[5] Journal of Endocrinology *169, pp. 205–231, © Society for Endocrinology (2001), reproduced by permission; from an original photomicrograph from Angevine[6] with markings overlaid. The original photomicrograph is itself reprinted from* Experimental Neurology *S2, by Angevine, J.B., Jr. "Time of neuron origin in the hippocampal region," pp. 1–70, copyright 1965, with permission from Elsevier.*

Because the majority of the limbic system is found at the medial ("middle") or mesial ("toward the midline") aspect of the temporal lobe, the term *medial temporal lobe* is often used interchangeably with the terms limbic brain or limbic system. The inclusion of the limbic brain within the temporal lobe is justified on anatomical and functional grounds – for instance, epileptic seizures originating in the hippocampus and amygdala prominently affect overlying temporal cortex.

There is no "one" definition of the limbic brain. The term was first used by the French scientist Paul Broca who originally associated it with the sense of smell, linking with the term *rhinencephalon* (from Greek *rhis*, nose; *enkephalos*, brain). Although the limbic brain is still involved with chemical sensing, it plays diverse roles in mood, emotion, memory, and motivation. And it is the limbic system which is believed to be centrally involved in the problems associated with ASD.

Hippocampal substructure

In cross-section, the hippocampus is subdivided into the CA regions, derived from another name for the hippocampus, Ammon's horn (cornu ammonis), as shown in Figure 5.3, and the dentate gyrus, a tooth-like pointed structure lying adjacent to the CA regions. Together, the CA regions with the dentate gyrus (DG), subiculum, and entorhinal cortex constitute the hippocampal formation.

Studying brain structure: techniques

Three basic techniques are employed to investigate altered brain structure in behavioral disorders. The first, histology (from Greek *histos*, tissue), is almost always restricted to post-mortem material, though in some conditions (perhaps not ASD) narrow brain punch biopsy samples can sometimes be justified. Though only a very limited number of post-mortem ASD brains have been studied, they have made a significant impact on the field. Second, structural imaging on the subject. X-ray procedures (CAT: computer-assisted tomography or computed axial tomography) are more rarely used because of the hazard they present; instead, magnetic resonance imaging (MRI) is routinely employed to look at regional differences in tissue density between conscious subjects and controls. Third, positron imaging examines the movement and distribution of radioactively labeled chemicals in the brain.

Histology

This most basic procedure involves slicing solid tissue (often frozen) into very thin sections that can be examined under the microscope, and usually employs chemical staining techniques to enhance contrast and assist cell-type identification (e.g. Figure 5.3).

Magnetic resonance imaging (MRI)

For this procedure the stationary subject, lying horizontally, is rolled into a large cylindrical magnetic field. Radio waves sent through the magnetic field are displaced and absorbed by brain tissue, sensors detect the radio-wave intensities, and a computer constructs an image of the brain based on the perturbations. The procedure can take as little as ten minutes, and permits high-resolution maps to be constructed throughout the brain.

Functional MRI (fMRI)

Oxygenated and de-oxygenated hemoglobins differ in their electromagnetic properties, and fine-tuning of the instrumentation allows inferences to be made regarding tissue activity and blood flow in different brain regions. Images can be produced in real time, as fast as one per second.

Positron techniques

Positron-emission tomography (PET) and a variant of PET, single positron emission computed tomography (SPECT), both rely on the introduction of radioactive chemicals into the blood that diffuse into the brain. Radioactive disintegration releases positrons that impact on adjacent molecules, producing gamma rays that can be detected by recording devices surrounding the subject's head.

PET

Depending on the compound that is injected, PET scanning can reveal blood flow and oxygen and glucose metabolism in different regions of the brain, with a high degree of neuroanatomical resolution (a few millimeters). The drawback of PET is that the radioisotopes most often used are very short-lived, limiting the duration of the scan.

SPECT

This technique uses more long-lasting isotopes, but the drawback here is that they are more limited in the kind of brain activity that can be monitored, and the resolution is poor (about 1 cm).

The following sections now consider structural studies on the brain of ASD subjects.

Morphometric studies: brain size

A series of reports, not discussed here in depth, have suggested that overall brain size might be increased in ASD, though others have failed to reproduce this observation. In systematic review Redcay and Courchesne[7] concluded that brain size is on average somewhat reduced at birth, increases substantially during the first year of life, but plateaus such that ASD individuals, as adults, are indistinguishable from controls. They suggest that later recognition of the disorder is associated with early pathological brain growth and arrest in ASD individuals.[7] Within the brain, there have been reports of global changes in gray-matter volume (comprising the neuronal cell bodies, in contrast to their white-matter axonal processes), ranging from increase[8] to a significant decrease.[9] Two recent papers focused on just one brain region, the corpus callosum, using this as an index of neural development and white-matter integrity. One reported reduced corpus callosum volume[10] but the other saw no differences in corpus callosum structure between ASD and matched controls.[11] The extent and significance of global changes in brain size and gray-matter volume are therefore unknown, and may be epiphenomenal to autism.

Histology: hippocampus, amygdala, cerebellum, cortex

Early histologic study of the ASD brain discovered subtle and widespread changes in several regions including the hippocampus, adjoining subcortical regions (subiculum, entorhinal cortex), other afferents to the hippocampus (septal nuclei and mammillary body), cortex, amygdala, and cerebellum.[12] A role for the limbic brain was postulated,[13] according with previous speculations based on functional deficiencies[14,15] and with DeLong[16] who proposed that ASD is a developmental syndrome of hippocampal dysfunction. Here key studies are dwelt upon; brain findings in autism have been reviewed.[17]

In brain samples from two infants with ASD, hippocampal neurons were clearly smaller with fewer local filaments (dendrites) connecting them to adjacent neurons.[18] In nine further brains examined, increased neuronal packing density was seen in the amygdala, with smaller and densely packed neurons in the CA subregions of the hippocampus, and also in linked regions including the subiculum and entorhinal cortex (see Figure 5.3). In all nine samples neuronal (Purkinje) cells of the cerebellum were reduced in number.[19] The most consistent changes were in the amygdala, hippocampus, and functionally related entorhinal cortex and mammillary body.[20] An increase in cell packing density in the hippocampus and prosubiculum was recently confirmed,[21] with a 23% increase in CA3 and 15% increase in the dentate gyrus.[22]

Imaging studies highlight the limbic brain

MRI studies also detect limbic abnormalities. Reduced volume of the amygdala was seen in 11–37-year-old autistic individuals, with lesser but significant reduction in hippocampal volume.[23] Another study saw small bilateral enlargement of the amygdala and hippocampus in 3–4-year-old autistic children.[24] Schumann *et al.*[25] report overall enlargement (9–12%) of the hippocampus at all ages (7–18 years) but amygdala enlargement (13–17%) only in the younger children (7–12 years); subdivisions of the hippocampus were not separately analyzed. Saitoh *et al.*,[26] in studies on affected and control individuals of 2 to 43 years, report a selective reduction in the cross-sectional area of the dentate gyrus of the hippocampus (see Figure 5.4). The largest deviation (–13.5%) was seen among the youngest autistic children (29 months to 4 years).

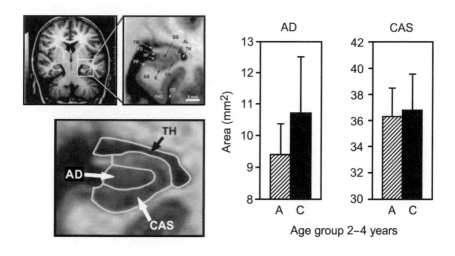

Figure 5.4 Reduced dentate cross-sectional area in ASD. Left: representation of the regions measured (AD, area dentata or dentate gyrus including the interpenetrating region CA4; CAS, regions CA1–3 of the cornu ammonis [hippocampus proper]). Right: mean cross-sectional areas of AD and CAS by age groups. Only the 2–4-year group is presented. A, autism; C, control subjects. Error bars are standard deviations. Over all age groups (pooled data; not shown) the dentate area was significantly smaller than in controls (p<0.05); significance remained both when normalized to CA1–3 area (p<0.01) or when dentate to CA1–3 areas were examined using total brain volume as a covariate (p<0.05). The cross-sectional area of CA1–3 did not differ from controls (p>0.1). Adapted from Figure 2 of Saitoh et al.,[26] published in Brain 124, pp. 1317–1324 (2001), by permission of Oxford University Press.

Another study revealed bilateral abnormalities involving the hippocampal formation, amygdala, and adjoining entorhinal cortex.[27] One study failed to find abnormalities of hippocampal structure.[28]

Also using MRI, bilateral abnormalities of the medial temporal lobes were observed, including enlargement of the amygdala.[29] MRI also pointed to deficiencies in the cortical region involved in the integration of sensory and limbic information, the superior temporal sulcus.[30]

Functional studies

Functional imaging, instead of looking at brain structure, examines blood flow and energy utilization in the brain. Many (but not all) studies confirm limbic/temporal lobe involvement. fMRI revealed reduced blood flow in the temporal lobes of autistic children;[31] in a further study using fMRI on subjects with Asperger disorder, there were significant abnormalities of functional integration of the amygdala with the parahippocampal gyrus.[32] It was concluded that functional connectivity of medial temporal lobe structures specifically is abnormal in Asperger disorder.

PET analysis revealed that regional blood was much lower in both the temporal lobes of ASD subjects.[33] The ubiquitous neuronal metabolite N-acetyl aspartate was reduced in both hippocampus/amygdala and cerebellum,[34] pointing to diminished overall activity in these brain regions. Using SPECT, relative blood flow in the right amygdala and hippocampus was positively correlated with a behavioral rating ("obsessive desire for sameness") typical of ASD. Ito and colleagues,[35] also using SPECT techniques, reported that blood flow is significantly reduced in the left temporal region in high-functioning autism, while a more recent study reported a correlation between reduced temporal lobe blood flow and the severity of the disorder. The more severe the autistic syndrome, the lower the relative blood flow in the left temporal lobe.[36] Overall, these imaging studies point to significantly reduced blood flow (hypoperfusion) of temporal regions including the hippocampus.

Cerebellum

There have been fairly consistent reports of cerebellar abnormalities in ASD. In studies on the post-mortem ASD brain patchy loss of cerebellar neurons and activation of brain immune cells (microglia) was seen.[37] The nature of the differences vary, however, ranging from dystrophy to enlargement.[24,38–41] Another study specifically argued against cerebellar involvement,[42] but though MRI scans failed to reveal abnormalities, SPECT analysis of the same autistic patients suggested that blood flow was reduced in this brain region.[43] Further fMRI studies revealed increased cerebellar activation that correlated with the degree of structural abnormalities.[44]

Some have suggested that the postural control system, associated with cerebellar function, is underdeveloped in ASD,[45] and this may be true. In a survey of children with mild motor disability (ataxia), some of whom also had ASD, there was an association between borderline ataxia and ASD.[46] It was proposed that ataxia may be one of many signs of early life events leading up to complex neurodevelopmental disorders including autism. But other work has failed to find deficits in skills and activities that require the cerebellum. Specifically, children with high-functioning autism have no deficit in an object-catching task that is markedly impaired by cerebellar damage,[47] perhaps arguing that cerebellar deficits are not central to ASD.

Nevertheless, despite the seeming independent function of the cerebellum, that there are direct connections from the cerebellum to the limbic brain[48] and cerebellar abnormalities could possibly contribute to the limbic deficits seen in ASD.[49]

Cortex

In addition to overall brain size changes, there have been some reports of localized enlargement of the frontal cortex in ASD. Carper and Courchesne[50] reported that some frontal cortical regions were significantly enlarged in young (2–5-year-old) autistic children. Casanova et al.,[51,52] using post-mortem histology, compared the morphology of neuronal cell columns in prefrontal cortex and temporal lobe of autistic patients and controls. Cell columns in brains of autistic patients were increased in number, but smaller and more diffuse, containing fewer neurons per column. Immune cell (microglia) activation in cortical regions has also been reported.[37]

Interpreting structural data

Despite the evidence for regional changes in the ASD brain, one must be cautious about the way in which these are interpreted. First, histological study of the post-mortem brain is by its nature restricted to those samples that are available, and these may not be representative of the wider ASD population. The work of Bailey and colleagues[53] highlights the difficulties in interpreting the results of post-mortem studies. Six subjects were investigated, all were mentally handicapped, and five of six were older than 20 years, and therefore unrepresentative of the recent rise in ASD prevalence. The youngest child (4 years) had a brain weight of 1.53 kg against a normal range (+/– 2.5 × SD) of 1.25–1.35 kg. Here the convolution pattern of the cortex was abnormal, with overlarge hyperconvoluted temporal lobes and upwardly rotated hippocampi. There were dispersed anomalies in other brain regions.[53] In this exemplary study, with just one case in the target age group, it is difficult to draw general conclusions.

Imaging studies in ASD are also to be interpreted with caution. Brain scanning is an onerous protocol for young behaviorally impaired children. Imaging volunteers therefore tend to be older (and less representative of the new phase) while early lesions may partly repair with time, at least at the level of resolution permitted by imaging: in one study[26] structural differences were most pronounced in the youngest age groups. Volunteers also tend to be high functioning, skewing the picture toward mild brain impairments, while adding a further complexity – high-functioning autism and Asperger syndrome, though diagnostically similar, may be distinct conditions,[54] and may further confuse the picture regarding the "typical" ASD subject.

It is likely that subtypes of ASD may be distinguished by brain imaging studies. Using MRI techniques, Hrdlicka and colleagues[55] attempted to categorize ASD according to structural data. They discerned four clusters: #1 had the largest increase in corpus callosum size; #2 the greatest enlargement of hippocampus and amygdala (and least epilepsy); #3 the smallest size of the hippocampus; while #4 had the smallest size of the amygdala and the highest frequency of epilepsy. Other biases were also observed, including pregnancy order and degree of facial dysmorphic features. The clusters did not differ in severity of ASD.

Consensus: limbic brain and overlying cortex, with lesser cerebellar effects

Cody, Pelphrey, and Piven[56] reviewing the literature, emphasize that different studies have pointed to changes in diverse brain structures, including cerebellum and other regions (cingulate gyrus, basal ganglia, corpus callosum, and brainstem), but concur that hippocampal and amygdala alterations are the most common. Extended analysis by Dawson et al.[57] concluded that abnormalities in the medial temporal lobe encompassing the hippocampal formation underlie the cognitive, perceptual, and language impairments of ASD.

Three imaging studies point to a correlation between ASD severity and limbic/temporal lobe abnormalities. Kates and colleagues,[58] in an MRI study of two identical twin boys (7.5 years) discordant for autism, reported that the affected twin had markedly smaller volumes of the hippocampus, amygdala, and caudate regions, as well as reduced cerebellar lobules, in comparison to his brother. Another study reported[36] that as ASD severity increases, so blood flow in the left temporal lobe was reduced. Finally, a significant correlation has been found between ASD severity (as assessed by parents) with limbic neuronal density, specifically at the amygdala–hippocampus–entorhinal cortex junction.[27] Further evidence specifically implicating the hippocampus and amygdala in ASD is debated in the next chapter.

It is not excluded that cerebellar (and possibly cortical) effects may be downstream of limbic dysfunction. There is no extensive evidence on this possibility, but cerebellar atrophy was seen in the famous patient HM (next chapter) who had undergone bilateral surgical removal of the hippocampus and amygdala.[59] This could suggest that cerebellar atrophy is a consequence either of his lesion or of his earlier epilepsy. And, one must consider, cerebellar damage could also feed back to affect the limbic brain.[48,49] However, cerebellar abnormalities could be indicators of the *timing* of insult[60] and be incidental accompaniments of limbic damage, unrelated to ASD development.

As noted earlier, much of the structural data reviewed here spans the period of changes in prevalence and evolution of presentation. However, one suspects that, if limbic damage was historically associated with ASD, the same brain regions will be centrally involved in more recent cases of ASD, even if the cause of damage is different.

In conclusion, the accumulated data suggest that the brain regions most consistently affected in ASD include the limbic brain, specifically the hippocampus and adjoining amygdala, and the cerebellum. It would require a quantum leap to infer that cerebellar damage could lie at the root of ASD, for the cerebellum controls posture and locomotion. While deficits can and do occur in conjunction with ASD, they are unlikely to be central to the diagnosis or cognitive features of the disorder. Instead, one must infer that limbic damage, with some involvement of overlying cortical regions (with which the limbic brain is intimately connected), is central to ASD. But, before one can conclude that limbic damage underlies ASD, it is first necessary to consider whether ASD features are consistent with limbic dysfunction. The next chapter addresses this specific question.

Key points

Studies on brain tissue show that the limbic brain, between the mass of the cortex and the brainstem, and including the hippocampus and amygdala, is most often abnormal in ASD, with increased packing density and smaller neurons.

Several imaging studies have showed reduced blood flow in this brain region, but imaging studies are to be interpreted with caution as they tend to select for high-performing subjects.

There are also consistent reports of cerebellar and cortical anomalies.

The consensus is that ASD is associated with the limbic brain (particularly the hippocampus and amygdala) and overlying cortical tissue in close proximity, with lesser cerebellar effects.

Chapter 6

Limbic Dysfunction Correlates with the Autistic Phenotype

Structural abnormalities in a central brain region, the limbic system, are seen in individuals with ASD. The question arises – could altered limbic function be the cause of ASD? The precise role of the limbic brain, particularly the hippocampus and adjoining amygdala, remains elusive. But different investigators have prominently highlighted the contribution of the hippocampus and amygdala to seemingly diverse and unrelated functions, including memory encoding, anxiety, and epilepsy.

These central roles are to be contrasted with the triad of impairments seen in ASD – impaired social interaction, deficits or marked abnormalities of language and communication, and a restricted and often repetitive behavioral repertoire. Such divergent views clearly must be reconciled before limbic damage (see Chapter 5) can be invoked as a plausible cause of ASD.

There are many examples in which damage to the hippocampus or amygdala, not only in rodents but also in primates including man, produces real and measurable behavioral changes. These are examined below, and compared with what is known of ASD.

It is important to state from the outset that the consequences of damage to the limbic system in early life (as inferred for the young cohorts of recent ASD) may be very different from the effects of damage sustained as an adult. For this reason, data on adult subjects are not easily extrapolated to ASD. With this reserve, this chapter addresses whether limbic damage is consistent with ASD.

Memory

Memory is considered first, reflecting the historic view that the hippocampus is centrally involved in memory. This idea became prominent through the renowned patient HM: bilateral removal of the hippocampus and amygdala was undertaken in an attempt to alleviate his epilepsy (the lesion also includes part of overlying entorhinal cortex).[1,2] This was successful, in as much as his epilepsy was controlled, but there was an unexpected side-effect: almost total amnesia.[3]

However, his memory impairment was not total, and some forms of memory remain intact. There are several clearly distinguished types of memory. For example, declarative (or episodic) memory relates to recall of events (or statements of events) such as: "I saw a yellow parrot yesterday." This form of memory is to be contrasted with procedural memory which relates to skills and habits, like learning to ride a bicycle. When the limbic system is damaged, as in HM, only declarative memory is abolished, while (skill) learning remains intact.[4]

A second distinction must also be made between recent and long-standing memory. HM has great difficulty in recalling events since his operation but, astonishingly, he can recall precise details from his earlier life.[5] Thus, the limbic brain is not the site of storage of memories, nor their site of recall, but would seem to be somehow required to boost the laying down of new permanent memories.

Then again there is another distinct type of memory, termed "working memory." This differs from the other types because it is transient; for instance, in conversation we remember precisely for a few seconds what has just been said to us (and what we have ourselves said) – all necessary to maintain a discussion. A few moments later we can recall the conversation, but not the precise words uttered. Fast working memory is still intact in patients like HM after limbic surgery.

Because of HM's renown in the field, over recent decades there has been a tendency to dwell exclusively on his amnesia. But, as Corkin[2] emphasizes, HM is a unique individual; it may be unsafe to draw too many conclusions from this one example. Specifically, we do not know what damage may have been caused by his intractable epileptic seizures prior to operation.

Other patients with moderately restricted limbic damage (RB and EH) seem to demonstrate profound amnesia for new information without other overt cognitive deficits,[6,7] just as in HM. Case IS, also having undergone bilateral removal of the medial temporal lobe, had no memory impairment[3] and though it was stated that the lesion was largely "sparing the hippocampal region," the patient "likely had as much direct damage to the hippocampus as did HM, based on Scoville's report."[8] This suggests that there is no one-to-one relationship between hippocampal lesions and amnesia. Indeed, in other amnesic patients (e.g. EP) the lesion includes large areas of overlying cortex,[7] and cortical damage may underlie the more severe memory impairment.

In animal models hippocampal lesions grossly impair memory. Here the memory disturbances following lesion to both amygdala and hippocampus are far greater than to either region alone,[9,10] pointing to conjoint activity of these two formations. Other work has highlighted the critical contribution of overlying cortex.[11]

One may conclude:

1. that lesions to the hippocampus/amygdala can impair memory, but the extent is variable between subjects

2. the hippocampus and amygdala play overlapping (conjoint) roles

3. overlying cortex, in close contact with the limbic brain, plays a role in determining lesion outcome.

Is there memory impairment in ASD?

A number of studies have noted distinct disturbances of memory function.[12–15] Some studies downplay the amnesic component of ASD, emphasizing deficits in attention and/or cognitive flexibility,[16–19] a role proposed for the hippocampus,[20,21] but subtle memory deficits do occur in ASD. Moreover, there is a slower rate of learning in ASD, particularly as task complexity increases,[22] mirroring effects of hippocampal lesions. A recent study on high-functioning ASD adults revealed impaired recall on a facial recognition task and impaired location memory.[23]

The most recent work, specifically investigating hippocampal-dependent memory function,[24] found a selective deficit in recall in ASD subjects, but hippocampus-independent memory was preserved. This provides further clear evidence implicating the hippocampus in ASD.

The barrier to learning, both in ASD and in hippocampal lesions, is not absolute. Repeat training in experimental animals with hippocampal lesions can improve performance to a level not statistically different from controls;[25] the same has been observed in ASD.[22]

Serial learning

Memory impairments in animals or subjects with limbic lesions become more pronounced when the complexity of the memory task is increased. For instance, rodents with hippocampal damage can learn, with repeat training, to remember the location of a hidden object. But once the object is moved to a new position they find it difficult to acquire the new position,[26,27] returning again and again to the original location.

This deficit was precisely replicated in a child with autism associated with lead poisoning. The authors relate: "While performing the computer-based Wisconsin Card Sorting Test, he quickly learned the rule needed to perform the task correctly. Once the rule was changed, he persisted in using the old rule and had difficulty in learning the new rule."[28]

Anxiety

ASD is often accompanied by mood disorders including anxiety and stress, depression, and obsessive-compulsive behavior.[29,30] In one study, 84% of autistic children examined met the criteria for an anxiety disorder.[31] ASD children are significantly more anxious than controls, but the severity of anxiety varied according to ASD subtype, with Asperger disorder exceeding PDD-NOS, and both exceeding autism proper (autistic disorder) on the anxiety rating scale.[32]

Anxiety is closely associated with hippocampal and amygdala function;[33,34] see also [35,36]. Induced anxiety in healthy male volunteers undergoing brain imaging (fMRI) specifically highlighted the entorhinal cortex of the hippocampal formation.[37] The patient HM, with bilateral lesions of the hippocampus and amygdala, is unable to sense anxiety,[34] though we see again that the mode and timing of the lesion is distinct from that encountered in ASD. But Prather and colleagues[38] report that young macaques (aged 6–8 months) with perinatal amygdala lesions display increased social fear suggestive of anxiety, suggesting that both hippocampus and amgydala contribute to anxiety. Other studies have confirmed a role for the amygdala in anxiety.[39]

Desire for sameness

ASD is characterized by a need for routine, with unexpected changes producing distress[40,41] as noted in the clinical behavioral rating "obsessive desire for sameness" employed by several researchers. This need for an unchanging environment may be an extension of the learning deficit with anxiety (above), perhaps accentuated by slow familiarization with a novel experience or environment, and linked to learning and memory impairments.

In experimental animals, failure to cope with change is a central characteristic of limbic/temporal lobe lesion; as Isaacson[8] properly emphasizes, a pioneer of limbic research, Heinrich Klüver, in a paper published almost 30 years after the start of his studies,[42] related other central characteristics of these lesions: specifically he stated, "The lesioned animals had difficulties in coping with any change in their experimental or environmental conditions."

This may cast light on a behavior known as "spontaneous alternation," which is exquisitely sensitive to hippocampal lesions. To explain: adult rats (but not pups), having experienced one arm of a Y-maze, and presented with a choice between a new arm and the arm already visited, systematically prefer the new arm. If the hippocampus is damaged, the spontaneous alternation disappears – animals lose the preference for the novel arm. In other words, preference skews toward sameness over novelty,[43] perhaps reflecting memory deficits or even anxiety.

Sameness is the inverse of novelty. The computation and response to novelty has been attributed to the hippocampus and the amygdala,[44,45] though this is undoubtably an oversimplification. Prather and colleagues[38] report that 6–8-month-old macaques with perinatal amygdala lesions display a lack of behavioral aversion to novel objects. Lack of appreciation of novelty has been reported in a patient with bilateral amygdala lesions.[46] No systematic studies on novelty perception in ASD have been done, but one autistic child seemingly failed to react to the presence of a TV film crew in the bath.[47]

Perception of facial emotion

Autistic subjects have a characteristic deficit in recognition of facial emotions.[48–51] This is shared by some patients with frontotemporal dementia[52–54] associated with limbic atrophy,[53,55–57] and by some patients with schizophrenia[58] where involvement of the hippocampus, amygdala, and overlying cortex has long been suspected.[59–61] Voeller[62] attributed face recognition to the temporal lobe.

Anxiety (above) is one aspect of emotionality, generally ascribed to the limbic brain. Eye contact in control subjects has emotional value and is often aversive;[63] the characteristic eye-gaze deficit seen in autism[64] could be because autistic individuals ascribe a higher negative value. Because eye direction and expression, particularly in the mother, are important early guides to training attention emotionality and language,[63] avoidance of eye contact might contribute to learning impairments, and further impact on the understanding (and perception) of facial emotion perception.

Social interaction

Impaired social interaction is a defining feature of ASD, and the known effects of limbic damage are consistent with autistic social deficits.

Few satisfactory studies have been performed on humans, but patients with bilateral lesions affecting the amygdala have impaired evaluation of social stimuli.[65] The situation in experimental animals is clearer. Rodents with hippocampal damage show deficits in social behaviors such as maternal care of offspring.[66] Social interaction, measured by the number of contacts between animals newly placed in the same cage, is adversely affected by hippocampal lesions,[67–69] with lesioned animals spending significantly less time in social contact. One study reports *increased* rather than decreased interaction[70] but this could reflect repetitive activity (above) rather than social interaction *per se.*

In monkeys, neonatal hippocampal lesions markedly reduce the time spent in social contacts with peers[71] while early lesions to the amygdala diminish social interaction in several models.[72]

The location and timing of the lesion is important. In newborn monkeys, bilateral removal of either the amygdala or hippocampus produces later-life socio-emotional disturbances.[73,74] Early damage restricted to the amygdala generated only some features of autistic-like behavior; stereotyped behavior was absent. Lesions restricted to the hippocampus caused socio-emotional disturbances but the animals were able to recover. The most severe autistic-like symptoms were produced by combined damage to amygdala plus hippocampus, probably involving adjacent cortical regions,[75,76] demonstrating co-involvement of limbic brain plus overlying cortex in social interaction.

Language

Language delay is a central diagnostic feature of ASDs with the possible exception of Asperger syndrome. Even here, in the original patients studied by Asperger, perhaps 25% had a delay in spoken or receptive language with a further proportion showing deviant modulation and articulation.[77]

Patients with limbic lesions also have language and speech impairment. Dlugos and colleagues[78] reported on five children (mean age 14 years) undergoing left temporal lobectomy for epilepsy; all exhibited significant loss of language but verbal IQ was only affected in one patient. Amnesic subjects HM and RB with limbic lesions both appear to have mild deficits in speech and vocabulary.[7,79] Schmolck, Stefanacci, and Squire[80] argued that lesions limited to the hippocampus do not affect language; linguistic impairments were only seen in patients with lesions extending into overlying temporal lobe, although there was no clear 1:1 relation.[81] However, 4 of 10 patients followed after left selective amygdalohippocampectomy showed a marked decline in linguistic functions.[82]

In review, Dawson and colleagues argued that both the social and language impairments of ASD are associated with deficits in the function of the medial temporal lobe, including the hippocampus and amygdala.[83] Specific involvement of the hippocampus and left temporal lobe in language processing is discussed further below.

Seizure

Limbic abnormalities are likely to underlie the epileptic brain activity seen in ASD. Seizures are recorded in up to 30% (population prevalence 2–3%), with two risk peaks, one before age 5 and a second in adolescence, as reviewed.[84] A 1996 survey of 187 children and adolescents with autism[85] detected 18.2% with epilepsy while more recent surveys have raised this to 35%[86] and 46%.[87]

Even in the absence of overt seizures, EEG abnormalities are common in ASD children:[86,88–91] more than 50% display abnormal traces, sometimes as high as 75%,[87] while EEG abnormalities have been associated with autistic regression.[92] In later life the elevation remains: a recent study recorded that 25% of adults with ASD have epilepsy[93] while this was 38% in another.[94]

Epileptic seizures most commonly have a focal origin in a small cluster of neurons firing uncontrollably – the activity of adjacent neurons is stimulated and a wave of abnormal neuronal firing spreads slowly through the brain, producing a fit. The sites of origin are most commonly associated with the limbic brain, particularly the hippocampus, amygdala, and adjacent sub-cortex,[95,96] with emphasis on the dentate gyrus of the hippocampus as a control point for the discharges.[97] Surgical removal of the epileptic foci can alleviate or cure the condition, as with HM.

One complexity, to be revisited later, is the reciprocal relationship between limbic damage and epilepsy. Damage can cause seizure activity, but recurrent fits can themselves *produce* limbic damage via persistent neuronal overactivation and local energy and oxygen depletion.

Sensory deficits

Sensory disturbances in ASD include both heightened and reduced responses to visual, acoustic, tactile, and pain stimuli, as reviewed.[98] Hearing deficits were seen in 8.6% and visual impairments of varying severity in 23%.[85] Sounds that are of marginal note to controls can be found aversive or unnotable to autistic individuals.[99] Another study reported increased perception of loudness in children and adolescents with autism.[100] Lack of response to adverse stimuli including pain, heat, and cold has been noted.[101] In 7 of 18 cases of infantile autism the medical notes stated explicitly "ignores pain" or "insensitive to pain."[102]

Few studies have been carried out on sensory processing in experimental animals or patients with limbic lesions, though a type of hearing "blindness" (auditory agnosia) was recorded in monkeys with bilateral temporal lobe/limbic lesions[103] and patient HM, with bilateral loss of the hippocampus and amygdala, has impaired perception of a painful heat stimulus.[104]

Stereotypy and repetitive/compulsive behaviors

Repetitive and restricted behavior is a diagnostic feature of ASD. To this one must add alternation between a restricted range of activities. In some children this could be linked to overlapping attention deficits, but autistic children do tend to move rapidly backwards and forwards between familiar activities, as if uncertain which to choose. This behavior is consistent with limbic damage.

For instance, rodents with hippocampal lesions display erratic and unstructured behavior, with "bursts and stops."[66] Locomotion is significantly increased: lesioned animals move about almost twice as much as controls.[68,105]

"Little and often" feeding behavior of animals with hippocampal damage is suggestive of autistic behavior. Clifton and colleagues[105] report "a striking behavioral syndrome in which the lesioned rats took smaller meals 2–3 times as frequently and showed a similar change in drinking," and continue: "lesioned rats alternated more frequently between feeding and drinking during a single bout of ingestive behavior" (see Figure 6.1). Similar behaviors have been reported in rats with fornix transactions – a major supply to the hippocampus,[106,107] confirming a role for the hippocampus in behavioral organization.

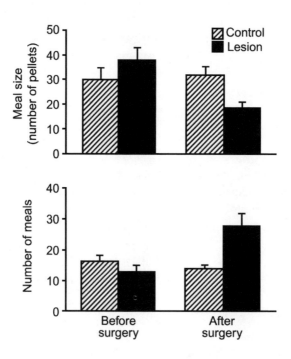

Figure 6.1 Little and often behavior in hippocampal-lesioned animals. Dark-time meal size and meal number were compared before and after surgery. Adapted from Clifton et al.[105] with permission of the American Psychological Association.

In monkeys, neonatal hippocampal lesions are reported to lead to locomotor stereotypies in adulthood.[71] Compulsive/focally-repetitive behavior is seen in humans with Klüver-Bucy syndrome (bilateral temporal lobe lesion).[108] Thus stereotypic and repetitive behaviors of autism are broadly consistent with limbic dysfunction.

Gastrointestinal (GI) effects and endocrine anomalies

The limbic brain is involved not only in cognitive processing (e.g. memory) but also in the control of body physiology, notably via regulation of endocrine (hormonal) secretions. Any damage to the limbic system would be expected to produce a wide range of regulatory problems. Chapter 8 deals with this in detail, but the conclusion is that ASD subjects clearly have a range of hormonal and physiological problems, including gastrointestinal inflammation, which parallel the effects of limbic damage.

Age of onset/maturation

Although the underlying deficit in autism is probably present much earlier, the condition is often first perceived as a problem by family members at pre-school stage (2–4 years). This is the age of onset of "adult-type" hippocampal function.

Overman[109] relates that infants as young as one year old can discriminate between objects as well as an adult, but fail dismally when picking an object *different* from one seen just a few moments before. Only at the age of 19 months did they begin to solve this task. Fitzgerald[110] reports that the first onset of the specific adult type of hippocampal-dependent memory (that of events and places) is usually between 3 and 4 years of age.

When faced with a repeated choice between two options an adult tends to choose the new or different option. A juvenile, on the other hand, tends to make the same choice over again. In rats, this is the basis of the spontaneous alternation test, dependent on the hippocampus. Douglas[111] described a critical period when a progressive switch takes place. There are individual variations, but in rats the transition generally takes place at around 4 weeks of age (accompanied by a new wave of gene expression[112]); in humans it occurs at 3–4 years.

The possibility merits consideration that ASD could reflect failure of this key transition of brain function. If limbic damage is already present, it might not be recognized before the switch from infant-type function (independent of the hippocampus and amygdala) to an adult type critically dependent on the integrity of the limbic brain.

Nevertheless, there may be a need to distinguish between congenital autism and regressive autism (childhood disintegrative disorder). In at least some children, autistic deficits can appear suddenly, and may correlate with infection and gastrointestinal disorders,[113] though these changes are hard to dissociate from the transition in brain function because they often occur at about the same time.

Table 6.1 overviews parallels between hippocampal/amygdala dysfunction and ASD (see also sections following).

Table 6.1 Similarities and parallels between autistic disorders and functional lesions of the hippocampus with adjoining amygdala

Property / deficit	Hippocampus (amygdala)	ASD
Structural/functional location	✓	Chapter 5
Anxiety	✓[33,34,114]	✓
Attention	[20,21]	✓
Epilepsy/EEG	✓	✓
Language processing	[83,115]	✓
GI effects	Chapter 8	Chapter 8
Memory	✓	[12, 24]
Endocrine regulation	✓[116]	Chapter 8
Repetitive behaviors	[66,105,108]	✓
Sensory abnormalities	✓[104]	✓[98,101]
Social behavior	✓[66,73]	✓
Age of onset/maturation	Infancy[111]	Infancy

✓ Generally accepted or defining feature. Only key citations are provided: for further literature see text.

Limbic lesions can produce ASD

A causal relation between limbic damage and ASD would be demonstrated if damage restricted to the limbic brain produces the behavioral impairments of ASD. In monkeys, this has been partially demonstrated, where the most severe autistic-like symptoms were produced by combined damage to amygdala plus hippocampus, probably involving adjacent cortical regions.[75,76] However, it may not be easy to extrapolate from monkey to man.

In human subjects, seven studies causally link limbic damage to autistic behavior. One early study reported that children with early infantile autism have a systematic anatomical pathology centered on the left medial temporal lobe and concluded: "we have suggested that dysfunction of the medial temporal lobe is a major factor in the pathogenesis of the syndrome of infantile autism."[102]

A further investigation examined a pair of identical twin boys of whom only one showed strictly defined autism. Imaging revealed that, in comparison to his brother, the affected twin had markedly smaller amygdala and hippocampus volumes[117] although other marginal brain differences were seen.

Another study reported[118] that as ASD severity increases, blood flow in the left temporal lobe including hippocampus and amygdala is proportionally reduced.

ASD severity was also found to correlate with limbic neuronal density, specifically at the amygdala–hippocampus–entorhinal cortex junction.[24]

In tuberous sclerosis tuber-like growths develop in the brain; associated deficits include mental retardation and epilepsy, but some children meet the diagnostic criteria for ASD. The location of the tubers correlates with behavioral phenotype. Eight out of nine patients with autism or atypical autism, but none of the non-autistic individuals, had tubers located in the temporal lobes, cortical regions proximal to and including the hippocampus.[119]

Chugani and colleagues[120] described 14 children (average age 2 years) with infantile spasms (seizure activity) and impaired hippocampal/temporal lobe metabolism as ascertained by PET analysis of glucose utilization. Though there was some cortical involvement in some children, only bilateral abnormalities in the hippocampus and adjacent brain (superior temporal gyrus) achieved statistical significance.

These children were followed for an average of three years because "this metabolic pattern had not been encountered or described previously." At the end of the study, all had developmental delay, minimal language development, and 10 of 14 met rigorous criteria for autistic disorder. One child was more widely impaired and could not be assessed for autism, while the remaining children had an autism spectrum disorder with communication impairment and stereotypic behavior. Thirteen out of fourteen children did not speak a single word; one child could say one or two words. The authors concluded that their findings are consistent with the hypothesis that autism is a syndrome of hippocampal dysfunction.

DeLong and Heinz[115] reported on four infants with bilateral damage to the hippocampus as ascertained by brain scanning. All were epileptic, failed to acquire language, and were severely impaired in social skills. They state: "bilateral hippocampal dysfunction in early life appears to be associated with a profound failure of cognitive capacities, including language learning and learning of

complex social and adaptive skills in general. The deficits correspond to the cognitive deficits of severe infantile autism."

The cause of hippocampal damage in these children was not known, but
three of four had perinatal insults; all had epilepsy that was subsequently controlled by medication. This study is particularly important because, as ascertained
by scanning, brain abnormalities were exclusive to the hippocampus.

One remarks that Hellmuth L, one of the original patients studied by Hans
Asperger, suffered from perinatal oxygen deprivation, a condition known to
cause specific hippocampal destruction (see Chapter 7).

These studies together argue most strongly that hippocampal lesions
underlie the brain and behavior disturbances of ASD. From the DeLong and
Heinz study (on infants with lesions exclusive to the hippocampus) one may
conclude, regarding autism, hippocampal damage fulfills the criterion of sufficiency.

Autism spectrum disorder is consistent with what we know of limbic function

The striking amnesia seen in the patient HM after removal of hippocampus and
amygdala is seemingly at odds with the pervasive social, linguistic, and cognitive
impairments of ASD. However, HM's profound memory impairment is not replicated in all other patients with similar lesions: hippocampal plus amygdala dysfunction does not equal frank impairment of memory function.[8] Even so, on the
one hand we have the historic association of the hippocampus with memory; on
the other we have language and communication deficits that are central to the
diagnostic ascertainment of ASD. Can these be reconciled?

First, the effects of limbic damage are critically dependent upon (a) the
timing and duration of the insult, (b) the type and extent of the lesion, (c) the par-
ticipation of neighboring brain regions.[121] In both amnesia and in ASD the role of
overlying cortex has been highlighted (see earlier). Amnesia can be produced by
damage in adulthood: but neonatal hippocampal lesions produce a syndrome
most akin to severe childhood autism.[115]

Second, the distinction between memory and speech and language retardation (as in ASD) is blurred. A body of thought has linked speech deficits to
specific memory impairment: "Sprachamnesie" or "aphasie amnésique," also
"semantic memory,"[122] and principally associated with the left temporal lobe.[123]
The left temporal lobe has been inferred to specifically deal with pitch/rate of
speech (prosody) and syntax, as reviewed.[62]

Third, clinical syndromes with ASD-like features including speech and language deficits are associated with left temporal lobe and hippocampal lesions (below).

Frontotemporal dementia (clinical Pick's disease)

The condition is characterized by abnormalities of personality, language, and social conduct,[124] often including aggression, while cognitive deficits are mild.[125] Face pattern recognition can be selectively affected,[52,126] as in ASD.[49] Histological abnormalities are most pronounced in hippocampus, particularly in the hippocampal dentate gyrus, and to a lesser extent in cortex.[127,128]

Alzheimer disease and dementia

The early signs of hippocampal degeneration are short-term memory loss, subtle language impairments, and personality changes, with only mild cognitive impairment.[129] Progressive speech and language loss in patients with semantic dementia is associated with temporal lobe atrophy.[130]

Hippocampal sclerosis (HS) and Reye

In children with bilateral HS associated with epilepsy or with bilateral limbic damage produced by herpes encephalitis, or Reye syndrome (acquired aphasia often associated with encephalitis and EEG abnormalities), marked memory deficits are typically accompanied by impairment of language development.[131–135]

Klüver-Bucy syndrome (KBS)

Attributed to bilateral temporal lobe/hippocampus/amygdala lesion, KBS is primarily associated with deviant hyperactivity and compulsive behavior[108] overlapping with inappropriate behaviors seen in hippocampal sclerosis dementia[136] and sometimes in ASD.[137] Speech deficits in classic KBS have also been recorded.

Overview and conclusions

The previous chapter argued that, on balance, limbic brain regions are most consistently abnormal in ASD. Other regions are also abnormal, including the cortex and cerebellum, but these are unlikely alone to explain the behavioral deficits of ASD. Here it is suggested that damage to the limbic brain fulfills the three key criteria of plausibility, necessity, and, most probably, sufficiency.

First, behaviors associated with limbic damage resemble autism in a long series of different categories (see Table 6.1). Second, the limbic brain is consistently abnormal (Chapter 5), while other brain regions such as cortex and cerebellum are only affected in some studies. Indeed, the cerebellum is generally held to govern movement and posture; these are not central diagnostic features of ASDs (though clumsiness is noted in some subjects). A crucial observation is that no studies report damage to only cortex or cerebellum in ASD, with an absence of any limbic involvement. Thus limbic damage is probably necessary for ASD to develop. Third, ASD is seen in subjects with selective limbic lesions, suggesting that limbic damage also fulfills the criterion of sufficiency.

It is therefore argued that the central impairments of ASD are consistent with damage to the hippocampus and amygdala, with variable involvement of overlying cortical regions.

Key points

The limbic system has generally been associated with memory, given the massive loss of new memory formation in some, but not all, adult patients with hippocampus and amygdala damage.

The outcome of brain damage depends on the age of the subject and the type of lesion.

Limbic damage could underlie ASD. Limbic abnormalities and ASD overlap in key areas including memory impairments, desire for sameness, anxiety, perception of facial features and emotion, social interaction, language, seizure, sensory deficits, and repetitive behaviors.

Seven studies in humans causally link limbic damage to autistic behavior.

Damage to the limbic brain fulfills the three key criteria of plausibility, necessity, and, most probably, sufficiency. Limbic damage is therefore likely to cause ASD.

Chapter 7

Environmental Factors, Heavy Metals, and Brain Function

All disorders have a cause. This can be purely genetic, a good example being the collapse of red blood cells due to abnormal hemoglobin in sickle cell anemia. The problem here is a mutant gene that causes production of anomalous proteins which in turn alter the shape of the red blood cells, impairing their function. Disorders can also be purely environmental – for instance, the drug thalidomide used by pregnant women to prevent morning sickness had the disastrous effect of producing severe physical deformities in the child. But, although both examples seem straightforward, they only tell part of the story.

One would expect that a gene causing faulty red blood cells would be quite rare since the sickle-shaped red blood cells do not carry oxygen and can cause blockage of small arteries. People with this gene mutation would be less healthy, leading to removal of the gene from the population. However, this mutation seems to be *beneficial* in malaria-infested areas – the parasite that causes malaria cannot reproduce in the altered red blood cells. People with the sickle-cell trait are protected and survive, and so carry the mutant gene into the next generation – a good example of the interaction of a genetic disorder and environmental factors.

Conversely, in the thalidomide tragedy many children of mothers taking thalidomide during the critical period showed no abnormalities. Although not well studied, one must presume that some mothers with favorable genes could degrade and detoxify the thalidomide molecule, preventing it from harming their children. And some children may not have been susceptible. Even a disorder like this, which appears to be entirely environmental, can be strongly dependent on genetic factors.

In considering autism, therefore, it would be unwise to look exclusively for an environmental or a genetic cause. Rather, one must consider the most likely scenario of an environmental trigger with an underlying genetic susceptibility. Given the evidence that autism and autistic spectrum disorders (ASDs) are becoming more and more common, and that changes in diagnostic criteria and awareness cannot completely explain this rise (see Chapter 4), there is a strong case to be made that something in the environment is at least partly responsible.

Environmental factors and ASD

Studies carried out over the 1980s to 2000s point strongly to the environment as a possible and plausible cause for the rise in autism. There are many well-documented instances in which exposure to toxins in the environment is known to contribute to the disorder.

For instance, it has been shown that living in a town compared to a rural area is associated with significantly increased ASD rates.[1] In Texas a study showed that the incidence of ASD in children growing up in an urban environment was over 4½ times that of the incidence of children growing up in a rural environment.[2]

Some environmental factors are shown to have their effect via the mother. Several drugs, when used by pregnant women, have been shown to increase the likelihood of the child developing ASD. Known specific exposures include maternal smoking[3,4] and thalidomide itself: 4% of Swedish victims meet the diagnostic criteria for autism.[5] Fetal exposure to maternal alcohol excess has also been linked to later development of autism.[6-8] An elevated ASD frequency (11.4%) is reported in children exposed to cocaine *in utero*.[9]

Prescribed drugs can also be a risk factor. Maternal anticonvulsant medication (specifically sodium valproate) has been linked to autistic behavior in offspring: in a systematic study 81% of children with fetal anticonvulsant syndrome were reported to display autistic-type behaviors; 77% had developmental delay.[10] In fact, fetal exposure to valproate has been employed in numerous animal studies to mimic the behavioral deficits seen in human ASD.[11]

These examples demonstrate that exposure to certain chemicals in early development can produce the behavioral signs of ASD in a significant proportion of exposed children. Given that ASD is associated with, and can be due to, neuronal dysfunction in and around specific brain regions (the limbic brain, centrally including the hippocampus and amygdala; see previous chapters), the question arises of what environmental agents might precipitate damage to these brain regions.

This chapter now considers the potential role of environmental toxicity, with specific emphasis on heavy metal exposure, in the causation of autistic spectrum disorders. The issue breaks down into several topics, each deserving of attention. Evidence is first reviewed that specific environmental toxicity is a known cause of ASD, before moving to consider whether heavy metals may be specifically implicated in the current rise in ASD prevalence. The contention is debated that the population, and ASD children in particular, is widely exposed to heavy metals. Because only some children are affected, the possibility is then raised that ASD children may be particularly prone to heavy metal toxicity through genetic susceptibility factors, perhaps affecting the mobilization and excretion of metals.

Consideration of the types of brain damage seen in animals and patients exposed to specific heavy metals and organometals leads to the conclusion that these are indeed very plausible candidates for the specific limbic dysfunction seen in ASD. The question of why the limbic brain might be peculiarly sensitive to heavy metals is then raised: this issue is debated further in Chapter 11.

Despite the special focus on heavy metals, it is clear that other insults can also cause damage to the limbic brain, and by way of conclusion it is suggested that new ASD may result from a cocktail of toxins, with metals playing a central role, but which together may cause more severe damage than any component in isolation.

Metals: evidence for exposure

With increasing industrialization, metals are becoming very much more abundant in our environment. Every ship that sinks, every rusting car, every unsealed mine, and every tin can in our refuse dumps all contribute to a rise in the levels of metals in seawater. Large quantities of metals are also launched into the atmosphere – by industrial processes, by incineration of domestic waste, and by the burning of fossil fuels. Metals in soils and oceans accumulate in plants, animals, and fish, and thereby enter the food chain.

Some metals, like iron, are thought to be relatively benign, while others are notorious poisons. Mercury and arsenic are well known for their toxicity, particularly on the brain. And exposure to these specific metals is increasing. In a recent California study the mean mercury level (in women) was ten times above an earlier government population survey; some children had levels 40 times the national mean.[12] The publicly debated decline in sperm counts in the population[13,14] has been correlated with heavy metal exposure.[15] It is possible that other disorders that are also increasing in prevalence, such as autism, could also be precipitated by exposure to toxic metals.

Historic evidence

A series of studies queried a possible link between lead exposure, ASD, and childhood neurodevelopmental disorders.[16–24] The first of these saw elevated blood lead levels in ASD children; 44% of cases had levels well beyond the normal range.[16]

This was however attributed to habitual mouth contact and odd food preferences called "pica," possibly deriving from the Latin word meaning magpie, reflecting this bird's peculiar eating behaviors. However, one suspects that this behavior is a consequence (rather than a cause) of heavy metal exposure. Often seen in pregnancy, pica describes the desire to consume unusual and even "abnormal" foods. These can include clay, coal, soil, and the desire is very troublesome to the subject. However, there have been studies in which mineral replacement (iron) has been able to suppress the pica behavior – and, though still hotly debated, the hunger is now thought to reflect a deficiency in nutrient metals.[25,26] In relation to heavy metal toxicity, exposure to abnormal heavy metals can block the uptake and metabolic pathways for nutrient metals like iron. Thus, pica can be a sign of metal poisoning, and not a cause. In fact, it has been argued that many children with lead poisoning first present clinically with pica.[27]

More recent work has implicated autism with exposure to lead – autism in children intoxicated with lead has been reported[28] and, in a cluster of Canadian children with an unspecified ASD-related disorder, elevated urinary levels of lead and other heavy metals were seen on treatment with a metal-mobilizing agent (cuprimine). Significantly, in this study heavy metal removal seemed to improve behavior.[29]

Lead is not the only contender. Superficial resemblances between mercury poisoning and ASD prompted the suggestion that mercury might also be causally involved.[30] We will see below that other heavy metals could contribute.

Metals in hair

Analysis of the hair of ASD children has been investigated as a means to address metal exposure. Hair is a useful indicator not only because is it easily sampled, but also because significant quantities of heavy metals from the bloodstream are actively secreted into hair. In rats given a single dose of methylmercury, 10% was transported into hair;[31] in humans mercury in hair reflects levels in internal organs.[32]

An early report on ASD individuals described elevated levels of lithium, but depressed hair levels of other metals including magnesium and manganese; no specific elevation of toxic heavy metals was observed.[33] One recent study of Chinese (Hong Kong) ASD children reported no difference in mean mercury levels.[34] Another study, in Kuwaiti children, reported significant elevations of metals in the hair of ASD children versus controls – lead (Pb) was two-fold elevated, uranium (U) three-fold, while mercury (Hg) levels were 15 times higher than in controls.[35]

However, these studies need to be interpreted with caution for hair metal levels do not adequately reflect exposure; and in fact abnormally low levels in ASD have been reported, as discussed below – suggesting that ASD children might be unable to secrete heavy metals into their hair.

Blood levels

In order to clarify these contradictions some studies have looked at levels in blood rather than in hair. One report[36] described high levels of mercury in red blood cells of ASD children. Total mercury levels were in the range 26–103 ng/ml (mean 68) against values in the range 11–34 ng/ml for control children (mean 20), a rise of just over three-fold. Another early study reported that mean blood levels of lead (Pb) were higher in ASD children than controls;[16] evidence of excessive exposure to lead, arsenic, and cadmium has been reported.[36]

Metals in teeth

Increased exposure to mercury is strengthened by an as yet unpublished baby-tooth study[37] describing three-fold increase in mercury in ASD samples versus controls.

Porphyrins

These are intermediates in the synthesis of heme, the red oxygen-carrying pigment of hemoglobin. Heavy metals are known to inhibit key enzymes in the synthetic pathway, and this leads to accumulation of precursors that are expelled from the body in the urine. Individuals exposed to heavy metals carry more porphyrins than usual and excrete the excess.[38,39]

Metals can be removed by absorbing them by a process termed chelation to specific metal-binding compounds, or chelating agents. The metal ions are then unable to react or to affect the body, and the inert complexes are then generally exported in urine or feces.

When heavy metals are removed by chelation then the amounts of porphyrins in the urine are reduced. Both in rats exposed to mercury[40] and in humans exposed to lead,[41] chelation (respectively with dimercapto-propanesulfonic acid [DMPS] and ethylenediamine tetraacetic acid [EDTA]) reduced urinary porphyrin levels.

One large survey has revealed that excess urinary porphyrin is a feature of autism (see Figure 7.1). In a group of French children mean urinary levels were 2.6-fold elevated in children with autism compared to the control group.[42] The elevation was very comparable to the increases seen in known arsenic (1.9-fold) or mercury (3.2-fold) exposure,[43,44] and was of high statistical significance (p<0.001).

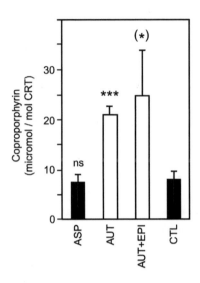

Figure 7.1 Excess coproporphyrin (a marker of heavy metal toxicity) in urines of children with autistic disorder. ASP, Asperger disorder; AUT, autistic disorder; AUT+EPI, autistic disorder with epilepsy; CTL, control group (unrelated conditions). Adapted from Nataf et al.;[42] ★★★, p<0.001; (★), p<0.1; ns, not significant.

A striking observation was that children of a similar age with Asperger disorder did not show any evidence of heavy metal exposure, while there was some evidence for elevated porphyrins in other ASD conditions, PDD-NOS and Rett's disorder.

Nevertheless, heavy metals are not the only agents capable of producing elevations of urinary porphyrins. Other toxicants and xenobiotics that elevate urinary porphyrins include polychlorinated biphenyls and dioxins.[45,46] Even so, the same study reported that treatment of a subgroup of these children with the chelating agent dimercapto-succinic acid (DMSA) reduced porphyrin levels toward control values,[42] suggesting that heavy metals are responsible. In addition, precoproporphyrin is a specific marker of heavy metal toxicity,[43] and is not found in chemical toxicity. Levels of this molecule were also systematically elevated in the urines of ASD children.[42]

Though this striking elevation of urinary porphyrins remains to be confirmed, the specific elevation of precoproporphyrin points to heavy metal exposure in these children. The relevance of porphyrin and heme pathways to the causes of ASD is discussed in more depth in Chapter 9.

Statistical correlations with mercury exposure

Holmes and colleagues found there was a link between ASD and the exposure of mothers to mercury while they were pregnant.[47] They compared ASD and control children for maternal mercury exposure via ethylmercury-containing Rho(D) immunoglobulin shots.

If a rhesus-negative woman (lacking a specific blood protein type) bears a rhesus-positive fetus (in around 10% of pregnancies) she risks mounting a damaging immune response against the "foreign" blood protein. Rho(D) or "rhesus" immunoglobulin is administered to the mother during pregnancy to prevent this immune response, and has been very effective. However, Rho(D) generally contains an ethylmercury preservative. The mean number of shots in mothers of ASD children was 0.53 versus 0.09 in controls,[47] and was of very high statistical significance. Another study has confirmed the link between rhesus incompatibility (and therefore Rho(D) administration) and the development of ASD.[48] These studies suggest either that rhesus incompatibility is an independent risk factor, or that maternal administration of ethylmercury in the immunoglobulin increases the rate of ASD development in the child.

Another study examined the association between autism prevalence in 1184 school districts in Texas (data from the Texas Education Authority) and local environmental release of mercury (as published by the US Toxic Release Inventory). For each 1000 pounds (1 pound = 0.454 kg) of environmental mercury release there was a 61% increase in the rate of autism.[2] Though the authors stress that a causal association cannot be determined from this study,[2] the study is also consistent with a causal link.

Metal release on chelation

Because heavy metals tend to become immobilized in body tissues, particularly on long-term exposure, blood levels do not adequately reflect heavy metal burden. Urinary and fecal export following chelation therapy is a more reliable indicator.

Significant quantities of arsenic were released in a clinical trial of heavy metal removal in ASD with the chelation agent thiamine tetrahydrofurfuryl disulfide (TTFD); increases in urinary cadmium, nickel, and lead were observed in some subjects, while mercury levels remained low.[49]

A further study[50] compared urinary metal levels in matched ASD children and controls following treatment with dimercapto-succinic acid (DMSA). After DMSA treatment, mercury levels were strongly elevated versus controls (factor of

5.94); in ASD, the rise was highly significant.[50] There was only a small increase in lead levels (1.5-fold), but the extent of release in some children was extremely high (18.2 +/− 43.3 µg normalized per g of the ubiquitous metabolite creatinine) compared to controls (11.8 +/− 8.6 µg/g).

Holmes and colleagues, following Hallaway and Strauts,[29] have suggested that heavy metal removal by chelation is associated with partial remission of ASD behaviors,[51] a challenging contention that requires validation.

Heavy metal susceptibility

If exposure to environmental heavy metals is widespread, one must ask why perhaps only some individuals develop autism. There have been recent suggestions that children who later develop ASD may be especially susceptible, and differ from other children in the way they process heavy metals. Specifically, it seems possible that they are unable to export metals, leading to toxic accumulation in the body.

Defective heavy metal mobilization: the Holmes study

Many families retain first baby hair as mementoes. This is sufficiently common to allow researchers to look back at heavy metal levels, specifically mercury, in samples from large numbers of children later diagnosed as autistic, as well as from normal children.[47] Using a first technique (inductively coupled-mass spectroscopy) it was discovered that, rather than showing evidence of excess exposure, to the researchers' surprise levels were abnormally *low* in the samples from pre-ASD children. This was in contrast to the samples from normal children – here mercury levels went up very much in line with exposure – as assessed by maternal fish meals, dental amalgams, and medications containing mercury (see Figure 7.2). Hair Hg values were: control children, mean = 3.63 parts per million (ppm, or µg/g); "autism," overall mean = 0.47 ppm; "severe autism," mean = 0.21 ppm. The comparison between autism and severe autism is particularly striking – the children later most severely affected had the very *lowest* levels.[47] This finding is reminiscent of the Seychelles study on over 700 children exposed to mercury, where the boys with *higher* hair levels performed better on some brain and behavior tests.[52] The same finding was made in the Faroe Islands, where developmental milestones were achieved earlier by children who, at 12 months of age, had *higher* levels of hair mercury[53] – in the same island population, blood (rather than hair) mercury at birth correlated with delayed neurologic development.[54]

Confirmation was provided by Hu and colleagues[55] who used a second independent technique (neutron activation analysis) on the same baby-hair samples previously analyzed, and found identical results. The results have been largely

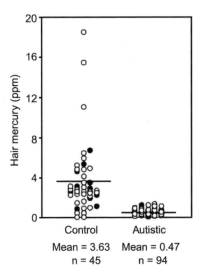

Figure 7.2 Deficient mobilization of mercury in ASD. Hair mercury levels in first baby hair of children later diagnosed as autistic were measured by inductively coupled-mass spectroscopy (ICP-MS). Adapted from Figure 1 of Holmes et al.,[47] copyright 2003, from International Journal of Toxicology 22, pp.277–285. *Reproduced by permission of Taylor & Francis Group, LLC, http://www.taylorandfrancis.com.*

reproduced by Adams and colleagues, on another series of autistic and control children, who reported median values in ASD children of 0.36 ppm (range 1–19 ppm) versus 0.85 (0.07–3.5) in controls[56,57] (J. Adams, pers. comm.). However, the Adams study (to be published) contrasts with the Holmes data in two ways. The low ASD values are broadly similar (median 0.36 versus 0.47 ppm mean); comparable levels were also seen in a further series of ASD children (n=18) where hair mercury was uniformly below 0.25 ppm (W.J. Walsh, pers. comm.). Nevertheless, values in the controls (0.85 ppm) seen by Adams were substantially below those of Holmes (3.63 ppm). Differences in calculating midline values (median versus mean) might explain part of the difference, but one suspects that the Holmes control population was more severely exposed.

A second difference: while the children studied by Holmes systematically gave low values for hair mercury (as did most of the children studied by Adams), a minority of the Adams subjects had strikingly high levels (to 19 ppm). This is not unexpected. If toxic metal accumulation is a prerequisite for development of the disorder, one can imagine two mechanisms: low-level exposure of children with an export deficit, or high-level exposure of children with no such deficit. A priori, one might expect a proportion of ASD children to display large elevations of hair mercury. This has been confirmed in yet another study – it was reported in a series of children in Kuwait that children with autism (mean age 4.2 years) had significantly (p<0.001) *higher* concentrations of lead, mercury, and uranium in their hair.[35]

A complexity here is that some studies look at current levels in autistic children, while others look at first baby hair. One cannot rule out the possibility that, for instance, metal detoxification and/or export mechanisms might be very different in babies and in older children. Indeed, it has been suggested that export of mercurials is particularly low in the first year of life.[58] Even so, the large baby-hair study teaches us that a majority of babies later to become autistic are abnormal in the way they mobilize mercury in early life. The deficit could extend to other heavy metals: an early study reported significantly reduced levels of cadmium in hair of autistic children.[18] If mobilization processes operate in other organs, mercury and related metals are likely to accumulate in a sensitive subclass of children to produce brain damage.

Genetic predisposition to heavy metal toxicity

It seems possible, if not probable, that many children developing ASD are especially sensitive because they cannot export mercury, and perhaps other metals too. There is a precedent for genetic predisposition to heavy metal toxicity. In a family exposed to arsenic only one individual, the daughter, presented with mental deterioration: she was found to have a deficit in an enzyme known as methylene tetrahydrofolate reductase, or MTHFR,[59] an enzyme required for efficient metal export.

It turns out that a variant gene (where the amino acid cysteine, C, at position 677 in the MTHFR protein, is replaced by threonine, T), known as the C677T allele, is widespread in the population. Importantly, the encoded enzyme is unstable and shows only partial activity,[60] and might be expected to sensitize to heavy metal toxicity. Studies have shown that roughly 12% of the North American population have two copies (i.e. are homozygous) of the low-activity C677T gene,[61] and could be especially sensitive. Several other polymorphisms have been described that are likely to affect the activity of the enzyme.[62]

An association between MTHFR genotype and the development of autism has been reported. In fetal anticonvulsant syndrome (drug-induced developmental delay), where autism very often develops in the children of mothers receiving anti-epileptic medication, C677T was found much more commonly, not in the children themselves, but in their mothers.[63] This suggests that the normal high-activity version (C677), in the mother, can protect the fetus against damage induced by the medication.

In ASD subjects themselves a significant bias in MTHFR alleles has also been reported:[64] 48% of controls had two copies of the normal C677 version (i.e. they were homozygous for the MTHFR C677 allele), but only 21% of ASD children. Conversely, homozygosity for the low-activity allele T677 was found in 23% of ASD versus only 11% of controls. This was of high statistical significance[64] – one can conclude that homozygosity for the low-activity C677T roughly doubles the risk of ASD development.

Other genes are likely to contribute. For instance, metallothionein (MT) is generally considered to be among the most important heavy metal binding and mobilizing proteins, and mutations affecting MT could render individuals susceptible to toxic metals. Nevertheless, despite anecdotal reports,[65] the specific involvement of MT alleles in ASD has not yet been confirmed.

Other metal-related genes and alleles whose frequencies are skewed in ASD subjects include the metal regulatory transcription factor (MTF-1) and a divalent metal ion transporter (ferroportin, SLC11A3).[66] One may also note that, like MTHFR, neither locus is located on the X-chromosome, and so cannot explain the elevated rate of ASD in males versus females.

A recent report has suggested that different alleles of a gene encoding a heme blood pigment synthesis enzyme (coproporphyrinogen oxidase) are likely to determine the extent of porphyrin excretion on mercury exposure, and could possibly determine susceptibility to the toxic effects of the metal.[67] Studies in autism and ASD have not so far been performed.

Overall, the toxicologic and genetic evidence suggests that children developing ASD are genetically distinct (but not abnormal – for instance, different MTHFR alleles are widely distributed in the population and one may suspect that, without heavy metal exposure, there would be no adverse consequences of bearing one or other allele). But, despite the focus on MTHFR, it is not yet known if allelic variants at this locus contribute to the hair export deficit described by Holmes *et al.*[47]

The next section addresses whether heavy metals, which perhaps accumulate to higher levels in ASD children, are viable candidates for the brain and behavior disturbances characteristic of autism disorders. Given evidence for both exposure and susceptibility, we face another central question – is it plausible that heavy metals might produce the brain damage and behavioral changes seen in ASD? Though preceding debate has focused on mercury, to answer this question we turn in the first instance from mercury to a different metal, tin, where an abundance of data regarding specific neurotoxicity has accumulated.

Heavy metal toxicity: the trimethyltin (TMT) paradigm

From rodents through to primates, exposure to organotin derivatives produces selective damage to the same brain regions abnormal in ASD – specifically the hippocampus with dentate gyrus, with some cortical and cerebellar involvement (see Chapter 5). This evidence is reviewed below, first in terms of the regional localization of damage, and then with regard to the associated behavioral disturbances.

In rats, diffuse TMT damage is seen in several brain regions including subcortex and amygdala,[68,69] but the hippocampus is most sensitive, with dentate damage being prominent.[68–77] The same profile is observed in mice[71,78,79] (see Figure 7.3). Exposure is accompanied by overproduction of several inflammatory cytokines IL-1α, IL-1β, TNFα, and IL-γ,[79,80] all implicated in toxic damage to the formation (see Chapter 9).

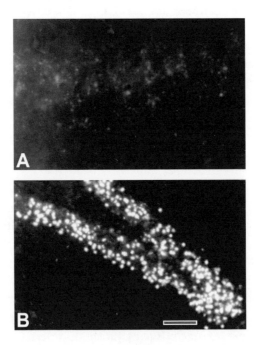

Figure 7.3 Neuronal death in the hippocampal dentate gyrus following trimethyltin (Me3Sn) administration. Brains of mice injected intraperitoneally with trimethyltin (2.5 mg/kg body weight) were examined three days post-challenge for DNA fragmentation on programmed cell death (white staining: technique was terminal transferase dUTP-fluorescein nick end-labeling [TUNEL]). The figure shows trimethyltin-induced DNA fragmentation in hippocampal dentate gyrus cells. A, control; B, TMT-treated mice. Scale bar, 76 um. Reprinted from Brain Research 912, Fiedorowicz et al.,[78] "Dentate granule neuron apoptosis and glia activation in murine hippocampus induced by trimethyltin exposure," pp.116–127, copyright 2001, with permission from Elsevier.

Although the doses in these models are high, such studies often employ single-shot administration to produce catastrophic damage to relevant brain regions. Diffuse damage (as seen in ASD) might occur in individuals with an export deficit on long-term exposure to low doses.

Exactly the same pattern of brain damage is seen in primates exposed to TMT. Single-shot exposure of marmosets (3 mg/kg by injection) resulted in bilateral neuronal loss in hippocampus and amygdala, with some damage to cortex and brainstem.[81] But, on chronic TMT exposure (0.75 mg/kg of TMT chloride for 24 weeks), adverse changes in the marmoset brain principally target the hippocampus and dentate gyrus.[82]

In a human male, sudden lethal TMT exposure produced specific and severe neuronal necrosis in the dentate gyrus of the hippocampus, with further damage to hippocampal CA regions, cortex, and the cerebellum.[83–85] In a female, after fatal TMT exposure, neuronal death was seen in the dentate gyrus of the hippocampus, with additional damage to the cortex and cerebellum.[86] Thus, TMT causes selective destruction of the same brain regions implicated in autism and ASD.

Organotins also demonstrate that toxicity is critically dependent on chemical formulation: tributyltin (TBT) produces swelling (edema) of neuronal filaments (axons) in rats while trimethyltin (TMT) causes bilateral alterations centered on the hippocampus, amygdala, and overlying cortex.[68] A third molecule, triethyltin (TET), produces brain and spinal cord edema.[87]

In cell lines cultured in the laboratory, exposure to TBT (and triethyltin) produced cell death at similar concentrations in all the lines tested. In contrast, TMT sensitivity was highly variable – some cell lines were resistant to TMT toxicity, others highly sensitive.[88] This concept of specific tissue susceptibility is revisited later in this chapter.

Behavioral consequences of TMT exposure

In rats, TMT toxicity (both chronic and acute) causes a spectrum of behavioral changes including hyperactivity, susceptibility to seizures, and impaired learning, but also with clear effects on vision, hearing, and pain thresholds (see Table 7.1). A similar spectrum including seizure susceptibility and hyperactivity is seen in mice receiving TMT.[89,90] One paper reported that TBT (rather than TMT) administration to newborn rats (but in this study by injection) produced hyperactivity at 4–5 weeks of age and, as with hippocampal lesions[91] implicated in ASD (see Chapter 6), hyperactivity was dependent on ambient illumination, only appearing during the dark cycle.[92]

Behavioral aspects of organotin toxicity have been reviewed.[87,93–96] These deficits are reminiscent of ASD. Swartzwelder and colleagues,[97] working with

Table 7.1 Behavioral and physiological consequences of hippocampal and wider brain damage induced by trimethyltin (TMT) exposure in rats and mice

Phenotype	References
Aggression	77,97
Auditory damage (ototoxicity)	98–100
Endocrine effects: hypokalemia and aldosterone excess	101
Growth retardation	74,102
Hyperactivity and hyperexcitability	68,69,72,97,103,104
Learning and memory impaired	73,77,105,106
Nociception (pain, heat, cold sensing) impaired	107
Seizure susceptibility	68,76,77,108,109
Social interaction depressed	92 (tributyltin)
Spontaneous alternation block (key phenotype of hippocampal damage in rodents)	110,111
Visual effects	112

rats, observed: "trimethyltin produced an autism-like behavioral disorder involving hyperactivity, perservation, aggressiveness and impairment in problem-solving and memory function." Though strongly reminiscent of ASD, it is perhaps unsafe to extrapolate too freely from rodents to humans.

Few systematic behavioral studies have been performed on the behavior of primates exposed to TMT, though the brain regions affected appear to be identical to those damaged in rodents. In marmosets, TMT exposure was associated with agitation and occasional fits.[81]

In adult humans, symptoms of acute TMT poisoning include headache, tinnitus, defective hearing, disorientation, sleep disturbances, depression, and aggressiveness,[83] with persistent memory deficits reported in one patient.[113] Behavioral and biochemical sequelae of TMT exposure have been reviewed.[85] Although in many respects TMT exposure resembles ASD, no confirming data regarding TMT exposure of children are so far available. Indeed, we will see below that there are reasons to suppose that the toxic effects on young children may be more intense and more long-lasting than in adults.

Developmental susceptibility

Rats are particularly prone to adverse TMT effects during the perinatal period; structural and behavioral changes can persist to adulthood. When exposed during gestation, postnatal changes were restricted to the hippocampus (CA3) and dentate gyrus,[73,74] while TMT administered to postnatal rats caused dose-related decrease in brain weights at all ages, with the hippocampus being the most reduced.[73] TMT produced hypoactivity early in development but this later converted to hyperactivity; deficits and hyperactivity persisted into adult life.[73]

Population exposure: excess and deficiency

The TMT paradigm demonstrates that heavy metals are plausible causal candidates for damage to the limbic brain regions implicated in ASD, even though doses were generally elevated in the data reviewed above.

Given this precedent, one must look more widely to different heavy metals and their derivatives to explore whether any, including tin, might contribute to the current rise in ASD prevalence. Here different metals (including lead, tin, mercury, and aluminum) and their derivatives are very briefly reviewed for their environmental distribution and potential to cause brain damage.

Lead (Pb)

Historically, lead exposure was widespread, through household plumbing, paints, and gasoline additives. Today, exposure is more likely through the diet – lead levels in fish up to 0.67 µg/g (= ppm) have been reported in Missouri,[114] a concentration compatible with toxicity. Lead levels may be elevated in ASD children.[36] The synthesis of blood cells in bone marrow is the classical target for lead toxicity, with the brain and kidney following.[27] Lead is clearly a neurotoxin: in rats, lead-induced behavioral deficits were ascribed to hippocampal damage,[115,116] though in rabbits the cerebellum was principally implicated.[117] Exactly as with TMT, the hippocampus appears particularly vulnerable to triethyl lead.[118] Developmental lead exposure in rats is associated with hyperactivity, decreased exploratory behavior, and impairment of learning and memory; later life anxiety is reported.[119] As discussed in the previous chapter, one characteristic of hippocampal damage is impairment in rule changing – it has been reported that children with low-level lead exposure have a tendency to repeat incorrect responses (perseverate) in tests,[120] and this impairment correlates significantly with blood lead levels. Lead-induced toxicity also includes abdominal pain, sometimes with diarrhea and sometimes with constipation,[27] as often seen in ASD (see Chapter 8).

Recently, two cases of children with autism-like behavior ascribed to lead poisoning were reported. Both boys showed loss of previously acquired skills, with decline of speech and communication, and met DSM-IV criteria for autistic disorder.[28]

Tin (Sn)

The ability of tin derivatives to cause selective hippocampal damage was discussed above. Like mercury (section following), metallic tin is a major component (12–16%) of dental amalgams. It is also found (as stannous fluoride and chloride) in some dental hygiene products including toothpaste; stannous fluoride is one of seven chemicals listed for use in water fluoridation programs.[121] Organotins are used as heat-stabilizers for PVC, catalysts for foam and rubber, and as biocides.[122] Tributyltin (TBT) is the most common organotin, but is converted in the biosphere to TMT (though phenyltins are also encountered). TBT was widely used as an anti-fouling paint on boats, but this has been largely discontinued, with a global ban on the application of TBT-based paint introduced in 2003 and declining levels of marine TBT have been recorded over the last few years.[123] However, TBT continues to be used in some applications, as does triphenyltin.

Overall, organotin (rather than just TBT) levels may still be rising. Organotin in tuna (muscle) was recently estimated at 20 ng/g (as reviewed[123]) but phenyltin levels may be much higher (up to 1.7 µg/g).[124] Unfortunately, there are as yet no data on tin levels in samples from ASD subjects.

Mercury (Hg)

Environmental exposure to mercurials is now widespread. The most common source is fish: industrial mercuric ion in water accumulates in aquatic life where it is converted largely to methylmercury;[125] there is a wide literature on this topic but, for illustration, total mercury levels, principally methylmercury, in Neckar (Heidelberg) fish were up to 0.8 µg/g;[126] maximum levels of 0.8 µg/g were seen in some Tennessee fish;[127] while mean freshwater fish levels of 0.7 µg/g were seen in Sweden.[128] These levels are reiterated in fish samples across the globe, with an average (of all means, ocean species, data from [129]) of 1.2 µg/g, and are comparable to those of Pb and Sn. In some localities, fish mercury levels were ten-fold higher.

Mercury release from dental amalgams (approximately 50% Hg) is a further source of exposure, but in the study of Holmes et al.[47] seafood consumption was not the major correlate of baby-hair levels in control subjects, with amalgams and medications containing ethylmercury preservative (Rho immunoglobulin, vaccines) playing a more important role. Then, when ASD development (rather than mercury levels) was studied, the most important factor (as assessed by statistical significance) was Rho immunoglobulin, suggesting that the risk of ASD in offspring is greater from injected ethylmercury than from maternal dental amalgams.

In adult humans, blood Hg correlates with seafood consumption: mercury levels reduce on avoiding fish (p<0.0001).[12] A prominent role for vaccine mercury in ASD development is thus debatable; one study reported a statistical link[130] while others found no such relationship.[131,132] However, vaccine and immunoglobulin mercury will be additive to other exposures and, most importantly, the route (injection) and timing (during gestation and infancy) would seem by far to be the most likely to be a risk factor for neurodevelopmental disorders.

Mercury, like lead and tin, is a neurotoxin. Phenotypic overlaps between mercury toxicity and ASD have been noted.[30] Prenatal exposure from a maternal diet high in seafood is known to impair later brain function in children followed up at 7 years[133] and 14 years.[134] Clinical manifestations of intoxication in children include excessive shyness, intolerance, irritability, and "difficult behavior."[27] The developing brain is very much more sensitive to toxic effects – in the Iraq 1971–72 incident infants born to mothers who ate bread contaminated with mercurials exhibited far more serious neurologic signs than their parent.[135]

Though one might suspect mercury as being a prime culprit in ASD, the neurologic signs of ASD are distinct from, though overlapping, those of mercury toxicity. In overt methylmercury poisoning, tremor and movement impairment (ataxia) are commonplace,[136] with marked kidney damage,[137] but these conditions are not typically recognized in ASD. ASD-specific symptoms have not so far been reported in tragic mercury/methylmercury poisoning episodes in Minamata, Japan, in the 1950s and in Iraq in 1971–1972, or in regions where increased environmental dietary exposure is suspected. Only occasional cases of acute mercury poisoning seem to manifest with developmental regression and autistic behavior.[138]

In fact, the physical signs of methylmercury poisoning are distinct from ASD. Overt methylmercury exposure produces distributed brain damage in humans, including different cortical and cerebellar regions, with no evidence of specific temporal lobe or limbic involvement;[139,140] similar results were obtained in adult rats exposed to methylmercury[141,142] and in young rats exposed during gestation and lactation.[142] However, the chemical type and route of administration are critically important.

Cicmanec[143] contrasted accounts of human exposures to mercury derivatives in Iraq, Seychelles, Faroe, and Peru. He noted that all four studies concerned Hg exposures in the range 0–40 ppm in maternal hair, but only the Iraqi study demonstrated overt neurological effects in this dose range (and it was unfortunately argued that outlying studies such as the Iraqi study "are aberrations"). Even so, in the three other studies the route of exposure was through consumption of seafood, while the Iraqi population was exposed through contaminated grain. Because extensive metabolic conversion takes place in marine organisms (but is perhaps less likely in fungicide-treated grain), the studies are not strictly comparable.

Mercuric ion versus organomercury: different toxicologies

TMT and TBT have different toxicological profiles, both in animals and in cultured cells (see earlier), with only TMT causing overt limbic damage reminiscent of ASD. Mercuric ion, methylmercury, and ethylmercury can therefore have distinct toxicologies.[144]

Only limited brain and behavior studies have been reported with ethylmercury, principally the work of Magos *et al.*[145] who restricted neurotoxicity studies to rat dorsal root ganglia and locomotor coordination (not directly dependent upon limbic function). Persistent behavioral effects consistent with hippocampal damage were seen in rat pups exposed prenatally to methoxy-ethyl mercuric chloride.[146] A more recent study[147] of ethylmercury in humans explicitly did not address neurotoxicity, while another study[148] addressed only cerebellar effects.

Different derivatives also decay at different rates. In a study on infant monkeys exposed to methylmercury versus ethylmercury there was a large difference in the blood half-life for the two derivatives. A much higher proportion of mercury was deposited in the brain (up to seven times more) of ethylmercury-exposed infants than with methylmercury exposure.[149] Outside the brain, methyl- and ethylmercury have pronounced immunosuppressive properties in mice while provoking auto-immunity; and here again mercuric ion, methylmercury and ethylmercury have distinct toxicologies.[150,151]

The route of administration is also important. In methodological contrast to these studies, Hornig and colleagues[152] reported that ethylmercury by injection, like dietary TMT, produces selective hippocampal damage in neonatal mice, with an increase in the number and density of neurons in CA1, distortion of the dentate gyrus, and generalized enlargement of hippocampal structures. Exposure was associated with reduced open field activity, a parameter dependent on hippocampal function. These toxic effects were only seen in one strain of mice (SJL); two other strains of mice (C57Bl/6j and BALB/cJ) were not significantly affected,[152] pointing to a major genetic susceptibility locus of unknown identity.

Other metals

Aluminum (like TMT) causes selective hippocampal degeneration, but particularly in the CA1 field of the hippocampus.[153] However, vaccine administration, a possible culprit, contains aluminum doses (adjuvant alum, typically hydroxide, 0.25–0.85 mg/dose)[154] below those needed to produce behavioral abnormalities in neonatal rats (1 mg/g diet[155] or 10 mg/kg body weight by injection[156]), though exposure from other environmental sources is possible if not likely.

Given that lead, tin, and mercury (in different chemical formulations) can all produce specific damage to the limbic brain, and behavioral changes suggestive of ASD, one must suspect that other toxic metals may do the same. In addition to mercury and lead, elevated levels of arsenic and aluminum were seen in some ASD children.[36] Arsenic may be a special case, because the average arsenic concentration of fish species in the UK was reported to be 4.4 µg/g,[157] higher than either lead or mercury. Specific roles of this and other heavy metals including antimony, cadmium, chromium, cobalt, molybdenum, nickel, thallium, tungsten, and uranium cannot be excluded; further assessment of the risk is needed.

A problem in defining specific risk factors, if they can be shown to exist, is that a child exposed to lead (for example) is almost certainly exposed to other heavy metals spread through the same industrial and food-chain processes. A specific combination of heavy metals could present a risk factor over and above single elements in isolation. In fact, there is a case to be heard that a combination of exposures might produce damage more extensive than any one specific exposure in isolation.

Natural heavy metal deficiency: zinc, copper, iron, selenium

There are two reasons to suspect that deficiency of some metals, rather than excess, might contribute to brain damage. First, some metals such as selenium are protective against heavy metal toxicity; deficiency could exacerbate sensitivity. Second, the brain is critically dependent on supply of natural heavy metals like iron, copper, and zinc – this supply risks being disrupted by toxic metals that interfere with uptake and delivery to the brain.

In rodents, zinc deficiency in pregnancy produces long-lasting behavioral deficits in the pups. Spontaneous alternation, a behavioral marker of hippocampal function, was disrupted,[158] pointing to hippocampal damage. There is anecdotal evidence for disordered copper/zinc ratios in ASD consistent with zinc deficiency.[65] Moderate copper deprivation during gestation and lactation causes structural deficits in the rodent hippocampus.[159] In ASD, low iron levels are reported;[160] and iron deficiency in animal models exacerbates limbic damage produced by other insults.[161]

Iron deficiency may also contribute to toxic metal uptake. Both in animals and in humans, higher lead (Pb) levels were consistently found in iron deficiency; population studies reveal a strong association between iron deficiency and elevated blood lead levels (see [162] for review and further data in support). It was also noted in this study that iron deficiency may correlate with calcium deficiency: and deficiency in calcium can increase toxic metal uptake.

Deficiency of selenium is also a plausible contributory factor: one-third of ASD children studied showed a deficit.[36] The element is increasingly depleted in the diets of some human populations, particularly in Europe.[163] Brain function is crucially dependent on selenium supply.[164] As we will see below, selenium plays a dual role. First, it is an essential component of key enzymes that prevent oxidative damage in the brain. Second, it is required for many processes of heavy metal mobilization and detoxification.

Selenium is unlike any other similar element because it is incorporated directly into proteins. In fact, the amino acid selenocysteine, a complex of selenium with the regular sulfur-containing amino acid cysteine, is an extraordinary addition to the genetic code. Specific unusually structured nucleic acid triplets (codons) drive the incorporation, into new proteins, of selenocysteine – the proteins containing this amino acid are termed selenoproteins. And selenium is essential for development and metabolism.

Humans make only about 25 selenoproteins.[165] The most important ones are probably the glutathione peroxidases (GPX1–4), for these play a crucial role in preventing oxidative damage[166] and regenerating cellular thiol groups necessary for metal mobilization. Another protein, selenoprotein P, is a selenium transporter[167] also involved in binding and mobilizing heavy metals such as mercury and cadmium.[168] Marked behavioral impairments are seen in mutant mice with a defective selenoprotein P gene.[169]

Selenium deficiency may be extremely important in determining the outcome of heavy metal exposure, for selenium is protective against mercury intoxication. In cell lines cultured in the laboratory, selenium supplementation can prevent mercury toxicity;[170,171] a similar protective effect has been documented in animals.[172] Conversely, selenium deficiency markedly increases the extent of neurodevelopmental damage induced by methylmercury.[173] This is most likely due to lack of glutathione peroxidase activity (dependent on selenium) because methylmercury toxicity was countered by glutathione supplementation.[174]

In ASD, levels of the key selenoenzyme glutathione peroxidase (GPX) in plasma and erythrocytes were found to be significantly depressed in subjects versus control children.[175] This is notable because selenium-dependent GPX deficiency in young children has been associated with seizure and recurrent infection that, in some accounts, show astonishing improvement on selenium supplementation.[176,177] Mice lacking selenoenzymes GPX-1 and GPX-2 demonstrate inflammation of the GI tract associated with changes in gut flora,[178,179] pertinent to GI disorder seen in ASD (see Chapter 8).

Although not yet confirmed, specific deficits in iodine, lithium, phosphorus, and potassium may also contribute in ASD.[180]

It is suggested that a combination of exposures contributes to limbic damage in new phase ASD, with environmental metals and other insults (see below) acting synergistically with dietary deficiencies.

However, an unresolved question concerns why damage to the limbic brain, principally the hippocampus and amygdala, might be most prominent in animals and humans exposed to toxic heavy metals. This is addressed in the following section.

Limbic susceptibility to toxic insult

At one level, one recognizes the fact that, while for instance exposed layers of the gut wall (if damaged by toxicants) can repair to restore functionality, neuronal loss in the brain, even if repaired, is unlikely to restore acquired behaviors (including memories and skills) that depend on the circuits of specific neurons. Thus brain and behavior may be sensitive indicators of rather more widespread damage. Within the brain, however, limbic regions appear exceptionally susceptible to toxic insults.

Peculiar sensitivity of the limbic brain

We saw above how exposure to organometals can produce selective damage to the limbic brain, and this can be exacerbated by deprivation for natural heavy metals.

The limbic brain is exceptionally sensitive to toxic insults of all kinds, and non-specific metabolic dysregulation often results in damage to these brain regions.

There are many examples. Bacterial toxins, exemplified by pertussis vaccine,[181] and the pneumococcus toxin pneumolysin,[182] are known to cause selective destruction of limbic regions. In Korsakoff (alcoholic) syndrome, specific damage to hippocampus and related limbic structures[183] is associated with vitamin B1 deficiency.[184] Excess blood homocysteine correlates with, and is likely to produce, a reduction in hippocampal volume.[185,186] Hippocampal dysfunction is seen in liver damage (hepatic encephalopathy).[187] Administration of excess L-cysteine (likely to boost homocysteine levels) to infant rats produces behavioral changes similar to those produced by selective hippocampal damage;[188] chronic administration of homocysteine to rodents impairs learning on a task critically sensitive to hippocampal damage[189] and can cause seizures.[190]

In general, environmental toxicants,[191] including heavy metals (above), infections (discussed further below), and deficiencies, all tend toward limbic damage.

This is starkly exemplified by the precise and selective neuronal loss in human hippocampus on brain oxygen deprivation (ischemia/hypoxia)[192] – and further illustrated by the hippocampal destruction in the autistic children studied by DeLong and Heinz,[193] and Hans Asperger's patient Hellmuth L, caused by perinatal hypoxia. The following sections address the issue of what biochemical processes underlie this differential sensitivity.

Heavy metal regulation

The brain depends on metal ions for function, and natural heavy metals in limbic regions are among the highest in the brain,[194] including zinc, copper, and iron. This could render the limbic brain especially sensitive to heavy metal poisoning. Some toxic metals accumulate in the hippocampus: lead is selectively enriched in the formation,[195] as is uranium at low exposure levels;[196] low doses of mercury preferentially accumulate in hippocampus and cerebellum.[197]

Despite evidence that some metals accumulate in the limbic brain, in the case of adult rats acutely exposed to TMT the organometal was uniformly distributed across cerebellum, medulla-pons, hypothalamus, hippocampus, and striatum,[198] but damage was restricted to the hippocampus. Selective destruction of the hippocampus must therefore reflect an underlying biochemical susceptibility.

Many regulatory metal-binding proteins are most prominently expressed in limbic regions implicated in ASD. These include Atox1 (copper),[199] hippocalcin (calcium),[200] metallothionein-III (zinc, cadmium),[201,202] stannin (tin),[203,204] transferrin receptor (iron, manganese, aluminum),[205,206] and ZnT-3 (zinc).[207] Of these, stannin is the most interesting.

Stannin

This is a short (88 amino acid) polypeptide whose function is still unknown. It appears to be associated with subcellular (mitochondrial) membranes but, most importantly, is crucial for heavy metal toxicity, at least for some tin derivatives.

In the laboratory, as we mentioned above, some cell lines are exquisitely sensitive to TMT exposure, but others extremely resistant. This prompted Toggas and colleagues[203] to perform a differential experiment (known as subtractive hybridization) to try to identify genes only expressed in TMT-sensitive cells. This culminated in the identification of stannin.

Expression correlates very accurately with sensitivity. When stannin expression was turned down (by antisense reagents) cell lines became resistant to TMT toxicity.[88] Conversely, when TMT-resistant mouse cells were engineered to express stannin, they became exquisitely sensitive to the toxic effects of TMT (and dimethyltin).[208] Thus, stannin expression sensitizes to toxicity. As an aside, induction of stannin expression by an important signaling molecule, TNFα (also implicated in ASD), is discussed in Chapter 9.

Although the function of stannin is not known, it is very likely that it binds to organometals: structural studies have shown that synthetic peptides based on semi-adjacent cysteine amino acids (in the motif cysteine-X-cysteine – CXC, or "vicinal thiols") from stannin polypeptide form stable complexes with a range of organotins. Furthermore, the stannin-based peptide is able to remove the organic methyl groups from TMT,[209,210] perhaps allowing toxic tin atoms to disperse inside the cell where they may cause further damage.

It is not known if stannin is tin-specific; one suspects that it may play a wider role in metal toxicology. Interaction with other metals or organometals seems highly likely. Peptides with the CXC motif (as in stannin) have a very high affinity for diverse metal ions, including Hg, Cu, Zn, and Cd.[211] The possibility deserves investigation that the stannin gene located on human chromosome 16 (region p13),[212] a region implicated in autism (see Chapter 4), might afford new susceptibility alleles for ASD.

In the brain, stannin is most abundantly expressed in hippocampus, with lesser expression in cortex and cerebellum;[204] elsewhere significant expression was seen in spleen. Because stannin expression seems to make cells sensitive to organometal toxicity, localized stannin expression in the hippocampus, and throughout the CA and dentate regions, will favor specific limbic organometal sensitivity including, and probably not restricted to, organotin derivatives.

Neuronal proliferation

Within the brain the hippocampus is also very distinctive because the production of new neurons (neurogenesis) continues even into adulthood. This has been demonstrated in the hippocampal dentate region not only in rodents but also in monkeys[213,214] and humans.[215] In addition to the olfactory system, significant late production of new neurons has been suggested to continue in some other brain regions, including the amygdala and temporal cortex,[216] and cerebellum,[217] all areas implicated in ASD, though in-depth studies have suggested that neurogenesis is principally restricted to the hippocampus and olfactory system in primates.[218] Abnormal olfactory responses in ASD[219] could reflect loss of olfactory neurons.

The formation of new neurons may be of crucial importance to understanding the sensitivity of the limbic brain. Dividing cells are critically sensitive to heavy metal toxicity. In fact, a platinum derivative (cisplatin) is widely used as an anti-cancer agent. Although DNA damage was thought to underlie its antitumor effects,[220] cisplatin, like methylmercury, interferes with microtubule assembly[221] to block cell division. Prenatal exposure of rats to cisplatin produces long-lasting behavioral effects;[222] damage to the production of new neurons in the dentate gyrus is anticipated. Inhibition of dentate neurogenesis was seen in rat pups exposed to lead acetate.[223]

At the molecular level, mercury causes destabilization of microtubule networks[224,225] involved in neuronal outgrowth, and microtubule abnormalities have been associated with mental retardation.[226] MeHg-induced dissociation of microtubules was observed at 1–10 uM[227,228] but toxic effects have been seen in model systems at concentrations as low as 0.1 uM,[229] a level consistent with current environmental exposures.

Metabolic demand

The hippocampus is also exquisitely sensitive to damage brought about by overexcitation and oxygen deprivation, as seen in stroke and prolonged epileptic seizure. In humans, transient oxygen deprivation (hypoxia) at birth is associated with hippocampal and cortical damage[230] while, in adults, transient brain deprivation produces highly selective damage to the CA1–3 regions of the hippocampus.[192,231,232] Carbon monoxide poisoning of an adult was blamed for hippocampal atrophy.[233] Although not demonstrated, the peculiar vulnerability to lack of oxygen could reflect higher metabolic activity than other brain regions.

Internal sensing and endocrine disruption

An important role of the hippocampus (and adjoining amygdala) is held to be as a sensor for internal physiological status. This is termed enteroception.[234] While not yet widely accepted, the idea was highlighted by Isaacson[91] because it reiterates the ancestral evolution of the limbic system.

The hippocampus receives signals from diverse hormones and metabolites, and it is likely to use these to guide motivations, hungers, and physiological adaptation. It has been strongly argued by Tracy, Jarrard, and Davidson[235] that the hippocampus plays a pivotal role in motivations including appetite. It is certainly true that the hippocampal formation is richly adorned with receptors for diverse molecules reflecting ion balance and blood pressure, immunity, pain, reproductive status, satiety, and stress.[234] Many of these receptors are selectively expressed in the hippocampus – for example, the primary receptor for stress steroid hormones (glucocorticoids), termed the mineralocorticoid receptor (MR), is almost exclusive to the hippocampus.

Specific destruction of limbic regions by, for example, bacterial toxins (above) could therefore reflect the selective expression and sensitivity of target receptors (including pro-inflammatory cytokine receptors) in this brain region (see Chapter 9).

In addition to causing microtubule disruption, heavy metals may also exert their toxic effects at specific target sites, and here steroid receptors are a case in point. Heavy metals disrupt hormone signaling, a process termed endocrine disruption, by binding to steroid receptors in the brain and other tissues.[236,237] Cadmium, lead, mercury, and tin all activate the estrogen receptor ERα in cell culture[238] and *in vivo*.[239] Cadmium binds to the hormone-binding domain of ERα and activates the receptor.[237] Endocrine disruption extends to the androgen receptor (AR). In mice, an environmentally relevant dose of cadmium (20 μg/kg bodyweight) activated the expression of an androgen-responsive gene *in vivo*;[240] the metal bound to human AR with surprisingly high affinity ($K_{eq} = \sim 10^{-10}$ M). Other relevant metals were not tested but, given that ERα responds to diverse heavy metals, the same may be true of AR.

Specific interference with heme metabolism and P450 activity (see below) may also be relevant: the cytochrome P450 hemoprotein CYP7B is selectively expressed in hippocampus[241,242] and acts to prevent excess activation of the second major receptor responding to estrogens, ERβ.[243,244] Interference with the activity of this specific limbic enzyme is expected to lead to endocrine disruption through ERβ overactivation. As discussed elsewhere in this volume, dysregulation of steroid hormones is an important but intermittent feature of ASD.

Limbic brain: summary of susceptibilities
The evidence suggests that the limbic brain, including (but not restricted to) the hippocampus, amygdala, and overlying cortex, is particularly and peculiarly sensitive to diverse toxic insults. Though there is some evidence for heavy metal accumulation in the limbic brain, this is alone unlikely to explain the selective damage seen in these brain regions. Instead, the limbic brain is biochemically unusual, possibly with higher metabolic demand, specific expression of metal-regulatory factors exemplified by stannin, the presence of diverse binding sites for soluble ligands including hormones, and finally the restricted location of dividing cells in the formation. Together these influences could render this brain region exquisitely sensitive to toxic agents (including infectious agents, below).

Nevertheless, because the limbic brain exhibits broad-spectrum susceptibility to toxic insult, it would be a mistake to conclude that any one type of toxin (e.g. heavy metals) acts alone to disrupt behavior.

Other environmental factors

Heavy metals are contenders for the damage seen in the ASD brain. But metals are not the only agents associated with specific limbic damage; chemical toxins and infectious agents could well contribute.

Chemical toxins

Like heavy metals, many chemical toxins interfere with steroid signaling (endocrine disruption) and produce overt reproductive changes, particularly on early developmental exposure.[245] Potential effects of xenobiotics including endocrine disruptors during gestation have been reviewed.[246] While in-depth discussion would be out of place here, these include bisphenols (plastics industry), dioxins (plastics, defoliants), DDT and related molecules (pesticides), and atypical steroids and related molecules.

Bisphenols have been shown to cause persistent reproductive changes in rodents while, in humans, two-thirds of children of dioxin-exposed women (Vietnam) had congenital malformations or developed disabilities within the first years of life.[247] Early exposure to DDT and relatives including DDE, DDD, and methoxychlor has been linked to precocious puberty.[248] Severe sperm abnormalities were seen in boys exposed to diethylstilbestrol.[249,250]

Attention has focused on reproductive alterations, but a growing body of evidence now points to non-reproductive behavioral changes (as reviewed[251]). Depressed exploration, motor activity, and anxiety are observed in offspring of gestating rats treated with estrogenic bisphenol A.[252] Males and females are very different in their susceptibility – it was suggested that environmental exposure is likely to contribute to the elevated rates of mental retardation (including severe ASD) seen in males.[253]

Effects of chemical toxins are most often seen during the developmental period, but there are adverse effects in maturity: in adult humans, dioxin exposure has been linked to stress and anxiety disorders.[254]

Levels of dioxins and PCBs in UK fish are in the range 0.06–13.8 ng/kg, with a broad mean of ~2 ng/kg.[255] In the brain, dioxins exemplified by 2,3,7,8-tetrachlorodibenzo-p-dioxin (TCDD) are thought to target the aryl hydrocarbon receptor, most abundantly expressed in hippocampus, with wider expression in cortex, cerebellum, and olfactory bulb.[256] In rats, exposure to TCDD produced oxidative stress in hippocampus and cortex, but not in cerebellum or brainstem,[257] and prenatal exposure impaired hippocampus-dependent learning.[258] A further series of studies has revealed impairments in hippocampal electrophysiology induced by dioxins. Bisphenols and DTT are thought to act at steroid receptors, particularly abundant in hippocampus.

In ASD, there is evidence for abnormal exposure to environmental chemicals, though the primary study did not specifically address endocrine disruption. Edelson and Cantor[259] studied 20 ASD subjects (3–12 years): 20 out of 20 showed a striking increase in a liver detoxification metabolite (D-glucaric acid) indicative of ongoing toxic challenge. Sixteen out of eighteen had levels of environmental chemicals exceeding adult maximum tolerance. In the two cases where toxic chemicals could not be found, levels of D-glucaric acid showed abnormal activation of liver detoxification.[259]

This study documented some remarkable levels of toxic chemical exposure: blood levels of trichloroethylene and toluene in two ASD children were respectively 19- and 100-fold in excess of adult maximum safe levels. Similar evidence of exposure to organic toxicants was presented by Audhya and colleagues,[36] where 67% of ASD children showed erythrocyte levels of hexane above the control range.

Infectious agents

Recent debate has highlighted the potential contributory role of vaccinal viruses and other infectious agents. It would be unwise to revisit the heated controversy associated with childhood measles-mumps-rubella (MMR) vaccination in any depth (gastrointestinal associations are discussed further in Chapter 8), but there is an established literature concerning a causal association between virus infection and ASD, noting cytomegalovirus, rubella, Epstein-Barr virus, and herpes viruses.

Multiple cases of congenital cytomegalovirus[260–264] or rubella[265,266] infection associated with ASD have been reported. Autistic behavior and seizure activity were noted in ~40% of pediatric/adolescent patients with a prior (historic) diagnosis of Epstein-Barr virus encephalitis.[267]

Of three children with acquired reversible autistic syndrome, one had a left temporal lobe lesion with elevated serum anti-herpes titer.[268] There are reports of ASD onset in adolescents (11 and 14 years old) with herpes encephalitis.[269,270] A male who contracted temporal lobe herpes encephalitis at 31 years went on to develop symptoms diagnostic of ASD.[271]

Reye syndrome (encephalopathy due to viral infection associated with probable underlying biochemical deficits) shares some features of ASD, with common speech and verbal memory deficits.[272,273]

The limbic brain does appear to be particularly sensitive to infectious agents, and the presence of dividing cells in the formation (as discussed above) provides a clue, for dividing cells are generally considered to be preferred substrates for viral replication (though inflammatory signals driven by peripheral infection may also contribute; see Chapter 9).

Histologic inspection of a patient with chronic herpes infection and intractable seizures revealed low-level active virus replication in hippocampus and overlying temporal cortex, principally in neurons.[274] Bilateral pathology of hippocampus, amygdala, and overlying cortex in an amnesic patient (known as EP) was attributed to herpes simplex encephalitis.[275] A rise in a new type of acute limbic encephalitis, attributed to a non-herpes virus,[276] is associated with bilateral abnormalities in the hippocampus and amygdala.[277]

Dentate destruction has been observed in experimental animals infected with bornavirus[278] though brainstem and hypothalamic nuclei were also targeted.[279] Bornavirus infection of the brain has been proposed as an animal model of ASD.[280,281]

It is possible, though perhaps less likely, that direct microbial (rather than viral) infection of the brain could also contribute: though dentate destruction was seen in bacterial meningitis,[282] and neuronal death in the dentate gyrus was seen in 26 out of 37 autopsy cases of patients with a prior history of bacterial meningitis,[283] the mechanism may be indirect.

There is so far scant evidence for a new infectious agent in ASD that could explain the recent increase in the prevalence of the disorder, though this explanation is not excluded.[284] Dyken[285] reviewed the association between subacute sclerosing panencephalitis (SSPE), due to aborted infection with wild-type measles virus, and the development of encephalopathy accompanied by autistic behavior ("neuroautistic encephalopathy"). He noted that the majority of these SSPE children may have been at risk because of an impaired immune system and also GI tract inflammation, surprisingly reminiscent of ASD (discussed in the next chapter).

The debate regarding MMR vaccine and ASD is not revisited in detail here, noting that autism prevalence continues to rise in Japan despite withdrawal of the triple MMR vaccine,[286] though with some reserves. Single vaccines of the same type have continued to be administered. It is also important to recognize that measures of ASD rates in immunized versus un-immunized populations fall short of testing the contention that a sub-proportion of recent ASD cases might be causally associated with vaccine administration. Specifically, only 4–20% of families have countenanced a possible link between MMR vaccination and development of ASD;[287] the higher percentage may have been influenced by recent publicity. A reasonable hypothesis is that around 5% of cases might be due to MMR vaccination, with impaired immunity a contributing factor.

The statistical challenge is then to detect an increase in ASD at this level. Population sizes in the order of one million in both the vaccinated and unvaccinated groups are needed, because below this the small increment could never achieve statistical validity. Smaller study groups, but at least 6000, are needed if analysis is restricted to the ASD population, and if for example ASD rates are compared prior to or post vaccination. Even so, recent studies on 473[288] or 5800[289] subjects fail to address the hypothesis that 5% of cases might be caused by MMR. One must remember, however, that massive loss of previously acquired skills, as in childhood disintegrative disorder, is rather rare – though the data do not exclude that a mild impairment in a child already at risk, for instance because of a weak immune system, is subsequently amplified on vaccination.

Heavy metals and other insults: a toxic cocktail in ASD

The combined data suggest that new phase ASD is associated with, and is perhaps due to, environmental heavy metal exposure. Many young ASD children appear to have a deficit, probably genetic, in mercury mobilization, and this could underlie the elevated body burden of metals including mercury and lead. Heavy metals target damage to the same brain regions that show dysfunction or abnormalities in ASD; trimethyltin (TMT) provides a compelling paradigm for the specific type of toxic damage that can be produced by metals and their derivatives. One may infer, therefore, that heavy metals are a plausible contender for new phase ASD.

It seems unlikely that a single metal is responsible. Seafood is the most prominent source of heavy metals, with lead, tin, and mercury all now achieving concentrations (in some fish products) up to roughly 1 μg/g – giving a total dose above 3 μg/g. Because different heavy metals interfere with biochemical pathways in slightly different ways, they may synergize in the type and extent of damage produced.

Back-of-envelope calculations predict significant toxicity. While the *in vivo* toxicology of organometals is largely unexplored, and will depend on multiple uptake, detoxification, and export processes operating in parallel, cell damage has been seen in model systems at concentrations as low as 0.1 μM (see earlier). If an individual should be unable to export toxic metals, 100 g of contaminated product (i.e. 0.3 mg organometal in seafood) consumed by each week for 10 weeks (a total of 3 mg organometal) by a young child of only 20 kg, provides a dose already exceeding the threshold level, and would rapidly approach 1 μM (roughly 4 mg organometal per 20 kg), at which point overt toxicity is expected, and predominantly in the limbic brain.

Nevertheless, heavy metals are not the only chemical toxic agents capable of causing limbic damage. Polychlorinated biphenyls, for example, induce toxicity via the same pathways encountered with heavy metal exposure, and most likely synergize with heavy metals in the extent and type of damage produced.[290] It is well known in the toxicological field that a combination of toxins can cause significant damage even when each is at subthreshold or "safe" levels.[291] It remains to be seen if heavy metals "alone" cause new ASD, or whether simultaneous toxic exposure to other chemicals (or infectious agents) is required to tip the balance toward ASD.

Overall, the evidence is in support of Rutter's proposal[292] that a "two-hit" mechanism (a combination of genetic liability with an additional risk factor) is required to take individuals from a milder and more diffuse phenotype to a seriously handicapping disorder. Children with ASD seem to differ from their peers in how they export mercury; heavy metal exposure and accumulation could explain both the brain damage seen in ASD and the rise in prevalence. Nevertheless, we cannot yet conclude that early life exposure to heavy metals is alone sufficient to produce ASD in a predisposed individual. But one might suspect that ASD develops only rarely in the absence of specific toxic insults including heavy metals.

In the next chapters we will see that the way in which the brain is damaged by environmental agents is not just by direct interference with neuronal growth and signaling. Brain damage induces peripheral dysfunction that, in addition to causing distress to the patient, feeds back to the brain to exacerbate the condition.

Key points

Cases of ASD due to early-life toxic challenge are well documented.

Subjects with autistic disorder show evidence of exposure to heavy metals; Asperger disorder is unlikely to be associated with heavy metal exposure.

Some affected individuals may have a deficit in metal detoxification.

Organometals, exemplified by trimethyltin (TMT), are known to cause limbic damage; heavy metal exposure affords a plausible mechanism for selective limbic destruction in ASD.

The behavioral consequences of TMT exposure resemble autism.

The biology of the limbic brain – neuronal proliferation, metal regulation, and internal sensing – may explain its sensitivity to organometals.

The limbic brain is particularly vulnerable to infectious agents.

Lead, mercury, and arsenic are implicated, though different chemical formulations can have very different toxic profiles.

Deficiency of protective metals such as selenium, zinc, copper, and iron may contribute.

A combination of toxins (metals and chemicals) may underlie autism, but predominantly in individuals who are genetically susceptible.

Chapter 8

Gut, Hormones, Immunity: Physiological Dysregulation in Autism

Limbic abnormalities and sometimes frank damage are seen in subjects with ASD. Because limbic dysfunction appears to fulfill the dual criteria of necessity and sufficiency regarding ASD, perturbed limbic function is very likely the explanation of the brain and behavior disturbances that define the disorders. However, the limbic brain plays a second role – it controls body physiology. If limbic dysfunction is indeed at the heart of ASD, altered physiological function is predicted.

The aim of this chapter is to explore physiological disturbances that accompany ASD. The treatment is necessarily technical – but it is worthwhile entering into the detail so as to underscore the fact that accompanying physiological disturbances are contentious, but the data, when properly scrutinized, are unambiguous.

Part of the difficulty in addressing this area lies in the fact that children with ASD are primarily referred to psychological, psychiatric, and educational services, all ill-equipped to assess physiological changes. Moreover, there is often too little understanding that the body and the brain are inextricably linked – and changes in one compartment have marked effects on the other.

Even so, it is hoped that the tide of opinion is changing, and neurological and psychiatric disorders are no longer always seen in isolation of the changes in physiological function they can produce (and be exacerbated by).

This change in perspective is in no short measure due to the work of Robert Ader and colleagues. In his seminal book *Psychoneuroimmunology*,[1] to give one example, he and his co-authors discuss a subject with severe allergy. To the astonishment of all, a plastic rose, or even a photograph, could precipitate a serious allergic attack. This graphically illustrates how perception can influence body function – in this case the immune system.

The limbic brain plays a pivotal role in this type of regulation. In another disorder of the limbic brain, Alzheimer disease, it has been suggested that the condition should not be considered primarily as a brain disease, but instead as a disease of physiological dysregulation.[2,3] Given the evidence for limbic dysfunction in ASD, one in fact must *expect* to see physiological changes in subjects with spectrum disorders. This chapter addresses whether ASD is accompanied by any such disturbances, and if so how often, and how severe. Before proceeding to examine this area, the evidence for limbic control of body physiology is briefly overviewed.

Brain to body signaling

Brain and body function are intertwined. For instance, psychological challenge – as in a perilous or threatening situation – leads to an instant increase in heart and respiration rate, with the release of stress hormones, and shutdown of digestion. The thought of a pleasant meal to come produces salivation and ominous rumbling of the digestive system. The sleep–wake cycle, controlled by the brain, entrains rhythmic changes in hormone levels that influence all aspects of physiology – and the unpleasant experience of "jet-lag" results when it goes wrong.

These physiological adaptations are largely controlled by the limbic brain acting via the hypothalamus. This small organ, just below the hippocampus, is intimately connected to the overlying hippocampal formation by direct neuronal relays. The hippocampus and amygdala modulate hypothalamic secretions that include stimulating factors. In turn these target another secretory gland below the hypothalamus – the pituitary. Finally, the pituitary releases activation factors that target body organs, for instance the adrenal gland, the source of stress hormones (see Figure 8.1).

This cascade – of sequential activation of the hypothalamus, pituitary, and adrenal – allows the brain to control the body. By this route perception of a threat causes the release of stress hormones from the adrenal gland. This has come to be known as the HPA axis (for hypothalamus–pituitary–adrenal). It should more properly be called the L-HPA axis, recognizing the role of the limbic brain in controlling the hypothalamus. Moreover, the axis is not restricted to the adrenal, and the thyroid, gut, and gonads are also controlled by the same mechanism (see Figure 8.1) – indeed activation of the stress response changes the activity of all these body systems, and the term "HPA" is very much too restrictive.

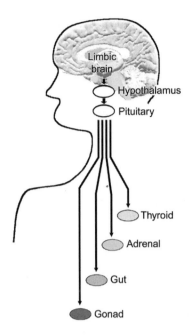

Figure 8.1 Sequential limbic control of the hypothalamus, pituitary, and downstream target organs.

Damage to the limbic system impairs the regulation of these target organs, with major effects on hormone levels and physiological function, including elevated stress steroid levels, impaired immunity, reproductive hormone dysfunction, and gastrointestinal inflammation.[1,4–6] Hippocampal (and amygdala) damage generally disturbs physiological function.

In ASD, where limbic damage is central, physiological effects are therefore expected. Consider, for instance, that a majority of autistic children meet the criteria for an anxiety disorder.[7] Anxiety is known to increase the risk of cardiac problems by almost five-fold, while gastrointestinal and genitourinary disorders are over twice as common as in controls.[8]

Before looking at more detail at physiological problems in ASD we will first look at the best specific example of brain-mediated physiological control – the gastrointestinal tract.

Brain–gut axis

Aspects of gastrointestinal (GI) function dictated by the limbic brain include GI mucosal immunity,[9,10] secretion, and motility.[11] This has led to the concept of the "brain–gut axis."[12,13] To illustrate the specific dependence of the GI tract on the limbic brain, the effects of stress and anxiety are considered.

From rodents to primates including humans, chronic psychosocial stress pre-disposes to GI tract inflammation[14] and bowel disease.[15] In rats, gastric ulceration is the result of stress produced by forced immobilization. The involvement of the hippocampus has been demonstrated – lesions to this tissue markedly *increase* the severity of the ulceration.[16–18]

The adjoining amygdala also plays a role;[19] chemical interference with amygdala function aggravates stress-induced stomach ulceration;[20] hormone administration into rat amygdala can alone induce gastric lesions.[21]

The same is true in primates, and probably in man, given the well-known association between stress and GI ulcers. Uno and colleagues[22] reported on a vervet monkey dying from unknown causes following social ostracization – a deeply stressful experience in this species. Post-mortem analysis revealed only two suspect features – hippocampal degeneration and severe stomach ulceration.

Control of GI function operates via the hypothalamus, the small organ just below the hippocampus (see Figure 8.1). Hypothalamic damage also affects gastric pathology.[23] Downstream of the hypothalamus, regulatory molecules include, in addition to the classic stress hormones (glucocorticoids and adrenalins), more than a dozen GI hormones. And, as we will see (Chapter 9), relay is not just by hormones, and the vagal nerves (that connect the hippocampus and hypothalamus to the GI tract) play a pivotal role.

Commencing then with the GI tract, the following sections consider the overall evidence for physiological dysregulation in ASD. Although the focus is on the effects of limbic damage on body physiology, one must also consider the pos-sibility that impairments could be due not only to toxic effects on the brain, but also by direct damage inflicted on different body organs.

Diverse physiological impairments in ASD

In ASD, there is widespread evidence of physiological dysregulation. Perturba-tions include immune abnormalities,[24] higher mean blood flow and lower periph-eral vascular resistance,[25] cardiac arrhythmia,[26] abnormal fatty acid profiles,[27] excess lipid oxidation products,[28] abnormal hepatic function,[29] altered reproduc-tive development,[30] with reports of polydipsia and aberrant thermoregulation. Unusual hormone and metabolite regulatory profiles in ASD have been observed for ACTH, beta-endorphin, glucocorticoids, growth hormone, insulin, interleukins (IL-1, -2, -6, -10, -12), IGF-1, melatonin, oxytocin, prolactin, purine metabolism, serotonin, testosterone, thyroid hormone, vasopressin. The list is not exhaustive.

Because these changes are widespread, affecting a diversity of body systems, it would be imprudent to attempt to provide comprehensive overview in each case. Some may be of major importance; others could be peripheral. Therefore, a judicious choice has been made in selecting and prioritizing areas for more detailed evaluation.

Subdividing physiological disturbances is not an easy task. All the different body systems interact with each other. Stress steroids (glucocorticoids) influence heart, kidney, and immune function. Immune anomalies predispose to allergy and GI inflammation. Impaired dietary nutrient uptake associated with GI problems will impact on hormone production. Therefore, the different sections below are not rigid subdivisions.

In the following selection, inspection of specific physiological aberrations in ASD dwells on abnormalities in GI function, serotonin pathways, hormone levels, the immune system, and finally the liver and kidney.

Gastrointestinal (GI) tract disorder

A growing body of evidence points to disrupted GI tract function in ASD, often covert, but sometimes severe. Inflammation, aberrant gut flora, decreased digestive enzyme activity, and other related gut abnormalities are commonly recorded in autistic patients, as reviewed.[31,32] Table 8.1 summarizes these reports; central findings are expanded upon and discussed below.

GI inflammation in ASD

Historically, autism and ASD were not obviously associated with any physiological impairments, though it is not known whether this was an oversight or due (perhaps equally likely) to a change in the pattern of presentation (see Chapter 4).

In the mid 1990s a group of parents expressed mounting vocal concern that their children, in addition to having behavioral disorders on the autism spectrum, were suffering from GI problems. Wakefield et al.[33] reported on a first series of 12 ASD children with loss of acquired skills, including language, but accompanied by diarrhea and abdominal pain. All were found to have GI tract abnormalities, ranging from inflamed intestinal lymph nodes (lymphoid nodular hyperplasia, LNH) to ulceration. Chronic colon inflammation (colitis) was seen in 11 and lymph gland enlargement in the ileum in seven. Some aspects of this paper have been challenged, but not the presence or absence of GI abnormalities.

Follow-up analysis[34] detected LNH in 93% of 58 affected children but in only 14.3% of control children with no behavioral signs referred to the same gastroenterology unit. Chronic colitis was identified in 53 of 60 (88%) of the children examined compared with 4.5% of controls. An elevated rate of colonic LNH was also present (30%).

Krigsman,[35] reporting on 43 autistic children, independently confirmed pathologic lymphonodular hyperplasia of the terminal ileum in 90%.

Table 8.1 GI tract abnormalities in ASD

Abnormality	First author (citation)
Reflux esophagitis	Horvath[41]
Gastritis	
Suspected gastric hypoacidity	Finegold[36]
Ileal lymphoid nodular hyperplasia (LNH)	Wakefield[33,34]
Reactive follicular hyperplasia	Krigsman[35]
Colitis, ileitis, colonic LNH	
Gut flora abnormalities	Finegold[36]
Ten-fold increase in clostridial titers	Parracho[42]
Increased intraepithelial lymphocytes	Furlano[43]
Epithelial IgG suggestive of gut autoimmunity	Torrente[44]
Mucosal immunopathology	Ashwood[45]
Specific mucosal lymphocyte subset elevation	Ashwood[46]
Reduced carbohydrate digestive enzyme	Horvath[41]
Altered intestinal permeability	D'Eufemia[39]
Antibodies to milk proteins	Lucarelli[47]
Behavioral improvement with dietary	Lucarelli[47]
modification	Knivsberg[48,49]
Impaired sulfation	Alberti[50]
Diarrhea or constipation	Horvath[41]
	Afzal[51]
	Molloy[52]
	Valicenti-McDermott[53]

Reduced stomach acid secretion may also accompany GI inflammation: of four autistic children typed for stomach pH, two had a significant *reduction* of acidity[36] that would impair digestion. Heightened levels of blood serotonin (section following) are also a marker of GI tract problems: the majority of body 5-HT is localized in cells of the GI tract where it controls gut motility.[37]

At heart, these reports confirm Wakefield *et al.*'s observations that many ASD children have GI problems. This is extended further below.

Gut permeability

Local inflammation can be accompanied by loss of intestinal barrier function,[38] and many molecules passing through the digestive tract are easily absorbed into the blood. After oral lactulose, a sugar that does not normally cross the intestinal wall, abnormally high levels of lactulose were found in 9 of 21 (43%) autistic patients *without* overt GI problems, but in none of the 40 controls[39] (see Figure 8.2a). This study is important because the ASD children tested had no known intestinal disorder, suggesting that GI abnormalities commonly go undetected. Increased immune reactivity to total cow milk protein[40] would seem to confirm that ASD subjects are more exposed to undigested protein, consistent with impaired barrier function.

Loss of barrier function in ASD could have important effects on the brain, as it could potentially allow the entry of toxic peptides, some resembling opioids, and underlies the opioid-excess theory debated in the next chapter.

Abnormal (toxic) gut flora

There is also good evidence for abnormal bacteria in the GI tract of ASD subjects. Stool analysis on 13 patients with regressive autism showed a dramatic increase in titers of the abnormal and potentially toxic *Clostridia*. The group of *Clostridia* is famously associated with severe disease including gangrene, botulism, and tetanus (depending on the particular strain). These specific hyper-toxic strains are rarely encountered in the GI tract; even so, *Clostridium difficile* is known to produce colon inflammation with abdominal pain and diarrhea, and is most commonly seen in patients treated with antibiotics that remove "normal" gut flora.

Finegold and colleagues[36] reported that titers of particular strains rose in ASD by up to seven orders of magnitude (10 million-fold) compared to controls. Titers of *C. ramosum* and *C. scindens* (identified by DNA sequencing) were respectively 6×10^7 and 9×10^7 in individual samples from autistic children but undetectable in controls; *C. symbiosum* titers up to 4×10^9 were recorded (highest titer in controls, 6×10^3). *C. difficile* itself was present in samples from ASD children, but was entirely absent in controls. Overall, the mean clostridial titer in stools of children with ASD was ten-fold greater than that in control children[36] (see Figure 8.2b).

Further abnormal gut flora patterns have been recorded in ASD children, with $46 \times$ excess of *C. bolteae* in feces of ASD subjects.[54] This has been confirmed by direct sampling of body fluids from ASD subjects – specific unusual bacteria (non-spore-forming anaerobes and microaerophiles) were totally absent from gastric and duodenal fluid from control children, but were found in four out of five samples from autistic children.[36]

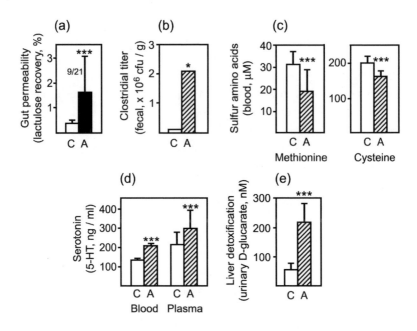

Figure 8.2 Physiological parameters in ASD. C, control group; A, ASD group. (a) Gut permeability and dietary lactulose uptake. Data on a 9/21 subgroup of ASD patients showing a diminished GI tract permeability barrier compared to controls. Data from D'Eufemia et al.[39] (b) Gut flora. Geometric mean titers of Clostridia species in ASD versus control children. Subjects were not matched for diet (e.g. gluten-free and casein-free). Data of Finegold et al.[36] (c) Sulfur amino acids. Blood levels of methionine and cysteine in ASD versus control. Data from James et al.[71] (d) Circulating serotonin (5HT) levels. Blood values from Anderson et al.,[72] plasma values from Naffah-Mazzacoratti et al.[73] (e) Urinary D-glucarate. This molecule is a marker of chronic activation of liver detoxification pathways. Data on ASD subjects from Edelson and Cantor[29] compared to reference values.[74]

A subsequent study reported excess *C. histolyticum* in ASD compared to normal controls.[42] *C. histolyticum* strains are known to produce toxins and are likely to contribute to GI tract inflammation in ASD. In this study, non-autistic siblings had a level intermediate between the ASD and unrelated control groups.

Recurrent diarrhea is often reported in ASD[41,52] but it is not known if this is a consequence of gut clostridial infection.

Gut flora abnormalities and GI tract inflammation are associated with an active immune response. Abnormal deposition of immune antibody (IgG) was found in GI biopsy samples (duodenum) from 23 of 25 ASD children.[44]

Elevations of inflammatory markers (IFNγ and IL1-RA; see Chapter 9) in whole blood cultures from autistic children[55] are consistent with an ongoing inflammatory response (see Figure 8.7d, later). However, another study failed to find any enhancement in inflammatory markers in ASD children, though the control group here was selected from other children also undergoing colon investigation.[56]

How common are GI disturbances in ASD? Record-based versus patient-based studies

It remains contentious whether gastrointestinal problems are indeed as frequent as these reports suggest, and some have challenged whether ASD is at all linked to GI problems.[57] Where studies have addressed specific GI pathology in ASD children referred for gastroenterological examination, surprisingly high rates of inflammatory disorders have been found.[33,44] But these children are unrepresentative, and such reports strictly do not address the prevalence of GI problems in ASD.

Data from medical records

In a wider investigation, Black and colleagues[58] examined prior physician records for 96 ASD children (mean age, 4 years) and contrasted them with records for age-matched controls. In this study, the same proportion (9%) of ASD children and controls had recorded signs of GI pathology in the period before ASD development. However, again this study did not strictly address possible GI co-morbidity with ASD because records pertained to the period prior to ASD diagnosis. The authors also state that the study excluded "less severe conditions of food intolerance and recurrent gastrointestinal symptoms" that did not appear in the practitioner's record.

Taylor et al.[59] consulted clinical notes from 278 ASD children (4–13 years). Bowel problems were excluded if records indicated they had lasted less than three months. Here 18% of autistic subjects had constipation, diarrhea, food allergy, or non-specific colitis. This study reported a significant link between these GI problems and regression: 26% of children with regressive autism were reported to have bowel problems versus 14% without regressive autism (p=0.002).

Molloy and Manning-Courtney,[52] also working with data abstracted from medical records, reported that 24% of 137 subjects with ASD (2–8 years old) had at least one GI symptom from a list including chronic diarrhea, chronic constipation, chronic reflux/vomiting, and chronic abdominal pain or gaseousness as reported by parents, the most frequent being chronic diarrhea. They note: "this approach may have underestimated the number of children with GI symptoms."

These three studies were based exclusively on clinical notes. This is noteworthy because sub-clinical disease is likely to be under-represented in the primary data.[32] Afzal et al.[51] used abdominal imaging to study ASD and control children referred for GI examination. The *actual* degree of constipation bore no relation to clinical accounts.

Thus, clinical records do not accurately reflect GI complications. There is little doubt that ascertainment is radically compromised in subjects with impaired communication skills. Equally importantly, ASD children are often pain-insensitive, and may not be in a position to volunteer their difficulties. This remains a major difficulty in evaluating the data.

Patient surveys

A higher prevalence has been seen in patient rather than record-based studies. Afzal et al.[51] found that 54% of referred ASD children, compared with 24% of co-referred controls, had moderate/severe bowel compaction, demonstrating a link between constipation and ASD. But the study population was again drawn from subjects referred for GI analysis, and may be unrepresentative of general ASD.

Krigsman[35] reported on 43 ASD children 2–10 years in age: 65% were found to have GI inflammation (colitis). A subgroup underwent coloscopy; of this subgroup 90% (36/40) showed evidence of inflamed lymph nodes. However, no data were presented on how subjects were selected.

Melmed et al.,[60] in a parent survey, reported a similar figure, 46%, for GI problems (chronic diarrhea, chronic constipation, or both) in unselected children with ASD, but in only 18% of siblings and 10% of controls. The excess in siblings deserves comment, for partial expression of ASD features in close relatives is very amply documented – siblings are not an appropriate control group.

Whiteley,[61] also using parent survey, reported that 35% of unselected ASD children had either diarrhea or constipation; the figure in autism proper was 43%.

Valicenti-McDermott et al.[53] compared 92 children with ASD (mean age 9.6 years) with control groups. Of the children with ASD, 59% had food selection, 14% chronic vomiting, 15% chronic abdominal pain, chronic diarrhea was present in 18%, bulky stools in 22%, fecal soiling in 23%, and chronic constipation in 40%. This was above the rates seen in the controls, and the difference was significant. Though many subjects had more than one of the above, if chronic diarrhea and constipation are exclusive, this points to 58% or more with GI problems.

These figures are broadly consistent with the study of D'Eufemia et al.[39] who reported intestinal permeability changes in 43% of unselected ASD patients with no history of chronic GI symptoms (see Figure 8.2a); the overall prevalence may be higher because this study excluded patients with known GI involvement. However, it is not known whether permeability changes correlate with GI problems including diarrhea and constipation, though barrier loss is often associated with stress and GI tract inflammation.

The findings reported in all these studies are reinforced by Finegold *et al.*'s studies,[36] discussed above, who reported a mean fecal clostridial titer more than 1 log greater in ASD than in controls. The authors stated: "all had gastrointestinal symptoms, primarily diarrhea and/or constipation." It was unclear whether the subject group was pre-selected for such symptoms.

Finally, a sulfation deficit was seen in 55 out of 60 (92%) of unselected ASD children examined:[50] defective sulfation is thought in part to reflect GI abnormalities (see below).

What can one reliably conclude from these data? First, that clinical records systematically underestimate GI pathology. This is perhaps understandable. Ascertainment is a particular problem in language-impaired children, often with pain insensitivity, and one suspects that medical records will tend to dwell on the primary behavioral problem (for which the patient was referred) rather than on ancillary conditions that may rarely be perceived as a problem by the physician.

Second, one can conclude that frequencies of GI problems in patient-based studies vary between 35% and 92%, averaging at around 60%.

GI problems therefore appear to afflict the majority of ASD subjects. Historically, it seems doubtful that GI symptoms were a common feature of ASD. There is a case to be made that GI co-morbidity may be restricted to recent (new phase) ASD; this point warrants further attention.

What causes gut abnormalities in ASD?

An answer to this question may be crucial to the understanding of ASD, but data are unfortunately limited. A first possibility is that disrupted limbic function directly impacts on the GI tract, via hormones and neuronal relays, to increase inflammatory reactions. Deficits in mucosal immunity are seen in animals with limbic damage – failure of immunity permits the overgrowth of toxic micro-organisms, such as clostridial species (and possibly viruses) that themselves cause the inflammation. There is a precedent for this – stomach ulcers are common in individuals suffering chronically from stress and, as first reported by Barry Marshall and Robin Warren, and much to the surprise of the scientific community, the ulcers are caused by a bacterium, *Helicobacter pylori* – the "ulcer bug."[62,63] Subtle immune impairments fostered by stress and anxiety could favor the overgrowth of this unusual micro-organism.

Infection with viruses is certainly not excluded, but the evidence for the involvement of vaccinal viruses (as in the live MMR vaccine) is contradictory. Although ASD children do appear to have an immune impairment – 5 of 13 autistic children had no discernible anti-rubella immunity despite vaccination[64] –

Singh and Jensen[65] reported that measles antibody levels (but not mumps or rubella) were higher in autistic children than controls. It is possible that reduced immunity, especially in the GI tract, might allow vaccine viruses to persist, just as with *Clostridia* and yeasts, and these could further contribute to local inflammation. But, as Jass observes,[66] regarding gut inflammation, "it is likely that the controversy regarding the role of measles/mumps/rubella (MMR) vaccination in the etiology of autism has overshadowed some additional observations that demand serious attention."

A second insult, perhaps operating in parallel, is by direct toxicity of heavy metals and other environmental agents. A major site of oral heavy metal accumulation is the ileum;[67] mercurials could be partly responsible for gut damage in ASD.[68]

The reciprocal relationship between mercury toxicity and selenium (see Chapter 7) is also informative – mutant mice lacking key selenoenzymes (and thereby sensitive to mercury toxicity) develop gastrointestinal inflammatory disorders dependent upon the nature of the gut flora population.[69,70]

Deficient sulfur pathways and the gut

ASD children have a deficit in circulating levels of two sulfur-containing amino acids, methionine and cysteine[71] (see Figure 8.2c), reflecting general depletion of sulfur-containing molecules.

GI inflammation is at the heart of it. Because sulfate is poorly taken up from the diet, the primary (but not exclusive) source for body sulfate is the amino acid cysteine (found richly in meat, fish, poultry, milk, eggs, nuts, and legumes) and alterations in the gut wall might impair uptake.

In the body, dietary cysteine is converted to sulfate. Impaired cysteine uptake is then expected to reduce tissue sulfate. This could be important for metabolic detoxification. Abnormal molecules including drugs are processed by the addition of different charged groups that "tag" them for excretion. One important tag is the addition of sulfate – the paracetamol painkiller (acetaminophen) is modified to paracetamol sulfate that is then sent for export in the urine. Sulfate is added enzymatically from an activated sulfodonor molecule, PAPS (phosphoadenosine-5'-phosphosulfate; see Figure 8.3). Sulfate depletion causes PAPS depletion, and prevents detoxification and excretion of drugs and toxins via the sulfate pathway.

There is evidence that this happens in ASD. On average, ASD children were deficient in the sulfation of paracetamol – after oral ingestion the amount of sulfated paracetamol excreted in the urine was reduced three-fold in 90% of subjects examined.[50]

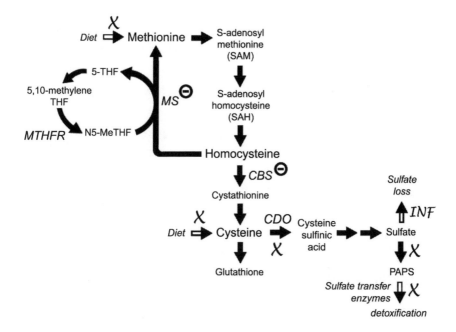

Figure 8.3 Sulfur pathways. THF, tetrahydrofolate; PAPS, phosphoadenosine-5'-phosphosulfate; enzymes (italic) are MS, methionine synthase, CBS, cystathione beta-synthase, MTHFR, 5,10-methylene tetrahydrofolate reductase. ⊖, enzymes thought to be inhibited on heavy metal exposure; X, steps inhibited by inflammation and dietary insufficiency; INF, a step promoted by GI inflammation. For further details see James et al.[71] and Strott.[78]

GI damage can also *cause* sulfate depletion by three routes. In the first, Murch *et al.*[75] reported that Crohn's disease and ulcerative colitis are associated with accentuated shedding of sulfated complex carbohydrates (glycosaminoglycans) into the gut contents, and excretion via the stool – thus GI damage in ASD accelerates sulfate loss. In the second route, GI inflammation inhibits the expression of the key enzyme that converts cysteine to sulfate (cysteine dioxygenase)[76] – GI inflammation will therefore deplete body sulfate supply. Finally, sulfate utilization will be impaired – in experimental animals, inflammation reduced sulfate transfer and PAPS synthesis.[77] Thus, overall, sulfate depletion is a marker of GI inflammation.

Heavy metal toxicity could also contribute, as this elevates sulfate excretion[79] and impairs sulfate transport,[80] to produce tissue sulfate deficiency.[81] Direct effects on key enzymes are also likely – both methionine synthase (MS)[82] and cystathione beta-synthase (CBS) may be inhibited (see Chapter 9) – further impairing sulfur-dependent pathways.

This section concludes that GI tract inflammation is undoubtedly a real feature of modern-day autism and autistic spectrum disorders, and warrants full investigation. However, one reserve is that GI involvement may evolve, perhaps becoming less severe with age (discussed toward the end of the chapter).

Serotonin elevation in autism

Abnormal blood levels of serotonin (known structurally as 5-hydroxytryptamine, 5HT) have been widely seen in ASD. Because serotonin/5HT is an important neurotransmitter in the brain, it could be connected to the behavioral disturbances of ASD. This section examines the origins and significance of the excess.

Serotonin (5-hydroxytryptamine) is derived from the essential amino acid tryptophan and also related to melatonin. In the brain, it regulates mood and behavior, and 5HT abnormalities have been linked to depression, aggression, obsessive-compulsive and feeding behaviors, and obesity.

Serotonin (5HT) is found principally in three body compartments – in serotonergic neurons of the brain, in enterochromaffin cells of the gastrointestinal wall, and in blood platelets – but the majority of body 5HT resides in the gut.

Blood serotonin is commonly elevated in ASD. Specific elevations have been reproducibly observed in whole blood from autistic patients (see Figure 8.2d). Mean 5HT levels were 205 ng/ml compared with 136 ng/ml in controls.[72] Elevation of 5HT was more frequently observed according to the severity of the disorder;[83] though levels did not correlate with behavioral score in one study,[84] a positive correlation was found more recently.[85] Though only modest (up to 50%), the elevation points to an underlying biochemical abnormality.

Serotonin is synthesized from the essential amino acid tryptophan (TRP), and degraded to produce 5-hydroxyindole acetic acid (5HIAA); it is also a precursor for the synthesis of the "jet-lag" hormone melatonin (see Figure 8.4). However, not all tissues are able to manufacture the molecule. Though both neurons and enterochromaffin cells synthesize 5HT, platelets take it up from the blood without significant local synthesis.

Separate brain and blood 5HT compartments

Brain 5HT is manufactured from dietary tryptophan (TRP): because human cells cannot synthesize TRP, dietary insufficiency (impaired digestive processes) will produce a deficit in 5HT. In mice, a tight link between blood TRP and brain 5HT was confirmed.[87] Here there was no correlation between blood and brain 5HT levels, suggesting that 5HT itself does not cross into the brain.

Therefore, blood 5HT is not an obvious source of brain 5HT, and instead 5HT in the central nervous system is produced by uptake of TRP from the

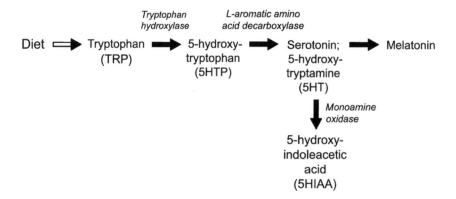

Figure 8.4 The tryptophan–serotonin pathway.[86] *This topic is discussed further in Chapter 9.*

circulation and metabolic conversion in the brain. When rats were injected with TRP, there was an immediate rise in brain levels of 5HT that persisted for over two hours.[88]

5HT in the gut

As in the brain, gut 5HT is also produced from TRP, principally sourced from proteins in the diet (see Figure 8.3). Approximately 95% of the body store of 5HT resides in the enterochromaffin cells of the GI wall.[37,89] Release of 5HT accompanies food consumption: release is initially within the gut wall; 5HT then appears in blood and probably also in the lumen of the tract.[90]

There is a logic to this pathway. 5HT is a potent regulator of GI function.[91-93] Administration of 5HT increases contraction amplitudes and motility in all GI regions examined,[94-96] and accelerates transit at the ileocolonic junction.[97] Thus, supply of dietary protein (TRP) attunes GI function to processing requirements.

However, in conditions with pathologic excess of 5HT due to disease, the excess could accelerate GI tract flow-through to a point that uptake of dietary nutrients is impaired.

5HT in blood platelets

Circulating platelets are another major store for 5HT. The majority (99%) of blood 5HT is held in platelets: blood levels are broadly in the range 100–200 ng/ml; platelet-free plasma levels are only 0.4–0.6 ng/ml.[98] But, unlike the gut and the CNS, platelets do not appreciably synthesize 5HT. Instead platelets have a specific uptake system that transits blood 5HT into intracellular storage organelles.[99] Platelet and free 5HT show different turnover rates: platelet 5HT turns over slowly while blood 5HT is immediately responsive to meal status.[100]

Excess 5HT in autism

Since the 1970s, specific 5HT elevations have been reproducibly observed in blood from autistic patients.[101,102] Given that platelets are the major blood repository of 5HT (though the major body store of 5HT resides in the gut), separate analyses have been performed on whole blood, plasma, and platelets, though a complexity is added because many studies did not explicitly address a relationship between meal status and 5HT levels.

BLOOD LEVELS

Eight of 27 (30%) ASD children had significant blood 5HT level elevations (hyperserotonemia), and excreted more urinary 5HT and its degradation product 5HIAA.[83] This result has been confirmed, with significantly higher 5HT in ASD children.[103,104] Mean whole blood 5HT levels were 205 ng/ml compared with 136 ng/ml in controls;[72] in another study[73] levels were 303 ng/ml (ASD) versus 215 ng/ml (control). Although blood 5HT levels decline with age (0–5 years)[105] no similar decline was apparent in ASD children.[106]

PLASMA LEVELS

In platelet-free plasma fractions 5HT levels appeared to be significantly reduced in adults with ASD[107] but another study, also in adults, reported a significant increase in post-meal 5HT in platelet-poor plasma.[108] However, truly platelet-free plasma levels of 5HT are very low (0.4–0.6 ng/ml).[98]

PLATELET LEVELS

A small (~25%) but significant increase is seen in platelet-bound 5HT in ASD. In ASD children the average level was 980 ng/mg protein, while in age-matched controls the concentration was 807 ng/mg protein.[102] This rise has been confirmed.[109–112]

These studies are to be interpreted with caution, for serotonin excess may only be seen in some subjects, while many studies present mean values across the sample group irrespective of individual differences.

However, the average increase in total blood 5HT (typically +50%) is not mirrored in platelet-bound levels (+25%). As no differences in total platelet counts have been reported, this discrepancy deserves explanation. Methodological issues may contribute: excess platelet 5HT release during sample preparation could be responsible, perhaps pointing to platelet fragility in ASD. In pre-eclampsia (pregnancy-associated hypertension), for example, increased serotonin is associated with platelet aggregation.[113]

5HIAA in autism

Serotonin (5HT) is broken down to 5-hydroxyindole acetic acid (5HIAA; see Figure 8.4) and excreted in urine. Because (unlike blood) there was no elevation of 5HIAA in cerebrospinal fluid (CSF, a fluid produced by the brain) in ASD subjects,[114] it seems unlikely that 5HT excess extends to the brain. There was nevertheless a significant increase in urinary 5HIAA in ASD,[83,104] confirming the 5HT excess.

Hyperserotonemia is familial

Excess of 5HT extends beyond the autistic proband: siblings and parents commonly (>40%) show similar increases.[115–117] A total of 70% of families with one hyperserotonemic member had two or more hyperserotonemic members.[118] There is no direct 1:1 relation between hyperserotonemia and ASD.

The importance of kidney handling

Dietary TRP is converted to 5HT in gut and brain; the kidney is a further site of 5HT synthesis.[119] Kidney 5HT is a regulator of fluid exchange[120] and may underlie the link between 5HT excess and elevated blood pressure. In patients with impaired kidney function there are marked elevations of blood 5HT (and 5HIAA) levels.[121,122] It is of note that kidney damage frequently accompanies environmental toxicity, both by heavy metals and organics (as reviewed[123]); porphyrin excess in ASD (next section) may be associated with kidney damage.

Origin of excess blood 5HT in ASD

Blood serotonin levels were not increased on seizure[124] – the excess is not a consequence of epileptic brain activity often associated with ASD. Instead, the gut is the most likely primary source.

In support, hyper-elevation of free 5HT following meal consumption has been reported in ASD.[125] In adult autistic patients, platelet-free 5HT response to diet is dysregulated compared with normal controls. Peak 5HT levels in adult autistic subjects were reached 1 hour after a meal, and declined after 2 hours. Normal controls showed a gradual linear increase over the entire period.[108] This could point to more rapid access of gut tryptophan to enterochromaffin cells, via accelerated transit or by impaired GI tract barrier function.

Role of gut damage and inflammation

Gut damage is a possible cause of the 5HT elevation. Inflammation and exposure to atypical gut flora produce long-lasting changes in the distribution of 5HT cells in the gut wall.[126] Bacterial toxins (exemplified by cholera toxin) also enhance 5HT release[127] and the overgrowth of clostridial species (above) is likely to contribute.

In addition to generalized GI inflammation, heavy metals may play a more direct role in releasing 5HT from the GI wall into blood. Both mercuric ion and methylmercury cause spontaneous neuronal release of 5HT *in vitro*.[128] Ethylmercury stimulates platelet serotonin release.[129] Copper administration produces nausea and vomiting: these effects were due to 5HT release as they could be prevented by agents that block the 5HT receptor, but the site of 5HT release and action was not determined.[130]

Other lines of evidence link the serotonin excess to GI problems rather than to the brain. First, urinary 5HIAA, the major breakdown product of 5HT (see Figure 8.4), is elevated in ASD. However, there was no excess of the same molecule in brain-derived cerebrospinal fluid (CSF).[114] Second, one 5HT study on ASD excluded all subjects with inflammatory, endocrine, allergic, or other chronic disease – in the remaining subjects no 5HT elevation was found.[131]

Even so, in this subgroup, oral administration of a 5HT precursor, 5HTP (see Figure 8.4), led to elevated blood 5HT in ASD subjects over controls. As the authors of this study[131] note, the enzyme converting 5HTP to 5HT (L-aromatic amino acid decarboxylase) is elevated by inflammation – more rapid conversion could reflect a GI tract inflammation.

Pointers from irritable bowel syndrome

So far it has been argued that the 5HT elevation in ASD is due to the gut, and not to the brain. Further insight comes from the condition known as irritable bowel syndrome (IBS) where 5HT is centrally implicated.[132–134]

IBS is characterized by abdominal pain, with diarrhea or constipation, often associated with disturbances of GI motility. Some 10–15% of the population is thought to suffer from IBS, but with enormous variation in severity, ranging from unremarkable to severe. As with ASD, a relationship between gut infection, altered local immunity, and subsequent development of IBS has been suggested.[135]

IBS is associated with 5HT abnormalities: 57 patients with diarrhea-predominant IBS had a mean blood level of ~300 ng/ml while the control mean (20 healthy volunteers) was ~100 ng/ml;[136] interestingly, the elevation correlated with anxiety, a condition commonly seen in ASD. Post-meal hyper-elevation of (platelet-free) blood 5HT is reported in IBS[125,137] as in ASD,[108] pointing to a primary dietary (TRP) origin in both IBS and ASD.

5HT: a marker of GI damage

There have been suggestions that abnormalities in serotonin transport might contribute to ASD. One study suggested that specific gene variants of the platelet serotonin transporter (SLC6A4) correlated significantly with 5HT levels in ASD.[138] However, several other large authoritative studies refuted any such correlation.

It is argued here that the 5HT elevation in the majority of ASD is due to GI tract inflammation, and is unrelated to the activity of serotonin neurons in the brain (though abnormal brain activity is likely to contribute to GI inflammation via a different route).

Hormones in ASD

This section now considers hormonal and endocrine abnormalities in ASD. These are many and diverse, but focus is on three categories. First, the stress axis (cortisol, and related hormones) in view of the prevalence of anxiety as a common companion to ASD. Second, oxytocin, "the social hormone," in view of the social and communication impairments of ASD. Then, gonadal steroids, because of the view that the autistic brain might be differentially masculinized – the extreme male brain theory of autism.[139]

Cortisol, ACTH, and beta-endorphin

These hormones are considered to be part of the stress axis – secretion is boosted under conditions of acute stress and they contribute to the fight or flight reaction. As described earlier, just under the hippocampus lies a small and richly innervated secretory organ, the hypothalamus.

On prompting from the higher brain (e.g. on perception of a threatening situation) the hypothalamus secretes a hormone (corticotropin-releasing factor, or CRF) that acts on the pituitary gland in turn immediately below it (see Figure 8.1). In response, the pituitary begins to secrete several peptide hormones into the blood including ACTH (adrenocorticotrophic hormone) and β-endorphin. These are produced by cleavage of a single large precursor molecule called pro-opiomelanocortin (POMC), as shown in Figure 8.5.

Both these molecules regulate the stress response. ACTH circulating in the blood binds to specific receptors on the adrenal gland cortex[140] to stimulate the release of stress hormones, particularly glucocorticoids.[141] Beta-endorphin (βE) appears to counter glucocorticoid activation and has been dubbed an "anti-stress" hormone; it may be important in switching off the stress response. While

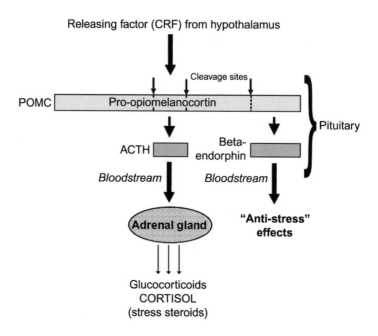

Figure 8.5 Production of ACTH and β-endorphin by cleavage of POMC in the pituitary.

glucocorticoids suppress the immune response (below), endorphins enhance the activity of immune cells.[142–144]

A caveat: glucocorticoids are not simply stress hormones. They play a much wider role, and modulate each and every body function including salt exchange, reproduction, digestion, and immune function. Moreover, the specific pattern of glucocorticoid secretion (high in the morning, low at night) plays an important role in attuning body physiology to circadian demand[145] – and abnormal patterning (below) could be linked to sleep pattern abnormalities in ASD.[146,147]

The limbic brain, acting via the hypothalamus and pituitary, regulates ACTH release and glucocorticoid production. Limbic damage is known to produce a chronic elevation of glucocorticoids.[148] This raises the question of whether the major stress glucocorticoid, cortisol, is elevated in the autistic disorders.

In ASD, paradoxical and sometimes irreproducible elevations of cortisol (and heart rate) have been seen in response to psychosocial and light physical stress,[149–151] amounting to cortisol hypersecretion in one study.[151] Cortisol release in response to insulin or a reproductive hormone (gonadotrophin-releasing hormone, GnRH, formerly called LHRH) was heightened in ASD subjects[152,153] (see Figure 8.7a). In this latter study, 6 out of 12 autistic patients displayed an atypical pattern of cortisol secretion following LHRH challenge but none of the controls. Another study failed to detect any differences[154] but a more recent study demonstrated frank cortisol excess following exposure of ASD subjects to a novel situation[155] (see Figure 8.6), and with increased variability in the night–day pattern of secretion.

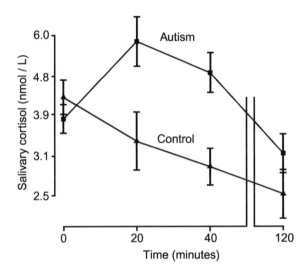

Figure 8.6. Excess secretion of a stress steroid (cortisol) in children with autism. Salivary values were determined before and 20 minutes, 40 minutes, and two hours following a non-social stress. Adaptation of Figure 2 from Psychoneuroendocrinology *31, Corbett et al.,[155] "Cortisol circadian rhythms and response to stress in children with autism," pp.59–68, copyright 2005, with permission from Elsevier.*

Other studies confirm defective control of adrenal cortisol production. Normally, when glucocorticoid levels are boosted artificially (by injection or by administration of a synthetic glucocorticoid like dexamethasone) there is a rapid drop in glucocorticoid production – this is because these molecules target receptors in the brain and adrenal to switch off production, a conventional feedback regulatory loop. This is impaired in ASD.

Nine out of 19 autistic children failed to downregulate cortisol on treatment with the synthetic glucocorticoid dexamethasone, while 26 volunteers and 19 schizophrenia patients all suppressed cortisol production.[156]

Although cortisol patterns are abnormal in autism, the defect is likely to be upstream (see Figure 8.5).

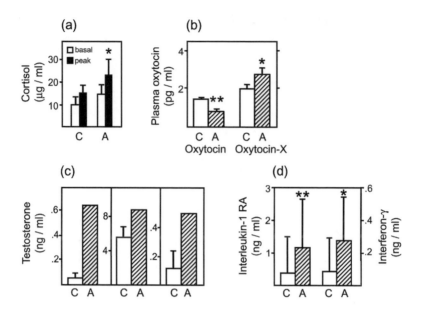

Figure 8.7 Hormone/cytokine parameters in ASD. A, autistic (ASD) group; C, control group. (a) Cortisol. Increased cortisol response to LHRH. Subjects were autistic patients with a matched control group of ADHD (data from Table 1 of Aihara and Hashimoto[153]). Both basal (pre-administration) and peak (post-administration) levels were increased. (b) Oxytocin. Mean plasma levels of oxytocin (OT) or OT-extended form (OT-X) in control and autistic children. Adapted from Figure 1 of Green et al.,[157] appearing in Biological Psychiatry 50, *"Oxytocin and autistic disorder: alterations in peptide forms," pp.609–613, original figure copyright 2001, with permission from the Society of Biological Psychiatry. (c) Testosterone. Plasma testosterone in three out of nine 8–17-year-old children. Single values from three individuals (from left to right: male, 10 years, pre-pubertal; m, 17, post-; f, 13, pre-) are compared with control children matched in each case for age, sex, and pubertal status; data of Tordjman et al.[30] (d) Inflammatory cytokines. Markers of inflammatory processes (interleukin-1 receptor antagonist, IL-1RA, and interferon-gamma, IFN-γ) are elevated in primary blood cultures from autistic and control children. Data from Croonenberghs et al.[55]*

ACTH and beta-endorphin (βE)

Both ACTH and βE may be elevated in ASD[154,158] including Asperger disorder.[159] No systematic studies have been done on ACTH, but detailed investigation has been carried out on βE.

Leboyer *et al.*[160] measured βE using antibodies directed against either the N- or C-terminal segments. The N-terminal antibody gave identical levels in controls and in ASD (9 and 7 pg/ml, respectively), while the C-terminal antibody revealed a ten-fold elevation of βE in ASD (70 pg/ml versus 8 pg/ml in controls). The specific elevation of the C-terminal segment was confirmed in a follow-up study.[161]

It is not excluded that ACTH/βE anomalies might be associated in some way with epileptic activity often seen in ASD: seizures are known to elevate neuroendocrine activity, with increased serum cortisol, prolactin, thyrotropin, and growth hormone accompanying epileptic seizure[162,163] and electroconvulsive therapy.[164]

Heavy metals could play a role. POMC processing is primarily performed by metal-independent proteases (subtilisin-type, PC1 and PC2) but highly selective expression of a metal-dependent enzyme (carboxypeptidase D) in cells producing ACTH could suggest that it processes POMC;[165] inhibition of this enzyme by heavy metals such as lead and cadmium might then contribute to dysregulation.

Overall, we see in ASD anomalies in the pathways governing adrenal stress steroid (glucocorticoid) secretion; the data suggest that the dysregulation is not simple excess or deficiency, but a rather more subtle impairment that is not yet understood. Paradoxically, although ACTH (and βE) appear to be upregulated, there are intermittent reports of behavioral improvement on ACTH treatment[166,167] but this could be due to direct (feedback) action on the limbic brain or control of subclinical seizure activity.

DHEA (dehydroepiandrosterone)

This is often referred to as the "anti-ageing" hormone, because of its fall-off with age, reaching very low levels in the elderly in primates including humans.[168,169] DHEA is a precursor hormone for the synthesis of a wide range of steroids including testosterone and estrogen. It is also the most abundant of all steroids in the blood, leading some to suspect that it also acts as a hormone in its own right. One emerging aspect of DHEA is that it has antiglucocorticoid properties, and may counter the effect of stress.[170] In many model systems, DHEA supplied at the same time as stress steroids depresses their adverse effects. For instance, while stress steroids (glucocorticoids including cortisol) are toxic to immune cells, DHEA (and its metabolic derivatives) prevents this,[171] and instead powerfully promotes immunity.[172] Whereas glucocorticoids damage hippocampal neurons, DHEA protects against this damage.[173]

In adults with autistic disorder, DHEA levels were reduced. Levels of sulfated DHEA (the major form in the blood) were reduced from 8200 nM in controls to 4800 nM in subjects, a significant 42% reduction. The free form of DHEA was also reduced, down from 54 nM in controls to 34 nM in autistic disorder, a reduction of 38%.[174] If confirmed, the reduction in DHEA could itself cause excess glucocorticoid action, contributing to adverse effects including immune deficits.

Oxytocin

This molecule has been dubbed the "social hormone" because it promotes social behavior including social bonding, reproductive pairing, suckling, and lactation.[175,176] Oxytocin, like ACTH, is produced by the pituitary gland in response to brain activation and, interestingly (like β-endorphin), may have marked anti-stress effects.[177,178]

Because impaired social interaction is one of the triad of critical impairments diagnostic of ASD, there has been great interest in the possibility that social impairments might be reflected, at the biochemical level, by deficiencies in oxytocin.

Oxytocin (OT) levels are depressed in autistic children (see Figure 8.7b),[179] and downregulation was accompanied by increased levels of the OT precursor polypeptide OT-X[157] suggesting, as with βE, a processing deficit.

This was confirmed by the age profile: OT levels rise with age in normal children; there was no such OT rise in autistic children. Instead, OT-X levels rise with age.[157] OT-X is robustly expressed in human fetal brain;[180] the OT abnormality in ASD could reflect incomplete brain maturation.

OT-X is a longer peptide than OT – normally the end of the molecule is trimmed off by a zinc-dependent enzyme (a carboxypeptidase B-related protease) to generate mature OT.[181] One wonders if interference with the activity of this enzyme by unnatural metals might explain the OT processing deficit.

In control children, increasing OT levels correlated positively with social skills, but in the autistic group the highest social skills were seen, surprisingly, in the children with the *lowest* OT levels.[157]

Thus, both OT production and behavioral responses seem to be distorted in ASD. Intriguing preliminary findings suggest that the repetitive behaviors of ASD may be markedly alleviated by infusion of OT,[182] though this result awaits confirmation.

Brain and plasma OT levels reflect release at separate sites;[183,184] only limbic (amygdala) exposure to OT is associated with social recognition.[185] Mice genetically deficient in OT do in fact show some social deficits such as in impaired social recognition (dependent on memory); social interactions are fully intact[185] and maternal care is also unaffected.

This argues that OT, at least in mice, contributes more to social memory than to social interaction *per se*. However, these mice also displayed increased anxiety-like behavior and enhanced glucocorticoid release following stress,[186] suggesting that an OT deficit could contribute to autistic behavior. A mouse OT-based model of ASD has been proposed.[187]

Gonadal steroids: male type behavior

Sex steroids (androgens in male, including testosterone, and estrogens in female, including estradiol) are typically produced by the gonads, though early and late in life significant synthesis takes place in other tissues including the adrenal. Gonadal sex steroid release is controlled by hormones of the hypothalamus and pituitary, under limbic control.

The role of the limbic brain in controlling sex steroid release has been demonstrated. In experimental animals, hippocampal lesions perturb reproductive hormone release.[188] It is of note that androgens are also regulated by stress, where the role of the limbic brain is amply documented. Androgen levels typically fall during stress (in males) but can achieve elevated levels on stressor removal.

No systematic studies on androgen regulation following stress have been reported in ASD. However, altered gonadal androgen levels have been observed in autistic individuals, and some ASD children and adolescents have impressively raised levels of testosterone[30] (see Figure 8.7c).

This excess could relate to some behaviors typical of ASD. It has been suggested that the autistic brain reiterates aspects of the male brain, particularly regarding "aloofness" and lateralization. This theory has been argued in detail by Baron-Cohen,[139] an extension of the work of Geschwind.[189]

Male behavior is implanted in the perinatal period by fetal testosterone and its aromatized (estrogenic) derivatives,[190,191] and this influence may extend to skeletal organization. The altered 2nd to 4th digit ratio is a sign of abnormal male steroid (androgenic) activity *in utero*[192–194] (see Figure 8.8), though androgens are clearly not the only hormones regulating this marker[195] and, confusingly, girls exposed to high concentrations of androgens during gestation do not display a male-type 2:4 digit ratio.[195]

The strongest support for the male brain theory of ASD derives from the altered 2nd to 4th digit ratio seen in subjects.[196] In another study, low 2:4 ratio in girls was related to hyperactivity and socialization deficits, while in boys a high 2:4 ratio was associated with emotional problems.[197] Children exposed to the highest levels of testosterone during gestation had the lowest score on a measure of "quality of social relationships" and, in boys, there was an increase in restricted interests.[198] Women with ASD also have an elevated frequency of disorders linked to testosterone excess, including excess body or facial hair (hirsutism), irregular menstrual periods in adulthood, and a history of severe acne.[199]

In normal subjects, the limbic brain is differently structured in males and females – in children (7–11 years) the hippocampus is disproportionately larger

2:4 ratio

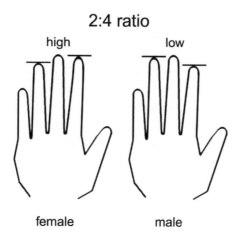

Figure 8.8 The sexually dimorphic 2:4 digit ratio; ratios in ASD subjects are biased toward the male ratio.

in females than in males, and the amygdala smaller in the female brain.[200] During development (4 to 18 years), hippocampal volume increases faster in females while amygdala size increases more rapidly in males.[201] In young adults, the hippocampus is, overall, larger in females.[202] This could relate to enhanced male susceptibility to limbic damage.

In considering whether androgen excess might contribute to the development of ASD, the inspection of other conditions is informative. For instance, early-life exposure to excess androgens is encountered in maternal polycystic ovarian syndrome, though enzymatic conversion in the placental wall may partly prevent overexposure of the fetus. But, in medical conditions where the fetus itself produces excess androgen, as in congenital adrenal hyperplasia (CAH), no link with autism has been demonstrated, even though the children develop some masculine behavioral preferences,[203] and there was a small increase in an overall self-administered autism score in CAH women.[204] However, as these researchers note, CAH is associated with glucocorticoid deficiency *in utero*, and possible excess on postnatal correction – both excess and deficiency have been associated with damage to hippocampal neurons,[205,206] affording a predisposition to ASD independent of androgen excess.

One must conclude that androgen excess may not be the direct cause of ASD-like behavior, though it does compromise neuronal integrity in the limbic brain, and the male brain is clearly more at risk – as demonstrated by the excess of males with problems of brain and behavior.

Instead, androgen excess may accompany other early-life stresses. For instance, perinatal infection is likely to contribute. In rats, female offspring of mothers treated with inflammatory agents were found to have significantly higher levels of androgenic testosterone and androstenedione.[207,208] Stress (restraint) of rat mothers skewed brain chemical profiles (hippocampus, amygdala, cortex) in female offspring toward the male pattern.[209] If this extends to humans, as seems likely, maternal infection or stress, or infection of the young child, may underlie the androgen excess and masculinization of females with ASD. Nevertheless, without any doubt the male brain is more "at risk" than the female brain, and factors biasing toward the male pattern will predispose to brain and behavior problems later in life.

Heavy metal toxicity can also contribute to androgen dysregulation (see Chapter 7). Lead, mercury, and tin are activators of estrogen receptor ERα in cell culture;[210] in vivo receptor activation by cadmium has been demonstrated;[211] while high-affinity binding and activation of the androgen receptor AR by cadmium has been reported both in the test tube and in intact experimental animals.[212]

It is possible, therefore, that the frank androgen excess seen in some children with ASD is a reflection both of early life stresses (including environmental toxicity) and abnormal limbic control. Nevertheless, it is intriguing that independent lines of evidence, from psychology to endocrinology, converge on the link between androgen excess and ASD, and further research toward an explanation is surely warranted.

Hormone metabolism

Modification of hormones and polypeptides by the attachment of a sulfate group is an important regulatory device, changing processing, activity, and excretion rate. There is evidence that ASD children are deficient in sulfur-containing amino acids and in sulfation pathways (discussed earlier), perhaps linked to impaired GI uptake and increased shedding that accompanies inflammation. This could have pronounced effects on hormone signaling.

POLYPEPTIDES

Sulfated polypeptide hormones include gastrin, where sulfation increases activity of the hormone,[213] and cholecystokinin, where sulfation is important for receptor activation.[214] Beta (β)-lipotropin, yet another small peptide product of pro-opiomelanocortin (POMC) processing, is partly sulfated.[215] Poly-sugars with sulfate groups are present on the pituitary hormones lutropin (LH), thyrotropin, and POMC. It is possible, but not demonstrated, that depressed sulfation in ASD might contribute to the POMC (ACTH and βE; see above) processing abnormalities discussed above. Reduced sulfate supply is likely to interfere with the activities of all these messengers.

STEROIDS

Many steroids have a specific hydroxyl (OH) group at the beginning of the molecule (3-position). These include estrogen (estradiol) and the "anti-ageing" precursor molecule DHEA (dehydroepiandrosterone); glucocorticoids and testosterone lack this group. In the body, estradiol, DHEA, and related molecules exist in two forms – the free molecule, and a derivative where a sulfate group has been attached by an enzyme (sulfotransferase) to the 3-OH group.

This modification changes the activity of the molecule. Estrogen (estradiol) sulfation is thought to represent inactivation of the molecule: loss of the sulfotransferase activity is associated with constitutive estrogenic stimulation of breast cancer cell lines.[216] For DHEA, sulfated and unsulfated steroids may target different sites[217] but it is generally thought that the sulfated steroid is less active than the free form, and sulfation may also enhance excretion.

Given that there is a sulfation deficit in ASD (see earlier in this chapter), it is likely that this would lead to an excess of both estradiol and DHEA – and both could contribute to excess masculinization in some cases of ASD. In fact, a significant reduction in DHEA-sulfate was confirmed in ASD, and though DHEA itself was diminished, the reduction was less significant.[174] It is of note that reduced steroid sulfation has been demonstrated in workers exposed to lead (Pb).[218]

THYROID HORMONES

These hormones play an important role in growth and development. The two most important thyroid hormones differ in the number of key iodine substitutions on the thyronine nucleus – triiodothyronine (T3) and tetraiodothyronine (thyroxine or T4) are released from the thyroid gland in response to pituitary-secreted thyroid-stimulating hormone, or TSH.

Sulfation is in important pathway for thyroid hormone *inactivation* during development, as reviewed,[219] but the effect of deficient sulfation *in vivo* on thyroid hormone levels is not known. Marked changes in thyroid hormone levels have not generally been reported in ASD,[220] but subtle thyroid hormone abnormalities have been recorded in autism with frank deficits in some rare cases.[221] Indeed, some ASD children appear to respond to the major thyroid hormone triiodothyronine.[222] Routinely, however, thyroid function is not examined in ASD.

Immune system

One of the primary targets of limbic regulation is the immune system.[1,223] In experimental animals, limbic lesions can cause reduced or increased responsiveness,[224] but generally depress reactivity – lesioned animals showed significant reductions in lymphocyte numbers[225] and lower immunoglobulin levels following vaccination.[226] An important component of this regulation involves the glucocorticoids, whose levels appear to be abnormally elevated in some cases of ASD and where subtle changes in the pattern of glucocorticoid release appear to be common.

Excess stress steroids (glucocorticoids, particularly cortisol) are known to have an immunosuppressive effect[227] – for instance, synthetic glucocorticoids are used to treat immune system excess in allergy and autoimmunity conditions including asthma, arthritis, severe allergic reactions, and systemic lupus.[228] Chronic cortisol excess can lead to profound depression of immunity, sometimes with adverse consequences.[229] Reduced levels of antiglucocorticoid DHEA in ASD,[174] see earlier, may also contribute to immune system dysfunction.

There are then several indications that ASD subjects might risk having immune impairments. Limbic damage and abnormal glucocorticoid regulation are expected to impair the immune system. Moreover, GI tract inflammation and abnormal gut flora point to impaired mucosal immunity in the GI wall. This section examines the evidence for impaired immunity in ASD, including allergies and autoimmunity.

General dysregulation of the immune system has been reported in ASD.[24,64,230,231] Five of 13 autistic children had undetectable anti-rubella immunity despite previous vaccine; all control subjects had normal post-vaccine immunity.[64] Ferrante and colleagues[232] observed a significant change in the spectrum of immune helper cells (CD4 positive), and a deficiency in a specific antibody type (immunoglobulin A) was seen in some subjects.[233]

There is evidence for altered immune responsiveness in primary blood cultures from autistic and control children (see Figure 8.7d).[55] *In vitro*, immune or white blood cells (lymphocytes) from autistic children were unresponsive when stimulated with a foreign antigen (phytohemagglutinin)[230] while other experiments recorded that lymphocytes from ASD children were hyper-responsive to a bacterial immunity-providing antigen (lipopolysaccharide).[234]

In addition to immune depression, there is evidence of heightened autoimmune and allergic responses. A high prevalence of digestive, respiratory, and skin allergies in ASD has been observed,[235] based on parent accounts.

Autoimmune disorders including diabetes, arthritis, hypothyroidism, and systemic lupus erythematosus are more than six times more frequent in close relatives of autistic patients,[236] though a recent study failed to find evidence of immune system abnormalities in relatives.[53]

Nevertheless, maternal immune problems during pregnancy, including asthma and allergy, represent a significant risk factor, while maternal psoriasis, a chronic itchy inflammatory skin condition, was significantly associated with ASD in offspring (risk factor, 2.7).[237]

Sweeten and colleagues[238] saw that blood titers of specific immune cells (monocytes) were raised in ~50% of ASD subjects, with parallel increases in a biochemical marker of monocyte activation (neopterin). Brain inflammatory processes in ASD[239] also point to immune system involvement.

The involvement of the immune system is strongly supported by the skewed distribution of immune markers (best known as transplantation or "histocompatibility" antigens) encoded from the HLA (human leukocyte antigen) chromosome locus. Several groups, but not all,[240] have reported highly significant HLA bias in ASD[231,232,241–243] suggesting that the immune response in ASD subjects is, if not frankly compromised, at the least atypical.

One must conclude that immune deficits in ASD are commonplace but, as with other physiological dysregulations, the alteration does not appear to be simple impairment. Instead the repertoire of the immune system is subtly altered – responses to foreign antigens are reduced, while at the same time reactivity to common self or dietary antigens is heightened. It must be emphasized that immune impairments may further contribute to GI problems: impaired mucosal immunity will allow colonization by adverse gut flora, while allergies to food components will be expected to provoke GI inflammation.

Liver and kidney

The limbic brain regulates liver function including acetate and glucose metabolism.[244–246] The extent to which the brain governs the function of the adjacent kidney is not known, although the organ is a major target for stress steroid (glucocorticoid) regulation of salt exchange, and limbic control of glucocorticoid release (and dysregulation in ASD) is well documented. This section explores evidence for altered liver and kidney function in ASD.

Defective hepatic detoxification

Detoxification of xenobiotics, metabolites, and hormones, principally in the liver, takes place broadly in two steps. In the first, termed "phase I," oxidative metabolism including demethylation is catalyzed by a range of cytochrome P450 enzymes. Typically, H atoms are replaced by OH groups, and this key step provides reactive hydroxyl groups on molecules that would often be otherwise unavailable for further metabolism. In the second, "phase II," the oxidized molecules are coupled to small molecular tags (sulfate, glucuronic acid, glutathione, and glycine) that are recognized by the body, directing the joint molecules toward excretion.

In ASD, problems with hepatic detoxification occur at both levels. In the first, heavy metal interference with heme synthesis (see the following section) may deplete the activity of P450 enzymes. Perhaps more importantly, the deficit in tissue glutathione, as recorded in ASD,[71] combined with the deficit in sulfate conjugation,[50] may reflect reduced ability of the liver to detoxify molecules.

Exposure to xenobiotics causes all these systems to increase, with raised levels of the liver enzymes responsible for both phases of detoxification. In ASD, liver detoxification is under pressure. Generally, urinary levels of D-glucarate (a metabolite of glucuronic acid involved in phase II detoxification) increase when phase II pathways are activated, affording a biomarker of toxic exposure.[247] Edelson and Cantor studied 20 ASD children (mean age 6.4 years) and reported systematic excess of urinary D-glucaric acid[29] (see Figure 8.2e). Most likely this is caused by excessive exposure to organic molecules that induce these pathways. There is indeed strong evidence for such exposure in ASD, with worrying levels of toxic organics including toluene and ethylbenzene.[29] However, one wonders if a general failure of either phase I oxidative metabolism or phase II coupling might lead to a defect in the removal of toxic substances – in which case abnormal persistence could cause the chronic elevation of urinary glucarate seen in ASD.

There are therefore good reasons to suspect that ASD individuals might be partly unable to detoxify environmental agents – not just metals (see Chapter 7) but also organics including pharmaceutical agents.

Moreover, there is a well-established link between metabolic deficiencies, oxidative metabolism, and toxic exposure. Reduced digestive assimilation (as often seen in ASD) could play a role, for phase I oxidative metabolism is depressed during malnutrition, leading to increased toxic exposure.[248] Deficiencies in sulfur-containing amino acids (as seen in ASD) exacerbate the metabolic effects of a chemical toxin (polychlorinated biphenyl, PCB),[249] presumably because hepatic detoxification via the phase II glutathione pathway is sub-optimal.

Chronic exposure to medications such as anticonvulsants, which induce the expression of phase I P450 enzymes designed to detoxify them, may increase demand for folate, and can itself produce folate deficiency.[250] Reduction in folate supply in patients receiving anticonvulsant medication has been widely described,[251] although another report confirming anticonvulsant-induced folate deficiency suggested that this might be by a mechanism independent of P450 induction.[252] Because folic acid (as tetrahydrofolate, THF) is a key cofactor for the sulfur-cycling pathway (see Figure 8.3), folate depletion on anti-epileptic therapy may also be associated with toxic homocysteine excess.[253,254]

In general, toxic exposure and detoxification deficits seem to come together in ASD, and no doubt contribute to brain problems, where both direct toxic action and biochemical deficiencies (including depleted folate) are potential routes to brain damage (see Chapter 9).

Heme pathways and ASD

Excess secretion of porphyrins in ASD urine was discussed in Chapter 7. These are related to the pathway of heme synthesis.

The essential blood pigment hemoglobin (and many other proteins) contains a tightly bound heme cofactor – a flat ring-like structure with an iron atom at its center. The iron, in this context, is able to bind molecular oxygen and activate it for key oxidation reactions. Heme is synthesized via porphyrin precursors in a sequence of steps (see below) in three principal tissues: liver, kidney, and in cells destined for the blood (erythroid cells). The liver and kidney are also sites of heme degradation, and liver and kidney problems could contribute to excess porphyrins in ASD.

The single large study discussed earlier reported excess urinary porphyrins in a large proportion of ASD subjects,[255] attributed to heavy metal toxicity. Levels of precoproporphyrin, a specific marker of heavy metal toxicity,[256] were also elevated in the ASD children examined, although this study awaits independent confirmation. The mechanisms underlying this phenomenon are reviewed below, asking whether brain damage or environmental toxicity could contribute.

Porphyrins and heme synthesis

Heme is synthesized from basic cell components (glycine and succinyl CoA) in a short sequence of enzymatic reactions (see Figure 8.9) – first to δ-aminolevulinic acid (δALA) that subsequently circularizes (three steps) to uroporphyrinogen, and then (in six steps) to protoporphyrin IX that finally accepts Fe^{2+} to produce heme.

Over 80% of heme synthesis takes place in blood precursor (erythroid) cells where it is used for hemoglobin production; of the remainder the majority occurs in liver and kidney where it is used for the production of cytochromes including P450 enzymes. Heme is subsequently degraded to bile pigments, both in liver and kidney, by heme-oxygenase.

In rat urine, the most prominent urinary molecule is coproporphyrin, with significant levels of heptacarboxyporphyrin and protoporphyrin. Other molecules detected include uroporphyrin and hexa- and penta-carboxyporphyrin, reflecting the most abundant molecules in the rat kidney cortex[257] and solubility:

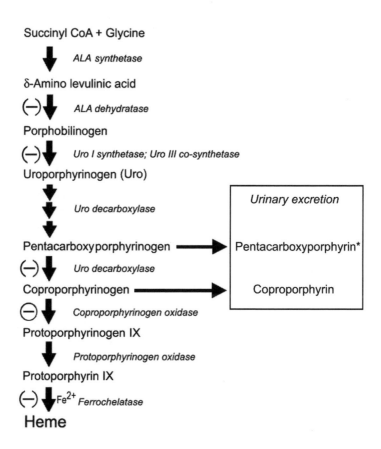

*Figure 8.9 Pathway of heme synthesis. (–), inhibition by heavy metals: ALA dehydratase, uro synthetase, coproporphyrinogen oxidase, and ferrochelatase are targets for heavy metal inhibition, with coproporphyrinogen oxidase ⊖ being the major target. Inhibition particularly by mercury leads to urinary excretion of coproporphyrin and pentacarboxyporphyrin; *this molecule is further converted to precoproporphyrin (also known as keto-isocoproporphyrin). For further details see Woods.[256,260]*

uroporphyrin and coproporphyrin are the most water-soluble and appear predominantly in urine (while hydrophobic protoporphyrin appears in bile and feces). In the lab these molecules are resolved by a chromatographic technique: the intensity of the peaks reflects the abundance of each molecule.

Abnormal elevations of urinary porphyrins are an established feature of heavy metal exposure,[256,258] thought to reflect kidney toxicity. On mercury exposure, urinary pentacarboxyporphyrin and coproporphyrin rise markedly, with a further diagnostic molecular peak termed precoproporphyrin, perhaps keto-isocoproporphyrin[259,260] appearing on the chromatographic trace. 6-, 7-, and

8-carboxyl porphyrins are not elevated.[261] Comparable results have been obtained in human subjects with occupational exposure to mercury.[262,263]

A causal relationship between heavy metal exposure and porphyrinuria was demonstrated through chelation studies. Both in rats exposed to mercury[261] and in humans exposed to lead,[264] chelation (respectively with dimercapto-propanesulfonic acid [DMPS] and ethylenediamine tetraacetic acid [EDTA]) markedly reduced urinary porphyrin levels.

Causes of porphyrin excess

How heavy metals cause porphyrinuria is not entirely clear, but inhibition of heme-synthetic enzymes has been documented. Enzymes inhibited by mercury include delta-aminolevulinate dehydratase,[265] uroporphyrinogen I synthetase,[266] uroporphyrinogen decarboxylase,[267] coproporphyrinogen oxidase,[268] and ferrochelatase[269] (see Figure 8.9). Inhibition of these enzymes leads to back-up accumulation of immediate precursors that, instead of being metabolized, accumulate in the blood and their oxidized derivatives are excreted at elevated levels in the urine.

Inhibition (tin, Sn) of the primary heme-degrading enzyme, heme oxygenase,[270] could also contribute to urinary porphyrin excess.

In addition to specific enzyme inhibition, heavy metals may cause generalized kidney damage. Methylmercury is known to damage the kidney[271] as do other heavy metals. Exposure to mercury, lead, arsenic, or cadmium injurs the kidney nephron and impairs central kidney functions including fluid and salt secretion and resorption.[272] Direct toxic actions of heavy metals on intracellular thiol-dependent metabolism, ATP generation, calcium release, and other enzyme reactions have been reported.[273]

Elevated porphyrin export could thus reflect generalized kidney dysfunction. Like heavy metals, polychlorinated biphenyls and dioxins can produce both kidney damage and porphyrinuria;[274,275] the kidney is a particularly sensitive target for xenobiotic toxicants.[123] Co-administration of bacterial antigens encountered in GI overgrowth and inflammation (lipopolysaccharides) can also markedly accentuate kidney toxicity[276] and may contribute to porphyrinuria.

Conclusion

We see, in ASD, a long list of physiological problems. These include dysregulation of physiological systems including the gut, the immune system, the kidney, and perhaps the liver. At the same time, abnormal control of glucocorticoids, oxytocin, androgens, serotonin, and heme metabolism is observed, which in turn can impact on other hormone and metabolic pathways.

While the GI tract is a focus of concern for the ASD subject, with enteric pain and other symptoms in a proportion (perhaps over 60%), the prominence of these signs conceals other problems, with covert but perhaps more worrying and widespread disturbances to body physiology. Other specific co-morbidities should not be overlooked, such as cardiac arrhythmia. Some of these may be consequent upon altered limbic function and environmental toxicity.

All in all, several physiological disturbances operate in autistic subjects, probably in the majority. But not all ASD cases have these specific biochemical and hormonal changes. An unsolved puzzle remains – how is it that some children have gastrointestinal inflammation, others serotonin elevation? Some have glucocorticoid excess, others extreme values of testosterone. Some have oxytocin deficiency. Can limbic damage explain these different problems? It is certainly possible that different types and timings of limbic damage, in conjunction with environmental exposure to more than one chemical toxin, might conspire to produce cortisol excess in one child and testosterone excess in a second. It is also possible that some of these markers go hand in hand – for instance, stress steroid excess in girls with adrenal hyperactivity has been associated with masculinization. For the future, biochemical subtyping in ASD will be essential.

It is also possible that the spectrum of physiological impairments evolves with age. It is certainly true that many children with ASD recover markedly as they get older, and though a majority retain a diagnosis of ASD through adolescence into adulthood, there are suspicions that the severity of the impairment declines. While the physiological disturbances could be in part a signature of a new type of autism that is increasing in the population, it is certainly not excluded that physiological problems decline with age. No studies to date have addressed this important question, and it may be difficult to address this issue empirically. However, there can be no doubt that physiological disturbances are a real feature of ASD, particularly in the younger child.

Before considering whether specific remediation of these changes is required, one must attempt to evaluate whether (and to what extent) these have adverse consequences for the subject – or are they merely benign accompaniments? The next chapter addresses the question – what do these physiological impairments mean for the brain, and could they contribute to the behavioral disturbances of the disorder?

Key points

Brain and body function are intertwined – the brain regulates physiological function through a cascade of sequential activation of the hypothalamus, pituitary, and adrenal (HPA axis).

The limbic brain is a key regulator of this pathway.

Regulation extends to other organs including the thyroid, gut, and gonads.

A brain–gut axis of control is well described. Limbic lesions accentuate gastrointestinal (GI) problems including impaired mucosal immunity and GI ulceration.

Diverse GI problems in ASD have been described, but the frequency depends on the type of study. Clinical records underestimate GI pathology. True rates may be as high as 60%.

Physiological impairments linked to GI problems include deficits in sulfur pathways (methionine, cysteine, and sulfate transfer) and serotonin elevation.

Dysregulation of hormone regulation in ASD includes the stress axis (elevation of the stress steroid cortisol with β-endorphin abnormalities), decline in dehydroepiandrosterone (DHEA), oxytocin deficit, and elevated gonadal steroids.

Immune impairments are common in ASD.

Defective detoxification and elevated urinary porphyrins point to liver and kidney damage, perhaps as a result of heavy metal exposure.

It is not yet known how physiological problems evolve as the child grows older.

Chapter 9

Body and Mind:
Impact of Physiological Changes
on Brain and Behavior in ASD

Just as the brain regulates the body, the body speaks back to the brain. A motivation – thirst – results from water depletion. A mood change – tiredness – is produced by exercise. Peripheral pain results in irritability and inability to concentrate. Sickness and infection make us disinclined to activity, conserving energy for the immune system. The brain is at the mercy of the body.

These are adaptive responses, but brain effects are also seen in medical conditions. In one 6-year-old girl complaining of severe migraine, with headaches and vomiting, a constriction was found in the aorta – the artery carrying blood from the heart to the body. On balloon dilatation of the artery the excruciating headaches abated instantaneously.[1]

A child with intractable epilepsy was found to have gut problems; when these were treated the seizures could be controlled.[2]

A 5-year-old boy presented with fatigue and speech delay, hyperactivity, and growth retardation. Thyroid problems were diagnosed; he improved markedly once these were treated.[3]

In these examples we see that a physiological or biochemical problem in the body can have a major impact on the brain. Could the same be true of autism?

One young girl, 9 years of age, from time to time developed the signs of an autism disorder, with social withdrawal, speech impairment, disturbed sleep, and gut pains. The autistic features were a result of intermittent porphyria (excess porphyrins in the blood);[4] when the porphyrins declined the autistic features vanished.

A 4-year-old girl with autistic-like features and occasional hyperactivity was discovered to have a biochemical disorder affecting urea metabolism with excess ammonia in the blood – once treatment was put in place all the autistic symptoms and hyperactivity disappeared.[5]

These may be isolated cases, but they well illustrate the principle that brain disorders, including ASD, are strongly influenced by body changes. This then asks the question – are the common physiological changes seen in ASD (see Chapter 8) just accidental companions, or do they lead the brain toward ASD?

Commencing with GI disorder, the sections following evaluate the differential physiology of ASD and whether it might contribute to the behavioral features of the disorders.

Gut and brain

Blood-borne hormones and chemicals can access the brain – illustrated by ammonia and porphyrins above. But from the outset one must emphasize a second route of communication, via neuronal relay, that plays an equally important role.

The brain is connected to the esophagus, stomach, duodenum, and colon via two major nerve bundles, the vagal nerves. In the brain, these access the brainstem, hypothalamus, and limbic system, notably the hippocampus.

These vagal nerves, which connect the limbic brain to the GI tract, signal bidirectionally. In one direction, vagal relay contributes to the GI tract ulceration seen in animals with hippocampal damage – when the vagal nerve was cut, gastric ulceration was abolished.[6]

The vagal nerves also signal in the other direction. Vagal stimulation can be used to treat drug-resistant epilepsy.[7] During evaluation of an epileptic patient, recording electrodes were introduced into the hippocampus during vagal stimulation. On gentle but rapid (30 Hz, but not 5 Hz) stimulation of the vagal nerve, hippocampal epileptic activity was abolished.[8]

Thus, vagal innervation permits rapid reciprocal modulation of body and brain. The specific involvement of vagal relay in ASD is emphasized below.

GI problems in ASD: brain effects

A substantial proportion of ASD subjects appear to have GI problems including chronic inflammation (see Chapter 8). GI problems could contribute to the behavioral phenotype of ASD including epileptic activity.

First, the link is entirely plausible – GI inflammation can have pronounced effects on the brain. In addition to the accounts presented above, a patient with chronic ulceration of the colon displayed severe neurologic signs that resolved on anti-inflammatory treatment.[9] A contribution of colitis to epilepsy has been reported in several case studies.[10,11]

Second, a causal role for microbial overgrowth in the gut in the development of ASD signs[12] is supported by the behavioral improvement seen in some autistic children receiving oral vancomycin antibiotic.[13] Antifungal and antibacterial treatments and dietary modification have been vigorously advocated as therapies for ASD.[14,15]

Third, impaired digestive processes may contribute. Wakefield and colleagues[16] reported parent accounts that certain foodstuffs including dairy products led to behavioral deterioration in their ASD children. Behavioral improvements in ASD have been seen with enzyme supplementation (caseoglutenase) to improve digestion[17] and, according to some accounts, dietary restriction in ASD can markedly alleviate symptoms.[18–20]

A contributory role of GI problems in ASD is therefore possible, but by what routes could gut problems impair brain function?

Gut-to-brain via the blood: leaky gut and dietary opioids

Perturbed GI function impairs digestion of dietary proteins; GI tract inflammation also predisposes to failure of the intestinal permeability barrier. The combination of the two could have an adverse effect on the brain.

The "leaky gut" theory postulates that impaired digestion, together with gut permeability, allow dietary peptides to access the blood and then the brain of ASD children. Debate has focused on opioid-like peptides, so-called because they target the same brain receptors as the opiates – a class of drugs (including morphine, heroin, codeine, methadone) that can be derived from the opium poppy plant. Exposure to these dietary components would appear to be increased in autistic patients.[21,22]

Natural opioid peptides include degradation products of maternal milk proteins. These neuroactive peptides cross the blood–brain barrier[23] and participate in subtle regulation of mood and appetite in both lactating mother and the infant.[24,25] They have also been implicated in postpartum psychosis.[26]

One such peptide, beta-casomorphin-7, suppressed anxiety when given to infant rats.[27] Brain signs can be rapid – behavioral changes were seen within 60 seconds of infusion;[28] effects on hippocampal neuronal activity were prevented by an opiate receptor blocker,[29,30] demonstrating that these peptides target classical opiate receptors.

Unnatural opioids and opioid-like peptides are also produced by partial digestion of common dietary proteins contained in milk and cereals. Given the permeability and digestive deficits in ASD, these foreign peptides could differentially enter the bloodstream and influence the brain in these subjects.[31,32] Indeed, there is some evidence that the profiles of peptides excreted in the urines of ASD subjects may differ from controls[33,34] though other studies saw no reliable differences.[35]

One double-blind study reported that dietary restriction, principally the avoidance of caseins and cereals containing gluten,[20,36] can be of benefit in ASD, with reduction of autistic behavior, and increased social and communication skills.

However, the mechanism may not be by the opioid pathway. First, opioids (like morphine) are generally regarded as inhibitors of brain activity, with sedative, analgesic, and anticonvulsant effects, at odds with the elevated prevalence of epilepsy and brainwave abnormalities in ASD. Instead, one suspects that immunological sensitivity to food components might exacerbate gut inflammation, and cause brain effects by a quite different route.

Dietary deficiency

GI tract inflammation impairs the uptake of essential amino acids and vitamins. Notable are the effects on tryptophan and sulfur pathways (associated with insufficient supply of tryptophan, methionine, and cysteine) not only through decreased uptake but also via depletion of essential cofactors including vitamins B6 (pyridoxal phosphate), B12 (cyanocobalamine), and C (ascorbic acid).

Gut-to-brain via neuronal relay

GI tract inflammation can signal directly to the limbic brain, stimulating local toxic cytokine production and neuronal damage.

CYTOKINES

These are small protein-signaling molecules, best described in the immune system, that are released from white blood cells to stimulate the activity of other cells immediately adjacent to them. Many different types of cytokine are known, including lymphokines, interleukins, interferons, and chemokines. The discussion here centers on four cytokines associated with inflammation: interleukin-1 (IL-1), tumor necrosis factor (TNFα), interferon gamma (IFNγ), and interleukin-6 (IL-6). Interleukin-1 comes in two varieties (IL-1α, IL-1β). All are known as "pro-inflammatory cytokines" because, in addition to being released on immune activation, they cause local inflammation and can be toxic.

CYTOKINES ARE UPREGULATED IN ASD

In ASD, two studies in post-mortem brain and/or cerebrospinal fluid[37,38] provide evidence for chronic elevation of pro-inflammatory markers that differentiate ASD from the control groups.

Vargas and co-workers[37] reported cytokine studies on post-mortem tissues from seven subjects as well as on brain-derived cerebrospinal fluid (CSF) from six living autistic patients. Only three post-mortem tissues were examined – middle frontal gyrus, anterior cingulate gyrus, and cerebellum. There was evidence of general cytokine upregulation in cortical regions but not obviously in cerebellum, though local activation of immune cells (microglia) was recorded in all three regions.

Cytokines were upregulated in both brain tissue and CSF (see Figure 9.1). The largest numerical increases were 30-fold augmentation of IL-6 in anterior cingulate gyrus and a 230-fold increase in IFN-γ in CSF.

Although the exact extent of the increase varied according to the technique used,[37] these results confirm a state of chronic immune activation in the brain of ASD subjects.

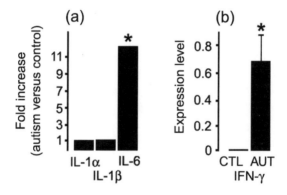

Figure 9.1 Elevated cytokine expression in the ASD brain. (a), anterior cingulate gyrus post-mortem tissue; (b), cerebrospinal fluid. In both (a) and (b) the increases were measured by a cytokine protein array method. CTL, control; AUT, autism. Adapted from Figures 3 and 5 of Vargas et al.,[37] with permission of John Wiley and Sons, Inc.

An independent study reported elevation of the tumor necrosis factor (TNF) receptor in cerebrospinal fluid of ASD subjects; the authors felt this was likely to be a marker of chronic brain inflammation.[38]

The Vargas study[37] is unfortunately incomplete because no central limbic region (hippocampus and amygdala) was analyzed – though the cingulate gyrus is not far away – but it seems reasonable to worry that upregulation of IL-1, whose receptor is most abundant in the hippocampus, could have been missed. Cytokine profiles are also known to differ between immediate and chronic long-term inflammation.[39] However, the absence of IL-1 involvement would be puzzling – this cytokine is centrally involved in both short- and long-term inflammation.[39] Zimmerman *et al.*[38] have highlighted the technical difficulty of detecting IL-1 in cerebrospinal fluid due to instability of the molecule.

In newborn rats exposed to bacterial infection, later life brain IL-1 production in response to immune stimulation was markedly *reduced* compared to controls[40] – the absence of IL-1 elevation in the ASD brain could be a marker of early life immune challenge.

CYTOKINE RECEPTORS IN THE LIMBIC BRAIN

The focus on the limbic brain seems justified because cytokine receptors are most prominently expressed in the hippocampus.

The receptor responding to IL-1β, termed IL-1R type 1, is expressed particularly abundantly in the hippocampus and adjacent regions including the choroid plexus, but with very highest expression levels in the dentate gyrus of the hippocampus[41-44] (see Figure 9.1b), a region implicated in ASD. In rats, receptor expression has also been seen in amygdala and the hypothalamus.[45,46]

The situation with TNF is more complicated because there are two major receptor types of different distribution, and although high-level expression is not generally seen for either, brain insult causes major cytokine TNF receptor upregulation in the hippocampus.[47]

For IFN-γ, as with the TNF receptor, insult causes remarkable upregulation of the IFN-γ receptor in hippocampus.[48]

Both IL-6 and its receptor are prominently expressed in hippocampus.[49-51]

Thus, brain upregulation of pro-inflammatory cytokines is likely to home in on the limbic system.

SYSTEMIC INSULTS INDUCE CYTOKINES IN THE BRAIN

Cytokine upregulation in response to local injury to the brain including stroke is well documented. Less well known is the upregulation of brain cytokine expression in response to systemic insults such as peripheral infection, generalized stress including glucocorticoid excess, and seizure.

PERIPHERAL INFECTION

Inflammation and infection in peripheral tissues provokes cytokine expression in the brain. One commonly used experimental tool is to cause inflammation by infection or with an extract of toxic bacteria. A potent activator of the immune system is a bacterial cell wall molecule, termed lipopolysaccharide (LPS) or endotoxin. Introduction of LPS by whatever route causes a massive inflammatory response, and simulates the effects of a peripheral bacterial infection. Also, many cytokines are themselves inflammatory, and inflammation can be caused just by blood injection of interleukins such as IL-1.

Infection, or artificially induced inflammation, causes striking increases in cytokine expression in the brain. Respiratory infection with *Bordetella pertussis* (whooping cough) or administration of broken *Shigella dysenteriae* (a cause of dysentery), both toxic bacteria, resulted in persistent hippocampal and hypothalamic expression of IL-1β and TNFα.[52,53] Administration of pertussis vaccine resulted in brain IL-1β release.[54]

Systemic administration of either LPS or IL-1 similarly boosts the levels of IL-1β in hippocampus and hypothalamus.[55,56]

STRESS AND OTHER INSULTS

There is a well-established paradigm of hippocampal damage in chronic stress. Over several decades a body of literature has accumulated to demonstrate that stress steroids (glucocorticoids), at persistently elevated levels, first impair neuronal function in the hippocampus, and eventually cause neuronal death.[57]

The toxic effects of chronic glucocorticoid exposure may involve local cytokine release. One study concluded that changes in IL-1β (but not TNFα) were central to the neurotoxic effects of severe stress (inescapable shock) in rats.[58] Thus, stress steroids may cause neuronal death through local cytokine production.

Insults operating through the cytokine pathway extend to irradiation and heavy metal toxicity. Partial body irradiation was shown to upregulate IL-1β in hypothalamus, thalamus, and hippocampus, and TNF-α and IL-6 levels in hypothalamus.[59] Organometal (TMT) treatment of the postnatal mouse results in specific elevations in hippocampal mRNA for IL-1α, IL-1β, TNFα, and IFN-γ.[60,61]

SEIZURE

Epileptic brain activity, common in ASD, may also contribute, noting that pertussis vaccine administration (in addition to upregulating IL-1β) increased seizure activity.[54] Seizures upregulate cytokine pathways in the brain including IL-1 in hippocampus[62,63] and IL-6 in hippocampus, cortex, and amygdala, and the IL-6 receptor in hippocampus.[64] Thus, epileptic activity activates many of the same toxic pathways as are induced by peripheral infection and inflammation.

However, the role of seizure is to be treated with caution, because brain cytokines can cause and not merely respond to seizure.

OBVIOUS BEHAVIORAL CHANGES

Excess cytokine production produces behavioral changes in experimental animals. These include depressed social interaction,[55,65,66] seizure activity,[54] and fever behavior.[67] Impaired memory was also seen.[68] IL-1 plays a central role – artificial blockade of IL-1 action systematically prevented the behavioral changes in these studies.

Gut to brain mechanism: vagal relay

GI tract inflammation and infection, in addition to other chemical or environmental challenges, signal to the brain to induce pro-inflammatory cytokine production, particularly the hippocampus and hypothalamus, and produce immediate changes in behavior. This relay operates via the vagal nerve cluster, and the vagus has been proposed as an immune–brain pathway.[69]

There is extensive and robust evidence that the vagal nerves, in response to peripheral infection or inflammation, transmit the signals that cause inflammatory cytokine production in the brain.

Electrical stimulation of the rat vagus induces hippocampal and hypothalamic IL-1β expression,[70] while inflammation produced by LPS activated the amygdala (and brainstem) – this was prevented by cutting the vagal nerves.[66] Inflammation (LPS)-induced upregulation of hippocampal and hypothalamic IL-1β was similarly blocked by cutting these nerves.[55] Brain IL-1 release induced by LPS (or IL-1) was consistently blocked by vagotomy, as was behavioral depression[55,65,66] (see Figure 9.2a).

Partial body irradiation increased levels of IL-1β in hippocampus and hypothalamus; vagotomy also prevented these responses.[59]

Thus, one may conclude that peripheral infection and other insults signal to the brain, particularly the hippocampus (but also amygdala, hypothalamus, and probably brainstem), to induce the expression of pro-inflammatory cytokines (and their receptors).

Cytokines are not good for the brain

Short-term cytokine production expression in the limbic brain is thought to be protective, but chronic high-level expression is very toxic.[71,72]

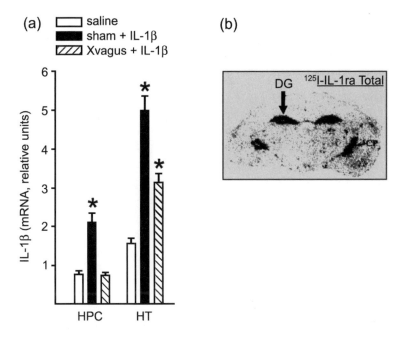

Figure 9.2 Brain IL-1β induction in response to peripheral challenge; abolition by vagotomy and receptor localization. (a) Effects of intraperitoneal injections of saline or IL-1β (0.5 μg/kg) on IL-1β expression in hippocampus (HPC), hypothalamus (HT) of sham-operated or vagotomized (Xvagus) rats two hours after the injection. Adapted from Figure 4 of Hansen et al.,[56] The Journal of Neuroscience 13, *with permission. Copyright (1998) by the Society for Neuroscience. (b) Selective expression of the IL-1β receptor in dentate gyrus of the hippocampus. Binding of radioiodine-labeled IL-1 receptor antagonist (IL-1ra) to mouse brain. Greatest binding recorded was to the hippocampus (principally the dentate gyrus, DG) and choroid plexus (CP), with significant diffuse binding in the cortex. From Figure 5 of Takao et al.;[43] a similar pattern was observed with binding of labeled IL-1 to mouse brain sections.[43,44] Panel reprinted from the* Journal of Neuroimmunology 41, *Takao et al. "Type 1 interleukin-1 receptors in the mouse brain-endocrine-immune axis labelled with ^{125}I recombinant human interleukin-1 receptor antagonist," pp.51–60, copyright 1992 with permission from Elsevier.*

Of these, IL-1 plays perhaps the most prominent role.[73] Lipopolysaccharide (LPS)-activated brain immune cells (microglia) are toxic to rodent neurons – toxicity was blocked by antagonists to IL-1β (but not to TNFα).[74] These mechanisms also operate in humans: the combination of IL-1β and IFNγ was potently toxic to primary human brain cell cultures; toxicity was dependent on local expression of TNFα.[75]

Genetic evidence also points to specific IL-1β effects on hippocampal neuronal survival: specific polymorphisms of the IL-1β gene (associated with hyperactivity of this interleukin) were significantly correlated to epilepsy with hippocampal inflammatory damage (sclerosis), but not to epilepsy in the absence of sclerosis.[76,77]

TNF is cytotoxic to hippocampal neurons.[78,79] IL-6 is also implicated: although neuroprotective in the short term, chronic excess is inferred to exacerbate brain damage;[80] overlaps with IL-1 signaling have been observed.[81]

Specifically regarding heavy metal toxicity, production of the sensitizing molecule stannin (which makes neurons sensitive to organotin and probably other organometals; see Chapter 7) is strongly amplified by TNFα.[82] This increase would therefore be expected to make the hippocampus, the central site of brain stannin expression, even more sensitive to heavy metals – heavy metals and GI inflammation would then combine to produce damage more severe than either alone.

GI infection and limbic damage in ASD

Vagal relay thereby permits peripheral infection and inflammation (including that in the GI tract) to signal back to the brain to upregulate toxic cytokines in the limbic brain.

Given emerging data concerning the prevalence of GI problems in a substantial proportion and perhaps the majority of ASD subjects, one must presume that this is accompanied by upregulation of toxic cytokines in the limbic brain. These have the potential to cause neuronal dysfunction and loss, and notably in the limbic brain. Therefore, GI tract infection and inflammation in ASD is likely to exacerbate limbic damage, and the behavioral perturbations of ASD.

Because hippocampal lesions themselves predispose to gastric ulceration, a feedback cascade could develop in ASD where hippocampal dysfunction and GI tract inflammation synergize to aggravate the disorder (discussed further below).

Nevertheless, the central role of IL-1 has not yet been confirmed, though massive upregulation of both IL-6 and IFN-γ in ASD was experimentally demonstrated.[37]

Serotonin – brain effects

Blood levels of serotonin (5HT) are elevated in many (perhaps 50%) but not all ASD subjects, and probably originate in the gut (see Chapter 8). The question then arises as to whether this elevation makes a significant contribution to the cognitive features of the disorder. Three lines of argument suggest that this is unlikely.

First, 5HT excess is often found in unaffected siblings and parents (40%). Therefore, 5HT excess alone is insufficient to produce the behavioral changes typical of ASD, and 5HT excess is not the direct (sole) cause of ASD. Nevertheless, a mild effect on cognition is not excluded: blood 5HT was significantly negatively associated with verbal-expressive/symbolic abilities across a group of 18 ASD probands and their first-degree relatives[83] but this may be a marker of GI inflammation, with rather more direct effects.

Second, brain 5HT is independent of the blood. As discussed (see Chapter 8), there is no correlation between blood and brain 5HT: blood 5HT does not contribute to brain serotonin pools.

Third, 5HT levels rise and fall with meal status (see Chapter 8) and it seems unlikely that these changes in 5HT (of a magnitude exceeding the excess seen in ASD) contribute to cognitive disorder.

Despite these compelling arguments that 5HT excess (alone) does not produce the cognitive signs of ASD, there are strong indications that 5HT abnormalities do contribute to a different disorder – depression.

As with ASD, there are blood 5HT elevations in depression, and more frequently according to the severity of the disorder,[84] though levels did not strictly correlate with behavioral score.[85]

Abnormal platelet 5HT uptake and release has been suggested in depression, and may correlate with mood, appetite, and anxiety changes in depressed subjects.[86] A 5HT uptake deficit in ASD is not yet excluded: one potential ASD contributing locus highlighted by computer survey of the genome was the serotonin transporter (SLC6A4/5HTT).[87]

Though a direct effect of blood 5HT on the ASD brain seems unlikely, significant endocrine functions have been attributed to 5HT that could impact on the CNS. In rats, infusion of 5HT brings an immediate increase in blood glucose, glucagon, and, after a delay, insulin,[88] perhaps through stimulation of digestion and uptake in the gut.

However, the effects on blood sugar and insulin could be prevented by adrenal surgery; these rises are unlikely to be due to immediate changes in gastrointestinal processing. Instead there is a more complex pathway, involving 5HT activation, vagal relay, and increases in pancreatic enzyme release.[89,90]

In addition to its action on the gut, serotonin is also a powerful vasoconstrictor. However, effects of 5HT administration are complex, with an initial rise in blood pressure followed by long-term depression.[91] Given evidence for reduced blood flow in parts of the ASD brain,[92–95] it is possible that 5HT excess is associated with reduced cranial blood supply. Therefore, a modest effect of blood hyperserotonemia on brain function cannot be excluded.

Tryptophan status: impact on brain function

There is better evidence that the precursor to 5HT, tryptophan (TRP), can exert directly modulatory effects on the brain.

TRP depletion, inferred to produce a fall in brain 5HT, is associated with negative changes in mood. In volunteers, ingestion of a TRP-free amino acid mixture produced a rapid lowering of mood and depressed performance on a proof-reading task.[96] Although the link may not be as clear-cut as first reported,[97] several studies have argued for a causal association between low blood TRP and depression.[98] As reviewed[99] TRP depletion in healthy subjects depresses mood while increasing irritability and aggression.

In ASD there have been suggestions that TRP levels are depressed. After normalization to other amino acids, TRP levels were significantly below the control mean in 35% of ASD children.[100] Although it has been suggested that the reduction might depend on medication status,[101] two further studies have confirmed the deficit.[102,103]

Depleted TRP is also associated with autoimmune conditions including arthritis[104] and systemic lupus, notable because of autoimmune and allergic conditions in ASD and first-degree relatives, and because of neuropsychiatric manifestations of lupus.

Low brain TRP availability could therefore contribute to the disorder. Notably, provoked tryptophan depletion in ASD led to a striking *increase* in repetitive behaviors.[105] These data do suggest that the brain TRP–5HT pathway is compromised in ASD but, it must be stressed, independently of the hyperserotonemia seen in blood.

Melatonin deficiency and quinolinic acid toxicity

Serotonin (5HT) is further converted, both in gut and brain, to melatonin. As argued above, blood 5HT is not the precursor for brain 5HT; instead 5HT production in the brain relies on blood TRP. If TRP levels are depressed (above), it is very likely that brain 5HT and melatonin levels are also reduced, despite the modest excess of blood 5HT (see Figure 9.3).

Significant reductions in overall melatonin levels have been seen in ASD[106] and disturbed melatonin regulation may underlie sleep disturbances seen in many ASD subjects.[107] Replacement has been reported to improve sleep patterns but not other behaviors.[108] Melatonin abnormalities may have consequences in the gut where it regulates GI function in concert with 5HT.[109]

While TRP is an essential precursor for 5HT and melatonin synthesis, it is also (>50%) converted peripherally and in the brain to kynurenines via an alternative pathway involving indoleamine 2,3 dioxygenase (IDO) or tryptophan dioxygenase (TDO) that open the indole ring. One downstream metabolite is

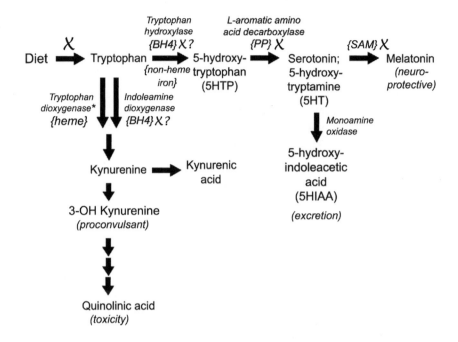

*Figure 9.3 Serotonin pathways impacting on the brain. Cofactors are: tetrahydrobiopterin (BH4); pyridoxal phosphate (PP, from pyridoxine, vitamin B6); SAM, S-adenosyl methionine. X, steps likely to be inhibited through GI tract maladsorption, driving brain tryptophan toward toxic quinolinic acid rather than toward protective melatonin. *Enzyme activity may be increased on Hg exposure.*

quinolinic acid (QUIN), that is a potent neurotoxin; both QUIN and its precursor 3-hydroxykynurenine predispose to epileptic brain activity.[110]

Regulatory pathways that upregulate this pathway, enhancing QUIN levels and neurotoxicity, include infection, LPS, cytokines, and other insults including oxygen deprivation, and these take place most prominently in the limbic brain.[110-114]

Therefore, limbic dysfunction and epileptic activity will be increased by QUIN released as a consequence of peripheral infection and inflammation, for instance in the GI tract. Brain levels of QUIN are increased dramatically in children with bacterial infections, as reviewed.[110]

The melatonin deficiency is of interest, because melatonin is effective against QUIN-induced neurotoxicity.[115-117] Therefore, GI dysfunction and inflammation could act on the brain in two ways – first, by restricting TRP supply, and reducing 5HT and neuroprotective melatonin; second, by increasing routing toward neurotoxic QUIN.

Cofactors

Serotonin is the result of two successive enzyme reactions, each with cofactor requirements. The first enzyme (tryptophan hydroxylase) requires tetrahydro-biopterin (BH4); the second (aromatic L-amino acid decarboxylase) requires pyridoxal phosphate (PP) (see Figure 9.3). The enzyme synthesizing melatonin requires S-adenosyl methionine (SAM).

Pyridoxal phosphate (from pyridoxine, vitamin B6) and SAM (synthesized from methionine) may both be depleted in subjects with maladsorption due to GI problems, and exacerbate deficiencies in the TRP–5HT–melatonin pathway. Pyridoxine supplied to rats increased both 5HTP and 5HT,[118] despite the fact that pyridoxine is not required for 5HTP synthesis. B6 supplementation has been trialed in ASD with some encouraging results.[119] Supplementation with sulfur pathway precursors has also been attempted.[120]

BH4 (tetrahydrobiopterin) is not a vitamin and is generally synthesized newly in cells using it. Levels of BH4 may be diminished in ASD.[121] However, inhibitors of BH4 synthesis do not diminish brain 5HT levels;[122,123] conversely, BH4 infusion into the brain did not increase 5HT.[124] Even so, a preliminary trial of BH4 in ASD gave encouraging results.[125] BH4 synthesis appears, in several systems, to be dependent on vitamin C (ascorbate) supply,[126,127] and dietary maladsorption of vitamin C could therefore deplete brain BH4 supply.

In each case, therefore, diminished cofactor supply due to GI problems is poised to compound the serotonin/melatonin pathway perturbations.

Finally, both the enzymes involved in TRP degradation toward kynurenine and quinolinic acid are modulated by a heme cofactor – as discussed later in this chapter, heavy metal effects on heme synthesis may increase the routing of TRP away from serotonin and toward neurotoxic quinolinate.

Summary: two separable phenomena relate 5HT to ASD

First, elevated blood 5HT most likely is a marker, possibly benign, of gut, kidney, and platelet abnormalities, perhaps brought on by exposure to environmental toxins. Second, TRP, pyridoxal phosphate, and SAM deficiency, perhaps themselves a consequence of GI tract malfunction, are likely to impact severely on brain 5HT release and melatonin production in ASD. In turn, this would accentuate limbic toxicity and contribute to the cognitive features of ASD.

Hormones and brain

Endocrine anomalies are common in ASD (see Chapter 8). This section addresses the possibility that endocrine effects could contribute to brain dysfunction seen in ASD.

Stress, glucocorticoids

Abnormalities of glucocorticoid regulation are seen in ASD, with frank excess in some studies. Severe psychological stress alone has been held responsible for ASD development in Romanian orphans subjected to extreme social deprivation.[128]

Excess glucocorticoids are toxic to hippocampal neurons and impair dentate neurogenesis.[129,130] Glucocorticoid excess may contribute to limbic damage in ASD.

In addition, the dysregulatory effects of glucocorticoids on immune function including GI tract immunity are well known[131] and promote pro-inflammatory cytokine expression in response to toxic metal (TMT) injury.[61] And finally, the deficiency of DHEA in ASD[132] is also likely to be harmful – DHEA has potent antiglucocorticoid activity[133] and the deficiency will increase the extent of neuronal damage in the limbic brain where glucocorticoid receptors are most abundant.

Limbic damage, in addition to affecting hormone levels and GI tract function, has adverse effects on immunity (see Chapter 8), and glucocorticoid excess is an important component of this pathway. Immune deficits will no doubt promote overgrowth of toxic micro-organisms in the gut, and lead to an increased incidence of infections of all types that one suspects, in other children, would not be nearly so frequent or severe. In turn, these infections can feed back to the brain to increase inflammatory processes that compromise neuronal integrity. By this route, glucocorticoid excess may further accentuate limbic damage.

Oxytocin

Defects in oxytocin (OT) maturation are common in ASD; the implied deficiency may impact on the hippocampus: OT is neuroprotective, enhancing synaptic transmission and modulating glucocorticoid receptor expression.[134,135] OT has been implicated in "stress coping" and glucocorticoid regulation;[136] defective production of mature-form OT (see Chapter 8) will compromise neuronal integrity in the limbic brain. Plausibly, OT abnormalities could overlap and synergize with glucocorticoid dysregulation.

Androgens

Excess androgen accentuates neuronal damage in the CNS: unlike neuro-protective estradiol, testosterone can be neurotoxic.[137] This could partly underlie the elevated incidence of ASD in males and, potentially, the association of elevated testosterone with ASD in the three children studied by Tordjman et al.[138] A contributory role for steroids is also suggested by symptom aggravation seen in some children at the onset of puberty, others showing improvement,[139] all potentially in support of the extreme male brain theory of autism.[140]

Sulfation deficit

Impaired uptake of dietary cysteine and increased loss of sulfated molecules in ASD (see Chapter 8) is thought to lead to a tissue sulfate deficit in ASD. This could contribute to the hormone imbalances. Reduced sulfation (see section later below) is likely to contribute to heightened activity of gonadal and adrenal hydroxysteroids: estradiol is inactivated by sulfation of its 3beta-hydroxy group, and depressed sulfation might lead to increased estrogen-dependent masculinization of the brain. However, this is unlikely to explain the very marked elevations of testosterone in some children with ASD (see Chapter 8).

Sulfur pathways and gene expression

The common sulfate deficit in ASD will produce a deficiency in the major sulfodonor, S-adenosyl methionine (SAM). This molecule, in addition to being required for serotonin synthesis, is also a key component of epigenetic regulation of gene expression. Specific regions of the human genome are modified by methylation, and this SAM-dependent reaction (which adds a methyl group to cytosine bases in DNA) can determine whether a particular gene will be expressed or not.[141,142]

The machinery that recognizes the methyl groups on the DNA, and earmarks the gene for switching off, includes a protein that binds specifically to methylated DNA, known as MeCP2 (for methyl-cytosine binding protein type 2). It is intriguing that genetic deficiency in MeCP2 is responsible for Rett syndrome,[143] a developmental disorder closely related to autism. Therefore, a deficit in sulfate availability would be expected to result in a disorder similar to Rett, where specific genes cannot be turned off, and continue to be expressed.

Even more exciting is the finding that MeCP2, critically dependent on nucleic acid methylation, may participate not just in gene activity, but also in the processing of the expression product. RNA copies of gene sequences are processed by "splicing" where parts of the RNA are chopped out – the remaining fragments are glued back together to generate the final messenger that codes for the protein product. Splicing is widely used as a regulatory device, so that a single gene can produce two or more different RNA copies (depending on which pieces are chopped out) – and they often code for different versions of an enzyme or a receptor. Termed "alternative splicing," this allows a single gene to make a range of products depending on tissue location or on metabolic demand.

Young and colleagues[144] looked for proteins binding to MeCP2, and discovered among them a protein known as YB-1. This is better known for its key role in alternative splicing. Young *et al.* then looked at the brain of mice engineered to have a deficiency, like Rett syndrome, in MeCP2 – and they found that alternative splicing is very much disrupted. It is not known how MeCP2 intervenes in alternative splicing – whether for instance it binds to methyl groups on RNA and not just on DNA. RNA methylation is well known – for instance, a protein involved in cellular stress responses (FtsJ) binds SAM and adds methyl groups to major cellular RNA molecules.[145] Thus, sulfate pathway deficiencies, at least potentially, could lead to defective splicing – perhaps this could explain the altered processing of molecules like oxytocin and β-endorphin (see Chapter 8).

Heme pathways – brain feedback

Porphyrin levels in urine are elevated in the majority (but not all) of ASD subjects.[146] No studies have yet been reported on blood, but levels in urine and blood go hand in hand in rodents with heavy metal toxicity. Blood protoporphyrin IX levels are increased in humans exposed to lead.[147] Elevated blood porphyrin levels, and disrupted heme synthetic pathways that cause the elevation, may well contribute to brain and behavior effects in ASD.

There are many precedents for brain and behavior anomalies in subjects with raised blood porphyrins. Neurologic symptoms are a prominent feature of acute intermittent porphyria, including generalized anxiety and elevated seizure frequency[148,149] with anecdotal ASD features.[4] Neurological disturbances in subjects with impaired liver function (hepatic encephalopathy) have been attributed in part to porphyrin excess.[150]

Variegate porphyria is due to a genetic deficiency in a key enzyme (protoporphyrinogen oxidase deficiency) required for heme synthesis, and is characterized by abdominal pain and constipation, psychiatric symptoms, and epileptic seizures.[151] Attacks are often induced by precipitating factors including drugs that interfere with liver function.

Molecular mediators and brain targets

Two molecular classes have been particularly implicated in the negative effects of heme pathway metabolites on the brain:[152] porphyrins and delta-aminolevulinic acid (δALA), their immediate precursor (see Figure 9.4).

Both interact with cellular targets for anticonvulsant, amnesic, and sedative benzodiazepines such as diazepam. Two such targets are known. First, the cell-surface receptor for the inhibitory neurotransmitter gamma-amino butyric acid (GABA); second, a mitochondrial membrane protein dubbed the peripheral benzodiazepine receptor (PBR). Functional coupling between these two receptors has been argued.[153]

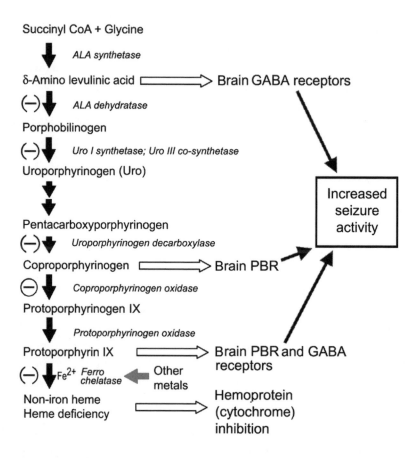

Figure 9.4 Heme pathway inhibition and the brain. (–), inhibition by diverse heavy metals and metalloids; porphyrins, oxidized derivatives of the porphyrinogens, target brain receptors: GABA, gamma-amino butyric acid; PBR, peripheral benzodiazepine receptor; both these receptors respond to the anticonvulsant diazepam.

Porphyrins and related molecules

Porphyrins are ligands of both PBR and GABA receptors. For PBR, protoporphyrin IX (Proto IX) has the highest apparent affinity;[154] this may reflect in part a natural function of PBR in translocating porphyrins across the mitochondrial membrane[155] to the interior where they are required to produce heme needed by mitochondrial cytochromes for energy generation by oxidative phosphorylation. Inferred brain concentrations of Proto IX are in a range consistent with inhibition of PBR function.[156] Proto IX is also a ligand of the major (A-type) GABA receptor and appears to stimulate receptor function.[150] The Proto IX precursor, coproporphyrinogen, also binds to PBR.[157]

Delta aminolevulinic acid (δALA)

The porphyrin precursor δALA is also elevated in blood and urine of subjects exposed to heavy metals.[147,158] δALA is a structural analog of GABA[159] and is an inhibitor of the major (A-type) GABA receptor.[160,161] Nevertheless, circulating δALA levels in lead-exposed workers (1–6 uM)[147,162] may be below the threshold needed for brain effects, and local levels of δALA in brain during heavy metal toxicity are unknown.

Proto IX and δALA target the same two receptors that bind the anticonvulsant and sedative diazepam, but their actions appear to be different. The major GABA receptor dampens neuronal activity in the brain, and activation of this receptor suppresses seizure activity. Proto IX is thought to activate the receptor (anti-epileptic effects) while δALA is an inhibitor (proconvulsant). But, paradoxically, δALA administration to rodents reduced seizure.[163] Unlike δALA, Proto IX also targets the second benzodiazepine receptor, PBR.

In porphyria, where genetic deficiencies in the heme synthesis pathway lead to large rises in heme precursors, seizure activity is common.[164] Similarly, seizure is a feature of heavy metal toxicity where heme synthesis enzymes are chemically inhibited. The biology is not fully understood, for Proto IX and δALA have paradoxical effects on purified receptors, but it appears, overall, that the outcome is an enhancement of neuronal excitability and an increased risk of seizure. Interference with the heme pathway could therefore underlie the abnormal EEG and seizure activity seen in ASD.

Because these metabolites also target the mitochondrial PBR, effects on cell growth are to be expected. Proto IX in particular inhibits growth and promotes cell death[165,166] – and could compromise brain repair.

Abnormal heme molecules

A series of brain and body enzymes are critically dependent on iron-containing heme groups for their activity. There are two routes by which heavy metals can impair their activity: first, by depleting available heme through inhibition of the heme synthesis pathway (see Figure 9.5, p.173); second, by replacing iron in the heme molecule.

The last step in heme synthesis involves the addition of an iron atom to the Proto IX nucleus. This is done by an enzyme, ferrochelatase. However, the enzyme is not entirely specific for iron, and in the face of interfering heavy metals such as lead, ferrochelatase will catalyze the formation of unusual heme-like molecules containing cobalt, zinc, or other metals instead of iron.[167]

These abnormal heme molecules are unable to bind oxygen; enzymes requiring heme are therefore wholly inactivated.

Cytochrome P450s and mitochondrial cytochromes

Among the best studied heme-requiring enzymes are the cytochrome P450s (also known as CYPs), richly expressed in liver and kidney, and they contribute to the vivid red-purple color of these tissues. These enzymes are required for oxidative metabolism of a wide range of molecules, including detoxification of foreign molecules and steroid synthesis.

In cultured human liver cells, heavy metals blocked the production of specific P450 enzymes – cadmium inhibited by 82%, arsenic and lead by 20–26%, while mercuric ion was a poor inhibitor, reducing activity only by 4%.[168]

Artificial non-iron heme molecules such as the tin (Sn) complex are potent inhibitors of P450s, and exposure of rats to the cobalt (Co) complex reduced tissue P450 content to less than 20% of normal levels.[169]

Hepatic detoxification is impaired in ASD (see Chapter 8), perhaps as a consequence of heme (and sulfur) deficiency, and could contribute to brain damage through failure to remove toxic molecules.

Specific P450 enzymes are expressed in the limbic brain, for instance the sterol and steroid metabolizing enzyme CYP7B.[170] In the brain, expression is substantially restricted to the dentate gyrus of the hippocampus,[171] with lower levels in cerebellum and cortex. The enzyme is thought to inactivate androgenic steroids[172] inhibition leading to excess steroid activity. At the same time, the product of the enzyme reaction (a particular 7-hydroxylated steroid) is suspected to have neuroprotective and immune-enhancing qualities.[170] Inhibition of this specific enzyme could contribute to limbic (and cerebellar) damage in ASD subjects with evidence of heavy metal exposure.

P450 enzymes, in addition to modifying natural molecules like steroids, are centrally involved in oxidative detoxification, principally in the liver, of foreign molecules including drugs. A liver detoxification disturbance has been recorded in ASD[173] but it is not known how this relates to P450 activity.

Mitochondrial cytochromes, also heme-containing enzymes, are responsible for intracellular energy generation. They are also critically iron-dependent, and heavy metal toxicity (e.g. organomercury) causes rapid inhibition of oxidative phosphorylation.[174] Mitochondrial damage is the major signal for programmed cell death throughout the body and also in the brain,[175] and organomercury-mediated induction of apoptosis has been recorded in human neuronal cells.[176]

Amino acid pathways and heme

Heme abnormalities may interact with impaired sulfur pathways, as discussed in the previous chapter. Impaired supply of sulfur-containing metabolites is a likely consequence of GI inflammation, but interference with heme metabolic pathways will also contribute, because two key enzymes (cystathione beta-synthase and methionine synthase) are inhibited concurrently with heavy metal impairment of heme pathways (see Figure 9.5).

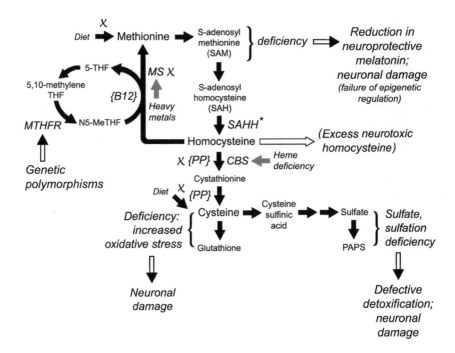

Figure 9.5 Inhibition of methionine pathways by heavy metal interference and heme deficiency. CBS, cystathionine beta-synthase; MS, methionine synthase; MTHFR, methylene tetrahydrofolate reductase; PAPS, phosphoadenosine-5'-phosphosulfate (phosphodonor); SAHH, S-adenosyl homocysteine hydrolase (*inhibition by adenosine, also elevated in some ASD subjects); THF, tetrahydrofolate; MeTHF, methylene tetrahydrofolate. Cofactors: {B12}, vitamin B12, cyanocobalamin; {PP}, pyridoxal phosphate, from pyridoxine (vitamin B6). X, steps inhibited by dietary deficiency, heavy metal toxicity, or heme deficiency.

Cystathione beta-synthase is a heme-dependent enzyme[177] and mercurials block the activity of the enzyme.[178] Methionine synthase is a metalloenzyme, requiring Zn for activity, and total inhibition of this enzyme was observed in the presence of organomercury.[179]

Inhibition of these two enzymes will have several consequences. First, reduced levels of sulfur-containing cofactors including PAPS (phosphoadenosine-5'-phosphosulfate) and SAM. Second, levels of homocysteine are likely to rise if onward conversion is blocked – and homocysteine is suspected to have neurotoxic actions, for excess correlates with reduced hippocampal volume[180,181] and impairs hippocampus-dependent skills in rats.[182,183]

In ASD, a sulfate deficiency has been recorded.[184] A wider study by James and colleagues[120] revealed a wider pattern of deficits. Children with autism had significantly depressed blood levels of methionine, SAM, cystathionine, cysteine, and total glutathione. Homocysteine was also depressed, but other reports suggest that homocysteine is most commonly elevated in ASD[185] (C. Skorupka, pers comm).

However, the profile is not entirely consistent with simple inhibition of methionine synthase (and CBS); James *et al.*[120] argue for secondary inhibition of the enzyme synthesizing homocysteine, S-adenosyl homocysteine dehydrolase (SAHH).

The reduction in glutathione may be of particular importance; this molecule is required for many different anti-oxidation reactions. It is possible to suggest that lack of glutathione (perhaps as a consequence of impaired dietary methionine uptake, sulfate loss, and enzyme inhibition) will be expected to promote oxidative damage in sensitive regions of the brain including the hippocampus.

Role of MTHFR

Because of the unique role of the methylene tetrahydrofolate reductase (MTHFR) enzyme in recycling homocysteine to methionine (see Figure 9.5), and maintaining the sulfur balance, common polymorphisms in the MTHFR gene might contribute to pathway defects.

A thermolabile variant with reduced activity[186] is present in the population at high frequency: roughly 12% of the North American population are homozygous for this C677T mutation;[187] several other polymorphisms have been described.[188] Reduced MTHFR is associated with elevated plasma homocysteine,[189] but dependent on folate status.[190] In one study, CC677 (high activity) homozygotes had 5.5 uM blood homocysteine: this rose to 7 μM in CT heterozygotes and to 12.1 μM in TT homozygotes.[191]

However, evidence is mixed for depressed MTHFR activity in ASD. In one study, mean plasma homocysteine levels in ASD were 5.8 μM compared to 6.4 μM in controls.[192] However, homocysteine can be difficult to measure, and a majority of ASD children examined by C. Skorupka (pers. comm.) were found to have homocysteine elevation, a finding confirmed in a recent report placing homocysteine at 9.8 uM in ASD compared to 7.5 μM in controls.[185]

Tryptophan pathways

Both indoleamine dioxygenase (IDO) and tryptophan dioxygenase (TDO), the enzymes that shunt tryptophan away from serotonin and melatonin synthesis toward kynurenine and neurotoxic quinolinate (see Figure 9.3), are modulated by a heme cofactor.[193–196] However, regulation is not just at the level of enzyme activity – when rats were treated with mercuric chloride the activity of TDO enzyme was markedly *increased*.[197] The tryptophan hydroxylase enzyme (which converts tryptophan onwards toward serotonin and melatonin) requires free iron, furnishing a further potential target for heavy metal toxicity, but is not dependent on heme. Interference with heme pathways is therefore expected to accentuate brain depletion of serotonin and neuroprotective melatonin, in favor of toxic metabolites including quinolinic acid, with effects on neuronal survival in the brain.

Do feedback cascades operate in ASD?

A feedback cascade is a regulatory malfunction in which an initial insult impairs the regulation, and spiraling damage results. A household heating system is turned off by a thermostat when the set temperature is reached. Should a faulty thermostat begin to malfunction when it gets too hot, then – as the temperature rises – it will fail more and more often. The result will be a cascade of thermostat failure and escalating temperature. What was a small and intermittent fault becomes catastrophic failure of the system.

This type of feedback was proposed to occur in Alzheimer disease (AD) in 1986. Sapolsky, Krey, and McEwen suggested that AD, also a disorder of limbic function, might be due to a cascade of stress steroid (glucocorticoid) excess.[198] They noted that the limbic brain, particularly the hippocampus, holds back production of stress hormones including the adrenal glucocorticoid cortisol – but at the same time is damaged by chronic excess of the same hormone.

Their theory proposes that initial hippocampal damage leads to a rise in cortisol levels, in turn provoking further neurodegeneration in the same brain region. Ever-increasing secretion of glucocorticoids and hippocampal damage becomes a neurodegenerative cascade, culminating in AD.[198]

There is circumstantial evidence in support of this cascade in AD, but the details remain to be clarified. However, the Sapolsky–Krey–McEwen cascade could provide a model for understanding other disorders affecting the limbic brain including autism and ASDs.

Given that the limbic brain is involved in regulating diverse aspects of body physiology, and not just the production of cortisol, several cascades potentially could link brain damage to disorganization of body physiology.

GI inflammation

A mechanism parallel to the Sapolsky *et al.* glucocorticoid excess pathway centers on gut infection and inflammation, with targeted cytokine production in the brain leading to hippocampal damage.

The limbic brain normally keeps GI tract inflammation in check. But peripheral inflammation feeds back to the brain via the vagal nerves, to induce neurotoxic cytokine expression in the brain. Thus, GI tract inflammation is likely to damage the hippocampus (and hypothalamus), and is a risk factor for the development of ASD. Because the hippocampus deters GI inflammation, a cascade of escalating brain damage and gut inflammation can be envisaged (see Figure 9.6).

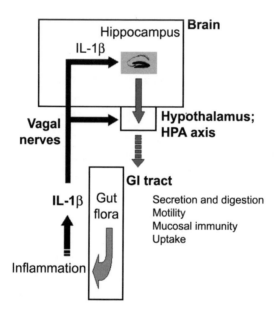

Figure 9.6 Brain–gut feedback loop.

There is a second minor aspect – gut deficits can lead to deficiencies in sulfur-containing amino acids and other essential dietary components: this is likely to lead to further brain damage, and also impair heavy metal handling where sulfhydryl binding is central to export.

Serotonin

Heightened 5HT seen in ASD is suspected as a sign of GI damage. Although unlikely to be directly neurotoxic (5HT enters the brain poorly) the 5HT elevation is accompanied by depletion of tryptophan and melatonin (and possibly quinolinate excess) that are all neurotoxic. These could also feed back to the brain to cause further limbic damage.

Heme precursors and metabolites

Abnormally high levels of urinary porphyrins, a marker of heavy metal toxicity, are a proxy for elevated levels of circulating δALA and protoporphyrin. These latter target anticonvulsant receptors, and can promote seizure *in vivo*. Seizure is a primary sign of heavy metal toxicity. In turn, seizure itself is a potent cause of limbic damage via excitotoxicity and oxygen depletion.

Porphyrins are produced principally in erythroid cells, liver, and kidney. In turn, the hippocampus regulates hepatic functionality including acetate and glucose metabolism (see Chapter 8): a brain–liver cascade could operate in some patients.

There is a further potential feedback cascade, the importance of which is unknown, via inhibition of P450 activity in the liver, kidney, and brain, which could lead to failure of detoxification of xenobiotics and promote damage by routes including limbic P450 inhibition.

Endocrine anomalies

In ASD there is evidence for changes in glucocorticoid production, but perhaps not in all subjects and the direction of the change is debatable. Nevertheless, glucocorticoid excess was most commonly reported, with likely toxic effects – as in the Sapolsky *et al.* cascade, excess will further damage the limbic brain. The large androgen excess seen in some subjects is also known to exacerbate neuronal damage. In those subjects with deficiency in anti-stress ocytocin, a parallel enhancement of neurotoxicity might be expected.

Other pathways

Immune deficits associated with limbic damage may also provide a cascade in view of the role of infectious agents in promoting peripheral inflammation (and brain cytokine release) and, at least potentially, direct infection of the brain.

Liver damage could also contribute. In an animal model of hepatic encephalopathy (HE) linked to hyperammonemia, brain damage was restricted to the entorhinal cortex, the principal afferent to the hippocampus;[199] hippocampal damage has been seen in HE patients.[200] In addition, because liver damage impairs detoxification reactions, the brain will be increasingly exposed to environmental toxins.

A complexity: seizure

The reciprocal relationship between limbic damage and seizure deserves comment. While hippocampal damage can clearly be the cause of epileptic activity, recurrent seizures can produce epileptic brain damage including hippocampal and temporal lobe sclerosis. These are seen in intractable temporal lobe epilepsy and in experimental animals where seizure activity is induced artificially.

As noted before, a large fraction (up to ~40%) of ASD subjects suffer from epileptic seizures, with a majority showing brainwave anomalies. In all the routes discussed here, one cannot exclude the possibility that biochemical and hormonal abnormalities impact on the brain to produce seizure activity, which in turn predisposes to limbic damage.

For instance, excess porphyrins have been implicated as a cause of epilepsy[164] and a range of other conditions have been associated with seizure activity.[201] Two interpretations are then available in subjects with epilepsy or brainwave anomalies: either that limbic damage causes the epileptic activity, or that seizure aggravates limbic damage. Under both interpretations, however, it is clear that epilepsy is both a sign of, and can exacerbate, damage to the limbic brain.

How good is the evidence? Assessment of different damage routes

In all the studies reviewed a complication is that few address the specific subjects affected, generally preferring to compare means across the ASD and control pools. This potentially could conceal a severe disorder that only affects a small number of individuals. Second, though some studies are very suggestive, not all are backed by evidence for an impact on the limbic brain, and a potential causal role in ASD has not been confirmed.

There is good evidence for a causal role in ASD for heavy metal toxicity, GI tract disorder, heme pathway abnormalities, and immune system abnormalities including chronic inflammation, all with established potential for toxicity in the limbic brain. The evidence for a causal role of excess serotonin, endocrine abnormalities, including impaired sulfation, is somewhat weaker, but not excluded in some ASD subjects. These potential feedback cascades are presented, in simplified form, in Figure 9.7.

It is argued that multiple interacting routes, including heavy metals and other environmental toxins, GI dysfunction, endocrine dysregulation, and genetic/metabolic deficiencies, converge on the limbic brain to produce neuronal damage and the behavioral signs of ASD.

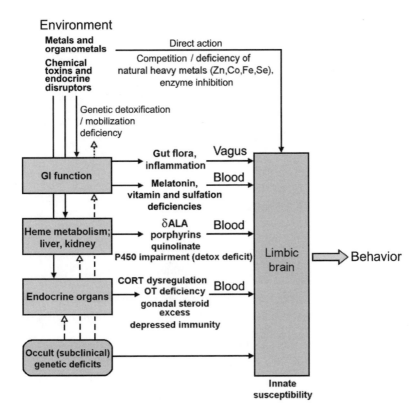

Figure 9.7 Environment, physiological feedback cascades, and the limbic brain: pathways. Summary of potential pathways causing limbic damage in ASD. ALA, aminolevulinic acid; CORT, glucocorticoids including cortisol; OT, oxytocin. Limbic damage feeds back on many of the physiological pathways presented.

Key points

Physiological changes can have adverse effects on brain and behavior.

GI inflammation signals back to the brain principally via the vagal nerves, heightening release of inflammatory cytokines in the hippocampus and adjoining brain regions. These are neurotoxic – GI inflammation is likely to exacerbate hippocampal damage.

Elevated brain cytokines are seen in ASD.

Elevated blood serotonin levels in ASD are unlikely to impact on the brain; instead tryptophan, serotonin, and melatonin deficiency, as a consequence of gut problems, is likely to damage the brain.

The stress steroid cortisol is also damaging to the limbic brain; other deficits such as in oxytocin and sulfation, and androgen excess, are also harmful.

Porphyrin excess, associated with heavy metal exposure, may also target key receptors in the brain, predisposing to seizure activity and neuronal loss.

Inhibition of key enzymes methionine synthase and cystathione β-synthase (through heavy metal toxicity) contributes to oxidative damage in the brain.

A feedback cascade of GI tract involvement and limbic damage may contribute to ASD.

Chapter 10

Biomedical Therapy: Typing and Correction

Toxicity, infection, and inflammation converge on the limbic brain. This, it has been argued, is responsible for the behavioral features of ASD. The question then arises of whether such damage can be reversed. Unlike most brain regions, the limbic brain has some capacity for repair. In most of the brain, neurons once formed lose the capacity to divide and, following damage, are unable to regenerate new neurons. In contrast, dividing neuronal cells are seen in the limbic brain until adulthood.[1,2] In monkey brains, neuronal division in the hippocampus was seen at the grand age of 23 years.[3] Even so, the rate of division was much lower than in the youngest animals examined, suggesting that repair capacity declines with age.

There are therefore prospects of some degree of recovery if the specific problem can be identified and treated. Whereas in high-functioning ASD it is questionable whether any therapy is at all advisable, in low-functioning individuals restorative treatment is clearly justified. There are many examples where remedial therapy can ameliorate the behavioral deficits. In one child with a urea cycle metabolic disorder, the autistic symptoms and hyperactivity disappeared on appropriate therapy.[4] Because neuronal proliferation in the limbic brain declines with age, therapeutic intervention should be put in place as early as possible.

What's wrong with my child? Subtyping ASD

There is an urgent need to match therapy to the specific deficits, and guidelines for good clinical practice, for instance as set out authoritatively by Filipek and co-workers,[5] recommend genetic testing and selective metabolic analysis. Clearly, each individual with autism is distinct, and underlying biochemical, physiological, and genetic risk factors are diverse. Only some children will have been exposed to specific toxins such as heavy metals. Other children will have an excess of a specific metabolite, while others will have a deficiency. Some will have precisely identified gene deficiencies, though the majority may not. There are children who will have extremely rare metabolic disorders that masquerade as ASD, and only a thorough understanding of the precise deficits will allow proper treatment to be put in place. For metabolic testing and approaches to therapy the works of B. Rimland and colleagues,[6] W. Shaw,[7] J. McCandless,[8] and more recently by J. Pangborn and colleagues[9] are recommended.

Subtyping

This is a major target of research. Autism and related spectrum disorders are not unitary conditions – there is emerging evidence that behavioral (and biochemical) deficits are distinct in different families or populations. One must side with David Amaral at the MIND Institute[10,11] that the phenotype needs to be broken down according to behavioral and biochemical markers.

One innovative study divided autism into two behavioral categories – a first type where repetitive and stereotypic activities predominate, and a second type characterized by resistance to change and need for sameness.[12] The validity of this distinction was demonstrated in a genetic investigation, where only the sameness-type showed linkage to a specific gene variant. The repetitive type showed no such association.[13]

More generally, diverse physiological impairments are seen in ASD. Altered brainwave patterns are evident in a proportion of subjects, ranging from EEG abnormalities (~50%) to frank epilepsy (~30%), while others show no such irregularities. Similarly, GI tract inflammation affects a substantial proportion of autistic children, perhaps exceeding 50%. Only some individuals with ASD have elevated blood serotonin. There are glimpses of marked endocrine changes in some, but far from all, affected individuals. How do these relate to each other?

It is possible, though not yet known, that these disturbances fall into specific clusters. Do subjects with EEG abnormalities have higher serotonin than others? Is GI inflammation related to endocrine changes? Are heme problems related to epilepsy? Future work documenting physiological changes in ASD will surely benefit from subclassification of subjects according to associated physiological conditions. There is therefore a major need to develop rapid methods for diagnosing biochemical and physiological abnormalities: only with accurate information can treatment be matched to the specific deficits.

Markers of environmental toxicity

The most commonly used markers of exposure are levels of porphyrins, δALA, and D-glucaric acid in the urine.[14,15] Porphyrins are markers of inhibition of the heme synthesis pathway, and elevations of specific metabolites including coproporphyrin point to toxic exposure to agents including heavy metals and certain organic inhibitors (see Chapters 7 and 8). The exact porphyrin profile is important, because some specific molecules such as precoproporphyrin can indicate specific exposure to mercurials[16,17] that inhibit later steps in the heme synthesis pathway. Exposure to lead (Pb), which inhibits an early step in the same pathway, is associated with elevation of δALA in the urine.[15] Finally, elevations of urinary D-glucaric acid point to abnormal exposure to xenobiotics that induce liver detoxification pathways (see Chapter 8).

Markers of GI tract involvement

As discussed earlier (see also Chapter 8), elevated blood serotonin (and a rise in urinary levels of its metabolite 5HIAA) is probably a marker of GI tract perturbations, but shows large variations and may be unreliable for diagnostic purposes. Inspection of GI wall biopsy samples is more accurate but ill-adapted for routine use. Non-invasive methods include direct analysis of stool flora for abnormal types including *Clostridia* and fungi; urinary organic acids including propionate, methylmalonate, butyrate, pyruvate, lactate, and beta-hydroxybutyrate are also markers of GI tract perturbations and abnormal gut flora including parasites. Intestinal permeability may be measured for instance by oral ingestion of lactulose and mannitol,[18] though several other methods have been used based on raffinose, rhamnose, and sucralose. Fecal calprotectin is a further marker.[19] Sonographic investigation of bowel compaction may be useful.

Metabolic markers

To address possible amino acid deficiency, particularly in sulfur-containing amino acids (cysteine and methionine), blood levels of these and related metabolites (glutathione and homocysteine) may be measured directly.[20] Sulfation of paracetamol (acetaminophen) appearing in the urine following oral ingestion is a further test addressing both sulfur supply and liver sulfate transfer.[21]

Genetic typing

This has a major role to play in assessing whether a given child is likely to have a particular biochemical deficiency. A range of single gene defects predispose to ASD (see Chapter 3). Some of these are frank deficits of specific cellular metabolic pathways, illustrated by phenylketonuria (failure to degrade the amino acid phenylalanine due to mutations affecting the key enzyme, phenylalanine hydroxylase, PAH), and so genetic typing of this and a range of other genes is an obligatory first step in order to put in place appropriate remedial therapy. However, single gene deficits of this type are encountered in under 10% of ASD cases; a wider trawl is warranted.

Examples of gene variants that influence accumulation and toxicity of metals include common MTHFR (methylene tetrahydrofolate reductase) and δALA dehydratase (ALAD) alleles (discussed in Chapters 7 to 9) respectively affecting sulfur and heme pathways: specific gene variants are major risk factors for toxic poisoning in the face of arsenic or lead exposure respectively.[22,23]

Low activity variants of the MTHFR gene are widespread, with 12% of the North American population having two copies (i.e. are homozygous) for the low-activity version.[24] In addition to MTHFR, James and colleagues[25] have recently reported additional associations between ASD and other sulfur pathway genes including transcobalamin II synthase reductase (TCII), catecholamine-O-methyltransferase (COMT), and glutathione-S-transferase (GST). Because heavy metals target methionine and trans-sulfuration pathways, particularly at the level of methionine and glutathione supply, all these gene variants could modulate susceptibility to heavy metal exposure.

For ALAD, there are two major alleles, ALAD1 and ALAD2. The ALAD2 allele, associated with *reduced* risk of lead toxicity, is found in around 10% of Caucasian populations, but is somewhat rarer in Asian and African-American populations.[26] Although the less common form ALAD2 appears to protect against lead toxicity, the activity of the two encoded enzymes is similar.[27]

For mercury, common variants in the coproporphyrinogen oxidase (CPOX) gene, encoding an enzyme required for heme synthesis (Chapter 9), can predispose to mercury toxicity.[17] Up to 15% of mercury-exposed subjects show an atypical (damage-sensitizing) response to mercury exposure, with abnormal porphyrin metabolism, ascribed to a specific variant of the CPOX gene (exon 4, N272H). This risk allele is also prevalent in the population, with 3% having two copies.

For most chemical (rather than heavy metal) environmental agents, detoxification is generally by the liver. Gene variants for specific detoxification enzymes are extremely common and widespread in the population[28] but have not been checked for linkage to ASD. An exception is the paraoxonase gene locus, required for detoxification of organophosphates – there was a significant association between ASD and particular paraoxonase alleles in North American (but not Italian) subjects.[29]

GABA receptors are another possible site of sensitivity and, because they play a central role in dampening brain activity, may relate to the epilepsy seen in ASD.

Seizure among domestic cats was among the very earliest signs of environmental methylmercury contamination at Minamata.[30] Mercury generally binds to GABA subunits[31] but only one key subunit, the beta-3 chain, modulates the binding of natural modulatory zinc (Zn) metal ion.[32,33] The gene encoding the beta-3 subunit is located within a major linkage site already identified in ASD (see Chapter 3) and has been specifically earmarked in at least one study.

Further genes contributing to heavy metal toxicity are discussed in Chapter 7, and for the future a panel of genetic tests will be required to ensure that the majority of known genetic risk factors are covered – including deficiencies, chromosome abnormalities, and predisposing allelic variants. There is no doubt that particular combinations of genes will, together, produce a risk of disease development far higher than any one in isolation.

Finally, mitochondrial DNA analysis may be warranted as defects in this non-genomic DNA have been suggested to represent a common cause of metabolic disorders that can underlie ASD.[34]

However, it would be a mistake to rely too heavily on genetic data alone. For example, Rett disorder has been considered by many to be a purely genetic disease, with deficiency in the gene encoding a chromosome-binding protein (methyl DNA binding protein MeCP2). But the severity of the disorder ranges from severe to asymptomatic,[35] suggesting an environmental contribution.

Two girls with Rett were examined for markers (porphyrins) of heavy metal exposure. On average, marker levels were the highest in Rett of all disorders examined.[36] Therefore, even in a "purely" genetic condition, biomedical intervention could be of enormous benefit because the genetic condition, as inferred for these two girls, may predispose to the toxic effects of environmental contamination.

Brainwave activity and epilepsy

Electroencephalogram (EEG) recordings are routinely provided by health services in cases of suspected epilepsy and, given the established link between anticonvulsant therapy and ASD development, it may be wise to confirm abnormal brainwave activity (and not another cause) before considering anti-epileptic medication (below).

Approaches to therapy

An obvious strategy is to diminish exposure to the minimum possible, bearing in mind that urban versus rural habitation is a major risk factor, and certain foodstuffs are known to have increased levels of toxicants. Because stress alone can damage the limbic brain, exposure removal should include exclusion from situations of social or psychological stress. The reported success of the Son-Rise program in at least some cases of ASD[37] may benefit from both these factors. Equally, peripheral infections that challenge the limbic brain are to be avoided, through vaccination and hygiene.

Pharmaceutical agents

Drugs have been notoriously unsuccessful in controlling the adverse features of ASD, but many have been trialed, with mixed results.[38–40] The aim has been to control the behavioral abnormalities, without addressing the underlying causes, and this approach is no doubt valid in cases of severe disease including self-mutilation, aggression, agitation, and uncontrollable anxiety or hyperactivity.

Detoxification deficit

From the outset it must be emphasized that some ASD subjects appear to be impaired in some aspects of drug detoxification (see Chapter 8), and this in some individuals may limit the use of pharmaceutical agents that rely on liver metabolism for excretion.

Haloperidol

There is a wide literature on the use of the classic neuroleptic (mood-stabilizing agent) haloperidol in ASD and related disorders. Significant reduction in repetitive behaviors has been reported.[41] But, unfortunately, only about half the children respond, and many have been unable to complete trials due to worrying side-effects.[42,43] The reason why only a proportion of children respond is unknown.

This molecule binds to a range of targets including serotonin, dopamine, and sigma receptors. This latter is of some interest, because the sigma binding site is closely associated in function with the peripheral benzodiazepine receptor (PBR) target for the analgesic, sedative, and anticonvulsant diazepam (which also activates the GABA receptor). Alterations to the synthesis and transport of metabolites including key cholesterol precursors, notably at the mitochondrial membrane, appear to be a central feature of sigma agents.[44] PBR is also a binding site for porphyrin derivatives that become elevated in heavy metal toxicity (see Chapter 9). Effects of haloperidol and diazepam on cell life and death in the brain have been demonstrated – because haloperidol enhances neuronal loss[45] it could be argued that long-term use in ASD could be detrimental. However, new generation ligands of the sigma receptor could merit evaluation in ASD and other neurodevelopmental disorders.[46]

Risperidone

This atypical neuroleptic targets serotonin and dopamine receptors, like haloperidol, and may also bind to sigma receptors.[47] Although reducing aggressive and injurious behaviors, it failed to correct the core features of ASD – social interaction, communication, and repetitive behaviors.[48] In one large study, irritability declined in risperidone-treated children with an overall improvement on a clinical global impression scale.[49] Risperidone is less neurotoxic than haloperidol[45] but has some side-effects notably including excessive appetite and sedation.[49] Many other atypical neuroleptics have been developed, but have not yet been systematically trialed in ASD.

Ritalin (methylphenidate)

An amphetamine-like molecule, but with diminished euphoric effects, has been used to treat the hyperactivity often encountered in association with ASD. But, again, only a fraction of children respond.[50] Efficacy has been demonstrated against the stereotypy and hyperactivity, but overall there was no change in the severity of autistic symptoms.[51] This study noted specifically that the drug had significant negative effects on many subjects: "this group of children seems to be particularly susceptible to adverse side effects."

Antidepressants

Three types of antidepressants have been studied in ASD. The older tricyclic drugs such as desipramine have been shown to control hyperactivity but the core features of ASD were unaffected.[52] More modern selective serotonin reuptake inhibitors (SSRIs) such as fluoxetine, and fluvoxamine, used to treat depression and anxiety, have been explored in ASD. Many studies have suggested beneficial effects,[53] particularly regarding repetitive behaviors, anxiety, and language usage,[54–56] although generally only a fraction of the subjects responded.[57] However, these drugs are subject to large variations in metabolic rates, and dosage needs to be monitored closely. Many SSRIs are also inhibitors of liver detoxification pathways[58] and may be contraindicated in ASD children with evidence of impaired hepatic detoxification. A newer drug, Remeron (mirtazapine), targets the brain serotonin system but is not a SSRI, and has been reported to alleviate problems with sleep, irritability, aggression, and hyperactivity.[59] Only 35% of children sustained a positive response.

Cholinesterase inhibitors

Drugs inhibiting the breakdown of the neurotransmitter acetylcholine have been widely reported to be of benefit in Alzheimer patients, another disorder of the limbic brain, and can slow progression of the disease. However, systematic review has failed to confirm their utility,[60] although they appear to be of benefit in some Alzheimer patients. In ASD children and adolescents two trials have been conducted, one with donepezil,[61] the other with rivastigmine.[62] Both reported improvements in expressive speech and modest reduction in autistic behavior. A third study in ASD adults, using galantamine, reported benefits for expressive language and communication.[63] These drugs are only rarely used in ASD.

Anti-opioids

The opioid excess theory (see Chapter 9) has prompted the evaluation in ASD of the opioid receptor inhibitor naltrexone. Intermittent descriptions of benefit have appeared[64–66] but, as with other agents, only some children appeared to respond.[67–69] Other studies failed to find any significant improvements.[70,71] Indeed, marked worsening of behavior has been seen.[72–74] Recent overview has concluded that there was no improvement of autism status and only marginal benefit in reducing self-injurious behavior.[75]

Adrenergic agents

Clonidine, sometimes used in ADHD, has been explored in ASD. There were small improvements on hyperactivity but drowsiness was reported.[76,77]

Anti-epileptic medication

Clearly, epilepsy must be controlled where possible, in view of the damage it can cause to the brain. However, many ASD children show impaired detoxification pathways (see Chapter 8) and it could be a mistake to administer a potentially toxic drug such as valproic acid, itself known to cause ASD in some subjects, without monitoring capacity for drug detoxification – the risk is that the drug and potential toxic metabolites might accumulate in the ASD child, with ever more serious effects on brain and behavior. The same is true of risperidone and Ritalin.

In addition, anticonvulsants impair folate (and methionine) metabolism[78] and folate supply is reduced in patients receiving anticonvulsant medication.[79,80] Adjunctive folate (vitamin B9) supplementation would seem justified, as has been recommended for epileptic women on anti-epilepsy medication.[81]

Newer anti-epileptic medications (including peptide adrenocorticotrophic hormone, ACTH [see Chapter 8], and its analogs[82]) have been trialed for the wider impairments of autism. There were clear improvements in some but not all children,[83] again pointing to a need to subtype subjects. This study did not specifically consider the epileptic brain activity seen in the majority of these children and the fact that ACTH may be effective against childhood seizures.[82]

Another approach that may be of particular utility in ASD is the ketogenic diet. Though the mechanism is unclear, the diet is high in fat, low in protein, and largely carbohydrate-free, and in at least some children can control epilepsy,[84,85] obviating the need for drug treatment.

Not all cases of ASD seizures are in fact epilepsy – in Rett syndrome epileptic fits were studied in subjects during electrical recording from the scalp; in many cases abnormal brain activity was entirely absent.[86,87] Respiratory or even cardiac anomalies could underlie these non-seizures, and failure to properly diagnose these conditions, where anti-epileptic medication would be damaging rather than restorative, has medicolegal implications.[88]

Rectification of biochemical deficits

Remediation centrally involves rectification of biochemical imbalances including inflammation. This section does not attempt a comprehensive overview; the interested reader is directed to excellent general accounts.[6–9,89]

Gut inflammation

Reduction of gut inflammation requires removal of toxic bacteria, particularly *Clostridia*, yeasts, and allergens. Antifungal and antibacterial treatments and dietary modification have been vigorously advocated as therapies for ASD.[7]

Antibiotic intervention with the oral antibiotic vancomycin (that only poorly crosses the gut wall) has been recommended in cases of recurrent gut *Clostridia* infection.[90,91] Sandler *et al.*[92] provide evidence that vancomycin treatment of gut infection can depress the behavioral disturbances of ASD. D-cycloserine is a broad spectrum antibiotic formerly used to control tuberculosis. One small trial[93] reported significant improvement in social withdrawal. However, antibiotics may increase mercury uptake. Administration of antibiotics to mice injected with methylmercury reduced excretion of mercury by 40%,[94] and reassurance may need to be sought regarding the absence of ongoing exposure.

Yeast infection is also recurrent in autism; a complementary approach is the oral administration of non-toxic "probiotic" micro-organisms that can outcompete and dilute the load of *Clostridia* and yeasts.[91] Probiotic supplements have been recommended as an accompaniment to chelation protocols.[95] Probiotic species include lactobacilli, bifidobacteria, and some types of *Streptococcus* and *Saccharomyces*.[96,97] In inflammatory bowel disease, marked reduction in pro-inflammatory cytokine production was reported on probiotic therapy.[98]

Specific antifungal therapy with nystatin or drugs related to fluconazole (Diflucan) appears to be effective in controlling yeast overgrowth including toxic *Candida* species[91,99] and may be of utility in ASD. However, the fluconazole-related group of drugs exert their actions through blocking key yeast cytochrome P450 (CYP) reactions. They therefore run the risk of depressing similar reactions in treated subjects, where liver P450 activity is centrally involved in drug metabolism and detoxification.[100] There is then a potential risk of treating ASD children with these reagents, where detoxification pathways in the liver may already be impaired.[101] Specific members of the imidazole group with reduced activity against human P450 enzymes are to be preferred.

Restricted diets (e.g. gluten-free and casein-free) have given some evidence of benefit[102–105] and the ketogenic diet used to control epilepsy is an example. Adams and Holloway[106] have reported that supplementation with a multivita-min/mineral preparation brought significant improvement of gastrointestinal problems.

Digestive enzymology

One goal has been to attempt to improve digestive processes through hormones and supplements. Secretin acts to stimulate pancreatic and stomach release of digestive enzymes. Following an early report of strong benefit in ASD a large number of controlled clinical trials were performed. Unfortunately, the utility of secretin was not confirmed.[107,108] Nevertheless, behavioral improvements have also been reported with enzyme supplementation (caseoglutenase) to improve digestion.[109] There are many anecdotal reports of behavioral improvement on long-term dietary supplementation with digestive enzymes, but these so far remain unconfirmed. It is of great interest that both tryptophan and melatonin (discussed below) act on the pancreas, though by an indirect route, to increase the release of digestive enzymes,[110] and so may be of major utility in ASD.[111]

Brain inflammation

Vargas and colleagues have argued for specific therapy of brain inflammation in ASD:

> because this neuroinflammatory process appears to be associated with an ongoing and chronic mechanism of CNS dysfunction, potential therapeutic interventions should focus on the control of its detrimental effects (while pre-serving reparative benefits) and thereby eventually modify the clinical course of autism.[112]

While treatment of the GI tract is expected to reduce brain inflammation, given the tight link between the two (see Chapter 9), it is also possible that separate treatment may be required, particularly in cases where infection of the brain might be suspected. Antagonists for inflammatory cytokines are being explored in other conditions of brain inflammation[113] – the same approach may be appropriate for ASD: IL-6 and IFNγ antagonists in particular merit attention because of evidence that these are specifically elevated in ASD.[112] General inflammation inhibitors include the docosahexaenoic acid (DHA) fraction of fish oil that may suppress cytokine production:[114–116] use in ASD has been suggested[117] but no studies have been reported. DHEA and its derivatives (below) may also be considered in view of modulatory effects on the stress steroid response.

Anti-oxidants and dietary supplements, including N-acetyl cysteine and vitamin E, may also be helpful. However, if the root cause of brain inflammation is peripheral infection and inflammation, particularly in the gut, direct GI tract intervention may be of most benefit.

Chelation to remove heavy metals

In subjects with clear evidence of heavy metal exposure, accelerated removal through the use of chemical agents that bind heavy metals seems obvious. Administered orally or by injection (or as suppositories), they accelerate excretion of heavy metals. Agents trialed include cuprimine (D-penicillamine), EDTA (ethylenediamine tetraacetic acid), DMSA (dimercapto-succinic acid, also known as succimer), DMPS (dimercapto-propane sulfonate), and TTFD (thiamine tetrahydrofurfuryl disulfide), all small molecules with high capacity for binding heavy metals. The exact affinity differs according to the element targeted, arguing that close inspection of biochemical markers such as porphyrins (whose profile depends on the exact metal or agent causing the toxicity) will permit matching of chelating agent to toxicity.

It must be emphasized that in no case has clinical benefit in ASD been proven beyond all doubt. Even so, several promising reports argue that systematic trials are justified.

An early report on a cluster of cases in Canada suggested that chelation therapy could be of benefit in ASD: though anecdotal, marked improvements were seen after chelation.[118] A 4-year-old boy with autism and ADHD and with elevated blood lead was reported.[119] On chelation therapy there was a decrease in both hyperactivity and repetitive behaviors. Evaluation of chelation therapy of autistic children is ongoing with encouraging results,[120,121] with the majority of younger children showing marked clinical benefit. A detailed protocol is available,[122] though chelation is a potentially taxing protocol[123] and strict medical supervision is required. Much more research in this area is needed.

The fall in urine porphyrin levels (a marker of toxicity) on heavy metal removal with a chelating agent (DMSA) is also extremely promising[36] and close porphyrin monitoring can distinguish children with frank heavy metal toxicity from unexposed children.

Nevertheless, two studies on DMSA (succimer) on cognitive performance in very young lead-exposed children (but without ASD) failed to find any improvement after chelation.[124,125] However, a concern was that DMSA might itself be toxic, potentially masking any benefit. Calcium supplementation during DMSA therapy has been suggested to improve heavy metal removal[126] and may diminish toxicity.

Unfortunately, chelation therapy is not without risk – by releasing bound metals from immobilized stores it can produce a swift rise in blood levels of toxic metals, resulting in acute toxicity.[123,127]

Even without specific chelation therapy, supplementation with protective and essential metals including zinc (Zn) and selenium (Se) is likely to be of benefit.[128] Calcium and iron supplementation is likely to be helpful, particularly because iron deficiency is associated with lead poisoning.[129] Melatonin may also protect against heavy metals,[130,131] and lipoic acid,[132] taurine,[133] and vitamin anti-oxidants[134] have been suggested to be of additional benefit in metal toxicity.

Amino acid pathways and cofactors

In children with excess homocysteine due to interference with sulfur pathways there are well-documented biochemical methods to reduce levels in the blood,[135] primarily based on accelerating removal by boosting the methionine synthase reaction (see Chapter 9) with cofactors and alternative methyl donors (below). However, James and colleagues[20] report that most ASD children do not have excess homocysteine. Nevertheless, a report has appeared describing elevations of homocysteine in ASD[136] and C. Skorupka (pers. comm.) also suggests that homocysteine is much more commonly elevated in ASD, noting technical difficulties in measurements of the metabolite.

The important James *et al.* study[20] focused instead on two protocols designed to rectify methionine pathway deficiencies. These included oral administration of folates (folinic acid) required for methionine synthesis from homocysteine, betaine (trimethylglycine) – an alternative non-toxic methyl donor in the methionine synthase reaction – and vitamin B12 (cyanocobalamin), a cofactor for the same enzyme. Marked restoration of methionine, cysteine, and glutathione levels was achieved[20] but behavioral improvements have not yet been addressed.

Dietary supplementation with purified methionine and cysteine (and perhaps tryptophan or the serotonin precursor 5-hydroxytryptophan), where deficiencies have been recorded, may not be advisable as the administration of chemical amino acids can sometimes be toxic. High protein diets (as in the ketogenic diet) plausibly could be of benefit, but this remains to be evaluated.

Supplementation with the tryptophan derivative melatonin in ⌐ trialled with evidence of benefit, particularly for sleep disturbance. with the condition; further studies are warranted.[111]

Pyridoxine (vitamin B6) is required for the tryptophan pathway, ⌐ conversion of 5HTP to serotonin (5HT) and melatonin, and may als⌐ epilepsy. Several trials with B6 supplementation in ASD have been perform. but despite encouraging results no overall conclusions have yet been drawn.

Tetrahydrobiopterin (BH4), another cofactor in the tryptophan pathway, ⌐ been explored in ASD with encouraging results[139] and, because BH4 synthes⌐ may be dependent on vitamin C supply,[140,141] supplementation with vitamin C may be helpful. A preliminary trial of high dose (8 g/70 kg/day) vitamin C (ascorbic acid) in ASD children found significant reduction in ASD severity.[142]

Biotin, also known as vitamin B7, is manufactured by gut bacteria and may also be obtained from meat and dairy products. Genetic deficiency in the biotin cofactor can lead to neurologic signs, and remission on biotin supplementation has been seen.[143] Improvements were seen in a subject despite lack of evidence for a genetic deficit.[144] Specific trials in ASD have not been performed.

Vitamin E (tocopherol), a powerful anti-oxidant, has also been demonstrated to prevent mercury-induced toxicity in several model systems.[145]

Generally, multivitamin and multimineral (including natural metals) supplementation has been recommended in ASD.[106]

Emerging cofactors

Recent attention has been given to a new group of quinine cofactors derived from tryptophan and tyrosine. These include PQQ (pyrroloquinoline quinine) and TTQ (tryptophan tryptophylquinone). The biology of these cofactors has not been worked out, but they are said to combine "some of the best chemical features of ascorbic acid, riboflavin, and pyridoxal cofactors into one molecule."[146] They are present in mammalian tissues including milk and improve growth in mice fed with chemically defined diets.[147] Dietary sources include fresh fruits and vegetables,[148] with the very highest concentrations of PQQ being recorded in human (but not cow's) milk and, oddly, cocoa.[146]

Hormones

Excess stress and anxiety are encountered in ASD, with elevated stress steroids (glucocorticoids) in several studies (see Chapter 8). Deficient dehydroepiandrosterone (DHEA) has been reported in another study,[148] important because the potent antiglucocorticoid action of DHEA has been debated over many years.[149] Hydroxylated derivatives of DHEA and related steroids may be even more potent.[150] Trials in ASD have not been reported.

Speech and behavior therapies

Very marked improvements in skills including language and communication have been seen in ASD children enrolled in intensive educational programs including applied behavioral analysis (ABA). This extremely important topic is discussed authoritatively elsewhere.[151,152]

Prevention

As with spina bifida, where deformities can be prevented by supplementation of the maternal diet with folic acid during early pregnancy,[153] it seems likely (though not proven) that many cases of ASD may be prevented by removal of toxic hazards and dietary deficiencies in the mother. An important preliminary report has described how, in pregnant rats treated with the anti-epileptic valproic acid (a model for autism associated with fetal anticonvulsant syndrome), supplementation with folic acid reduced, and perhaps eliminated, the adverse effects of prenatal valproic acid in the pups.[154] If confirmed, this would argue that some cases of ASD in offspring may be avoided by modification and supplementation of the maternal diet.

There are also suggestions that calcium supplementation during lactation may reduce mobilization of lead (Pb) and reduce exposure of breast-fed infants;[155] the same is most probably also true during pregnancy.

The consumption of seafood would seem to be counter-indicated. Though the beneficial effects of fish oils are well established, the risk of heavy metal (and other pollutant) contamination is not to be underestimated. An environmental warning has been issued by the UK Food Standards Agency stipulating that fish products are to be minimized during pregnancy.[156] Similar warnings are current in other countries.

The analysis undertaken here provides pointers that biomedical therapies may be of clinical benefit in ASD. The field is however fraught with uncertainty because very few logical therapeutic approaches have been evaluated in a systematic manner, despite the enormous cost to society of these disorders. A problematic area is that specific drug therapy is the approach favored by the pharmaceutical industry, with resources to carry out large placebo-controlled studies, while relatively low-cost therapies (such as those discussed here) fall back on limited public finance. Nevertheless, some remarkable successes have been reported on remedial therapy of disorders of brain and behavior.

The Gesch and Walsh studies

Some 231 males at a UK young offenders institution were supplemented with vitamins, minerals, and fatty acids. A control group received a placebo. Over a five-month period the number of incidents of violent or antisocial behavior fell by 26%.[157] Biochemical markers in these subjects were not studied, but the authors recommended that future investigations should include blood analysis.

Researchers in the USA studied a range of biochemical markers in 207 patients with violent behavior including physical assaults and destruction of property:[128] 75% had an abnormal copper/zinc (Cu/Zn) ratio indicative of improper metal handling; 38% had elevated blood histamine, a marker for methylation deficiency; and 33% elevated urinary kryptopyrroles, markers of environmental toxicity. Some 18% had elevated heavy metals in blood or hair. Other disturbances were also common.

Biomedical rectification was put in place, attuning the treatment to the precise imbalances observed in each individual patient. Specifically, this involved zinc, cysteine, and manganese for abnormal Cu/Zn ratio; methionine, calcium, magnesium, and vitamin D for undermethylation; and natural heavy metal supplementation with pyridoxine and selenium for toxic metal exposure. Three-quarters of the patients complied with the treatment. In the treated group, violent behavior was reduced in 92%, and 58% achieved complete elimination of the behavior.[128]

This remarkable research demonstrates beyond any doubt that some behavioral problems can be alleviated, in the majority of study subjects, by rectification of biochemical imbalances. Though these studies did not overtly include ASD subjects, the indications are that biomedical remediation is likely to be of major benefit in autism and autism spectrum disorders.

The final chapter includes discussion of other adjunct behavioral therapies that may further promote neuronal repair in the limbic brain.

Key points

There is a need to subtype ASD according to genetic and biochemical factors.

Pharmacotherapy in ASD has not proven effective against the key features of the condition, but some control of damaging behaviors has been achieved.

Intolerance to pharmaceutical agents, including anti-epileptic drugs, may be a particular problem in ASD.

Treatment of GI problems includes control of inflammation with antifungals, antibiotics, and probiotics, with restricted diets.

Heavy metal removal with chelating agents could be justified but further trials are needed.

Remediation of biochemical deficits includes vitamin and cofactor supplementation.

Prevention, by maternal supplementation and dietary precautions prior to and during pregnancy, may reduce child rates of ASD.

Chapter 11

The Environmental Threat: From Autism and ADHD to Alzheimer

More than 50 years ago the Edinburgh geneticist C.H. Waddington performed an experiment. He exposed eggs of tiny fruitflies (*Drosophila*) to a brief period of elevated temperature ("heat-shock"). Among the adults emerging from these treated embryos were, perhaps not so surprisingly, a number of flies with developmental abnormalities – such as anomalies of wing and body structure.

The surprise came when he bred these abnormal flies together, for the phenotype (the visible expression of the insult or deficiency) was soon expressed in offspring without any heat-shock. In other words, an "environmental" effect had somehow become "genetic."[1,2]

The interpretation of this experiment is interesting. Waddington deduced that the flies carry a series of mild genetic impairments that, under normal conditions, give no discernible phenotype. Low-activity variants of developmental genes persist in the population because there is no selective pressure for their removal. But stress interferes with the activity of these genes just a little, enough to produce visible developmental abnormalities.

Then, when the abnormal male and female flies with subefficient gene variants are crossed, similar low-activity genes come together in the offspring. In these flies, now with a double dose of low activity, the same developmental abnormality appears, but without the stressor – uncovering what Waddington called an "occult" or hidden phenotype.

Other stresses have exactly the same effect. When newly-laid eggs were treated with ether, and the emerging adults were intercrossed, Waddington wrote: "individuals exhibiting the phenotype began to appear in samples of the selected stock which had not been subjected to the unusual environment."[3] The same happened with very different stress conditions – such as a food source containing an excess of common salt[4] – and, in each case, the visible anomalies depended on the stock of flies used and the nature of the stress.

McLaren[5] has pointed out that such gene–environment effects extend to beetles, plants, toads, mice, and foxes.

The unexpected phenomenon was confirmed by an unusual but even more convincing route. Flies have a major protein called HSP90 (heat-shock protein, 90,000 being its molecular size) that is induced by stress. Its role is to "chaperone" unstable enzymes and signaling proteins, protecting them against structural collapse and denaturation. Rutherford and Lindquist[6] examined flies in which HSP90 had been partially inactivated by mutation or by drug treatment. When these flies were subjected to heat-shock, as was done by Waddington, a series of developmental abnormalities was uncovered, including malformations of wings and body structure. But now the frequency was at least ten-fold higher.

Again, the nature of the malformation depended on the laboratory strain used, and intercrossing once more generated individuals whose phenotype was maintained even when HSP90 was no longer blocked.

This work has established a central principle – stress during early development uncovers new phenotypes, but the nature of the disturbance depends on hidden genetic predisposition.

Could the same be true for humans? There is no reason to think that the gene–environment interactions operating in humans differ fundamentally from flies, toads, mice, or foxes – Anne McLaren (pers. comm.) states: "As for human populations – I don't think we're so different from all the rest." Subjecting the population to stress will uncover new phenotypes.

That this is undoubtedly true is illustrated by two specific examples. In the late 1950s and early 1960s thalidomide was widely given to pregnant women to alleviate morning sickness. This produced limb deformations, but only in some children. Exposure to other chemical agents including alcohol has also been linked to upper limb abnormalities. It is known that the same deformations can be produced by mutations in key genes,[7] implying that the chemical agents interfere with the same pathways, and children with suboptimal gene variants are most at risk.

Spina bifida, one of the most common human malformations, is associated with toxic exposure. Though the cause is not usually known, maternal valproic acid anti-epileptic medication has been blamed in some cases.[8] The majority of these malformations can be prevented by maternal supplementation with folic acid during early pregnancy,[9] demonstrating that a biochemical deficit is the underlying cause.

Because the brain is the most complex of all body systems, at least in terms of the number of genes it requires for proper function (perhaps half of the entire genome is expressed in the brain), behavioral phenotypes are expected to be common.

Environmental effects on later-life behavior have indeed been seen in humans. In Germany, in the children of mothers exposed to the horrors of the closing stages of the Second World War, the frequency of homosexuality was unexpectedly high.[10] For children born of the wartime famine in Holland, the so-called "Dutch hunger winter" of 1944–45, the rates of schizophrenia were significantly elevated.[11] It was concluded that prenatal nutritional deficiency was responsible.[12] This was confirmed in a large study in China, where David St. Clair has discovered that children of the 1959–1961 famine have been more than twice as likely to develop schizophrenia as those born either before or after.[13]

Nature and timing of the insult

Most cases of ASD are recognized early in development, usually by the age of 3 years, and the insult must have taken place at or before that time. Several studies have looked in detail at children who later became autistic, and uniformly recorded abnormalities as early as the first year of life. Effects during gestation are likely – both in thalidomide cases and in children of mothers receiving the anti-epileptic drug, the incidence of ASD is markedly elevated. Depending on the timing of exposure, the same kind of insult can produce either malformations or autism.

Ongoing postnatal exposure is likely to contribute. Bauman and Kemper[14] state the position – at least some of the abnormalities observed in the autistic brain are of prenatal origin, but "the underlying neurobiological processes may be on-going and...postnatal factors may also be important."

Well-established risk factors for ASD development include medical problems in the immediate postnatal period.[15] The association between early life psychosocial stress and severe behavioral impairment is well documented in young Romanian orphans subjected to extremes of social deprivation,[16] and supports the idea that both pre- and postnatal insult can contribute.

Though the focus has been on heavy metals, it seems unlikely that these alone are responsible. The human population is increasingly exposed to stresses of diverse types, many chemical. Heavy metals, polychlorinated biphenyls (PCBs), dioxins, and phthalates (the list is not exhaustive) are all rising in the environment. Children developing ASD show clear evidence of heavy metal exposure (see Chapter 7) but they will have been exposed too to other chemical residues that accumulate, along with metals, in industrial and urban wastes and in seafood.

For instance, breast milk from mothers consuming large amounts of seafood contained both mercury and PCBs. There is emerging evidence that exposure to non-metal toxicants may contribute to ASD – there was a significant correlation between ASD and gene variants causing inefficient organophosphate detoxification.[17]

Diverse impairments – from autism to Alzheimer disease

One interesting outcome of the Paris study[18] exploring metal toxicity in French children (through the urinary porphyrin marker) was the diversity of phenotypes in the high-exposure group. Although exposure was most significant in the specific ASD subtype "autistic disorder," other diagnostic categories were well represented. At the very highest levels of exposure, autistic disorder, PDD-NOS (pervasive developmental disorder – not otherwise specified), hyperactivity, cerebral palsy, epilepsy, Rett, and non-specific mental retardation were all present.

In fact, the highest marker value among the 269 children assessed was in a boy with PDD-NOS, and alongside, in the top five, were cerebral palsy (two girls) and, in boys, hyperactivity disorder and autism.[18]

One infers, in these "highly exposed" individuals, that the developmental presentation is the expression of inherent but concealed genetic susceptibilities. It seems likely, as in Waddington's fruitflies, that the deficits in these children would not have emerged had it not been for the environmental stress.

All the children in the Paris study were referred for examination because of neurodevelopmental disorders. Therefore, if other distinct conditions emerged in some similarly exposed children, the study would not have picked this up. Depending on individual genetic make-up, and perhaps the type of toxicity, exposure could lead to other conditions, and not just neurodevelopmental disorders including autism.

This has been confirmed. A diverse range of disabilities and disorders are associated with heavy metal exposure.

Attention deficit hyperactivity disorder (ADHD) has been associated with heavy metal exposure. In Dutch children, attention problems correlated with hair lead (Pb) levels.[19] In Denmark, attention, language, and memory problems related to mercury exposure in 7-year-olds[20] while, in US schoolchildren, there was a striking dose–response relationship between hair lead levels and ADHD.[21]

Cerebral palsy is a known manifestation of prenatal methylmercury intoxication.[22]

Hair from dyslexic children showed significantly higher concentrations of cadmium, aluminum, magnesium, and copper than hair from control subjects; the cadmium concentration exceeded safe limits.[23]

In 1984 an association was found between heavy metal levels and disturbed social interactions in schoolchildren.[24] A large study on delinquency then looked at bone lead (Pb) levels in children. At 11 years of age, there was a significant correlation between bone lead and delinquent and aggressive behavior, and with social and attention problems.[25] A later study confirmed a causal association: delinquent and antisocial behavior correlated strongly with maternal and postnatal exposure to lead, assessed by blood levels.[26]

Heavy metal toxicity is also implicated in Gilles de la Tourette syndrome, a childhood-onset disorder accompanied by motor tics and vocalizations. Ten out of 80 patients were found to have low copper levels (a possible sign of heavy metal toxicity). Two such subjects were examined in detail. Both had deficiencies of copper handling, with abnormally fast removal from the blood but delayed liver uptake.[27] This is reminiscent of the mercury handling deficit in some cases of ASD (see Chapter 7).

Anxiety is also associated with mercury exposure: anxiety was the most prominent feature of a group of patients referred for low-level mercury exposure.[28]

Opler et al.[29] investigated whether environmental lead exposure might be associated with schizophrenia. Looking at archived maternal blood serum samples (1959–1966) they compared levels (assessed using another marker of heavy metal exposure, δALA; see Chapter 7) in the mothers of children later becoming schizophrenic and controls. There was a correlation – children whose mothers had evidence of high levels of exposure were more than twice as likely to develop the condition.

For years there have been suspicions that adult-onset Alzheimer disease might be linked to heavy metal exposure, notably to aluminum and mercury. Studies on blood (rather than hair) metals in Alzheimer disease have revealed elevations. Blood plasma levels of aluminum, cadmium, and mercury were increased.[30] Mercury levels were twice as high in patients compared to controls, and in early-onset Alzheimer disease blood mercury was almost three-fold elevated.[31]

Though the relationship between Alzheimer and heavy metal toxicity is strongly debated, in ASD the association can be with either low levels – in individuals with a processing deficit – or (one infers) with high levels in those who do not have this deficit; the same may be true of Alzheimer disease. Excretion of heavy metals is a normal mechanism for preventing toxicity. One significant route is into hair – in rats given a dose of methylmercury, 10% is transported into hair[32] while, in humans, hair mercury levels reflect internal levels.[33] Surprisingly, hair mercury levels of children becoming autistic are often *reduced*[34] rather than elevated. The inference is that these children cannot remove mercury by export pathways, and so it accumulates in the body to cause brain damage (see Chapter 7).

Alzheimer disease has repeated the same finding – in a Japanese study of hair aluminum in Alzheimer patients, levels were significantly *lower* than in controls.[35] It is possible that, in Alzheimer too, a deficit in the export of heavy metals is a major risk factor.

Intriguingly, in newborn rats exposed transiently to lead (Pb) in drinking water, when followed over their lifetimes, there was a striking upregulation of the key Alzheimer molecule (amyloid precursor protein, APP), but only once the animals entered old age.[36] One may suspect, in humans, that early life exposure to an excess of heavy metals including lead and mercury predisposes to Alzheimer disease in the elderly.

Beyond the brain

The effects of environmental toxins are likely to extend well beyond the brain, though the brain may be more affected because memories and skills, unlike skin and muscle, are not easy to repair.

Deficits associated with toxicity are diverse. Nakagawa[37] measured hair mercury in the general Japanese population. Levels in subjects recently deceased were compared with age-matched healthy controls. In subjects with conditions including asthma, dementia, cerebral infarct, osteoporosis, hypertension, and diabetes, mercury levels were all significantly higher. The much publicized decline in semen quality also correlates with parameters of heavy metal exposure.[38]

The association between asthma and heavy metals is well documented, particularly in workers in the metal industry.[39,40] In children, hair copper levels were significantly higher in subjects with asthma or eczema.[41] In a large US study, high blood lead (Pb) levels were a significant risk factor for the development of strictly defined asthma.[42] This study is of interest, because the risk was confined to Caucasians. When African-Americans were examined as a separate group there was no relationship between blood lead and asthma, pointing to an underlying genetic susceptibility that differs between populations.

Co-risks and co-disorders

The data point to an "uncovering" of subclinical genetic deficits by exposure to environmental toxins. Depending on their genetic make-up, some individuals will veer toward ASD, others to conditions including, for example, asthma or eczema. If this is true, a proportion of children may unfortunately have acquired susceptibilities for more than one common condition. Given the prevalence of both ASD and asthma, one might expect to find children who have both conditions.

There is a significant association between child ASD development and asthma in their mothers.[43] And, in children, the US National Health Interview Survey (1997–2003) of 65,000 children revealed that 20% with strictly defined autistic disorder have been diagnosed with asthma (J. Drew and D. Hogan, pers. comm.) – the population prevalence in all children is generally in the 5–12% range depending on severity.[44]

Concerning brain and behavior, children with pervasive developmental disorders – PDD (i.e. ASD) – have a surprisingly high frequency of non-ASD conditions. Sverd[45] relates: "it is being increasingly recognized that individuals with PDD are at risk for a wide array of psychiatric disturbances, including affective disorders, anxiety disorders, schizophrenia-like psychoses, aggression, antisocial behavior, and Tourette's disorder." Without exception, all these specific conditions have also been linked to limbic damage and environmental toxicity.

Environmental toxicity only produces disease in predisposed individuals

As with Waddington's fruitflies, the nature of the deficit revealed on early stress is dependent on a pre-existing genetic susceptibility. That can be either in the target tissue (as with the wing and body phenotypes) or in genes (like HSP90) which make the individual hypersensitive to challenge.

Genes contributing to human susceptibility are discussed in earlier chapters; many deal with heavy metal toxicity. However, biochemical markers of heavy metal contact may merely reflect more widespread exposure to environmental toxins. A combination of exposures (e.g. heavy metals with polychlorinated biphenyls) will produce more severe damage than each agent alone.

This has been demonstrated. In young children, cognitive performance was most adversely affected in subjects with evidence of dual exposure to polychlorinated biphenyls and mercurials.[46] The combined insult scenario is emphasized by the absence of autism as a primary diagnosis in overt heavy metal toxicity, though sporadic reports have suggested an association.[47-50] Therefore, predisposing factors are unlikely to be restricted just to heavy metal pathways.

There is ample evidence for toxic chemical exposure in ASD. Some 16 out of 18 young ASD children had levels of toxic chemicals such as trichloroethylene and toluene that exceeded adult maximum tolerance, some by massive margins.[51]

The association between organophosphate detoxification (paraoxonase gene) and ASD is a case in point – there was a significant association between ASD and particular paraoxonase gene variants. The association was only found in North American subjects, and not in Italy, where household organophosphate use is far less than in the USA.[17]

Other environmental stresses contribute. Severe psychological stress early in childhood has been invoked as a cause[16] and can produce ASD in the absence of any other known predisposing factors. Genes and receptors involved in all aspects of the stress response are candidates – oxytocin is a further case in point, as it would appear to play a role in dampening the stress response and improving social behavior. A positive association between an oxytocin receptor gene variant and ASD was reported in a Chinese population,[52] suggesting that reduced oxytocin activity is a risk factor for ASD development.

Finally, many environmental pollutants may only exert toxic effects in individuals with an underlying dietary problem – for instance, selenium protects against mercury toxicity.

Sociobiology of the limbic brain: convergence

In Waddington's flies, stresses produced a diversity of new phenotypes. But, in children exposed to environmental stress including toxicity and psychosocial deprivation, a restricted range of behavioral deficits emerge. These include ASD, epilepsy, and anxiety, but also affective and schizophrenia-like conditions, all associated to a greater or lesser extent with the limbic brain.

There is therefore a paradox. In humans, unlike flies, stresses converge on the limbic brain (though behavioral phenotypes in stressed flies have not yet been examined). In children, perinatal oxygen deprivation is a major risk factor for ASD, with selective damage in the hippocampus. Chronic psychosocial stress causes restricted hippocampal destruction, as does peripheral infection and inflammation. Chemical, physiological, and psychological insults all selectively target the limbic brain (see Chapter 7). Bruce McEwen uses the term "allostatic load" to describe limbic wear and tear as a result of stress, poor diet, or a disrupted sleep–wake cycle;[53] additions to the list include infection and environmental toxicity.

The peculiar susceptibility of the limbic brain then demands an explanation: why has evolution determined that such a crucial brain region should be so exquisitely prone to damage, while other body and brain functions remain intact?

The answer may lie in the sociobiology of brain and behavior. The argument runs like this. In any social grouping, decisions about home site, preferred food-stuffs, and group behavior are made by one or more high ranking or "dominant" individuals, either males or females, whose personal choice or choices extend to the group as a whole. This is true in all social species, from birds to primates including humans.

There is a tight linkage between social dominance and health. In mice and rats, stress, infection, toxicity, and nutritional inadequacy contribute to low social status, while the highest social status is enjoyed by individuals with physiological equilibrium.[54]

This is for very good reasons – it favors individuals with the most positive preferences: for the most nutritious foodstuffs, the sites most removed from sources of infection or predators, the best hygiene. In short, the fittest lifestyle. Few would question that the fittest take precedence in making choices on behalf of the group; conversely, that the most unfit and unhealthy rarely assume positions of social dominance.

A good example, in humans, arises from observations made on artificial depletion of the essential amino acid tryptophan (TRP) – this depresses mood while increasing irritability and aggression;[55] the authors of this study suggested that a TRP-rich diet (with add-on benefits for brain biochemistry) promotes social interactions by increasing dominance and decreasing aggression.

TRP balance is one signature of a balanced diet; there are many others. The specific effects of deficiencies in essential dietary ingredients (or excesses of toxic metabolites) on brain and behavior is a central theme of this book (Chapters 7 to 9).

The tight linkage between diet, health, and social status is soundly established, but the mechanistic explanation is rarely discussed. Physiological impairment leads to social impairment. Regarding diet alone, is there a mechanism whereby individuals with excellent nutrition assume dominance, or, conversely, is there a negative mechanism to block dominance in individuals whose nutrition is poor?

Both appear to operate. The key brain region is the hippocampus (with adjoining amygdala). Because of its sensory capacity, it can respond rapidly to body physiology, and a primary and immediate effect of hippocampal and amygdala damage is aggression and loss of social status.

This has been amply demonstrated. In a striking early (1954) study on macaque monkeys, Rosvold, Mirsky, and Pribram[56] performed small selective amygdala lesions on individuals in a social hierarchy. The outcome was revealing – all animals became more aggressive but, in two out of three cases, the operated individual, once in a position of dominance, fell to the bottom of the pile. The exact extents of the lesions were hard to record, and some included part of the hippocampus.

One easily measurable correlate of social status is the rate of production of new neurons in the limbic system. The hippocampal dentate gyrus is most unusual because it contains, unlike most other brain regions, dividing cells even into adulthood.[57-59]

Physical activity is important because it influences the number of dividing cells in the dentate gyrus. In rodents, high-ranking males are boisterous; those at the bottom of the pile are lethargic and depressed.[60] Increased activity directly stimulates the rate of new neuron formation in the dentate.[61] Many more new neurons are seen in the dentate gyrus of dominant rat males compared to subordinates.[62] In mice, dominant males have an increased number of dividing neurons.[63] New neurons improve learning skills in a very significant way; in turn, learning skills contribute positively to social status.

Conversely, when such positive influences fail, as in stress or infection, low social status is the outcome. Loss of hierarchical status may be a consequence of prenatal exposure of mice to endocrine disruptors.[64] As with toxic organometal exposure, the dentate gyrus is the first to suffer.

The conclusion is tangible: the exquisite sensitivity of the limbic brain (and neuronal replacement processes) to toxic insult is the result of an evolutionary design – a "self-destruct" mechanism – that ensures that individuals exposed to toxins lose their social dominance. For the group as a whole, choices are made by dominant individuals whose own preferences have kept them away from any such exposure.

Following this line of argument, one would expect, in human populations, that the same mechanism boosts social dominance in the fittest, and an identical, but destructive, mechanism reduces social skills in the least fit.

This may be what is happening in autism. Perhaps we are seeing an elevated incidence of conditions where social skills are impaired, precisely because the physiological system is designed to impair them.

A parallel hypothesis, advanced by David St. Clair (pers. comm.), is that when the population is challenged, for instance by starvation (as in the Dutch hunger winter or the Chinese famine), the children are more likely to develop schizophrenia and related disorders (which reflect, by implication, genetic risk factors). They may then have a selective advantage if the behavioral change predisposes them to overcome social and physical barriers as adults – so as to forage, disperse, or migrate – and with an improved chance of re-establishing a new population.

Both scenarios prompt a debate – are autism and related disorders the logical consequence of "when it all goes wrong" as a result of pervasive environmental contamination? If, in the closing paragraphs, I might offer an opinion, I would suggest that this is indeed the case.

Promoting neurogenesis: potential for therapy

Because the primary deficit is argued to be in the limbic brain – the hippocampus with adjoining amygdala – restoring limbic function could benefit from techniques that promote neuronal repair. Rectification of biochemical deficits (see Chapter 10) is a first step, but a second follows on.

Cell division even into adulthood is a unique feature of the limbic brain. Proliferation is presumed to allow restoration of new neurons, and the process is under environmental control. Correction of biochemical deficits and inflammation (see Chapter 10) will undoubtedly have beneficial effects on dentate neurogenesis, but other influences also weigh in.

In experimental animals, positive stimuli include exercise[61] and environmental enrichment,[65] with remarkable stimulatory effects on neuronal proliferation in this region of brain. Indeed, rats with early brain damage (fetal valproate exposure, a model for ASD) have been reported to respond positively to a rich and stimulating environment;[66] prospective use in ASD was discussed. It seems likely, though unproven, that interventions specifically promoting neuronal division in the dentate gyrus, including exercise and environmental enrichment, will be of benefit in ASD.

Indeed, the observed efficacy of antidepressant medications in ASD (see Chapter 10) could operate in exactly this way – their behavioral effects have been attributed to their ability to promote neuronal proliferation in the hippocampus[67] (though chemical toxicity argues against their specific use in ASD). The remarkable recovery of one child from ASD, though anecdotal,[68] given the central focus on stimulation and reward, could have profited from this specific mechanism.

What causes autism?

The increase in rates of autism argues strongly for an environmental contribution to ASD. Even so, there is unlikely to be a unitary cause for autism. Each individual is unique. Some single gene conditions are major risk factors for ASD, but more generally environmental toxicity and physiological dysregulation, underscored by genetic susceptibility, converge on the limbic brain to exploit the peculiar sensitivity of this brain region to insult. For the majority of autistic children, limbic damage is linked to a combination of factors, some environmental, some genetic, that combine to tip the balance toward ASD development.

The roles of heavy metal exposure and GI inflammation have been emphasized. However, these do not completely explain the recent rise, perhaps ten-fold, in the prevalence of ASD. The problem is this. Our populations have been exposed to heavy metals over decades if not centuries. The rise in ASD is new.

Therefore we must search for a new causation. Two hypotheses may be considered:

1. **Trigger factor theory**. *A new risk factor, on a background of environmental and genetic challenge, triggers the development of ASD.* If there should be such a hypothetical trigger factor, what do we know about it? First, exposure must be widespread in the population. Second, it is relatively new: exposure has risen markedly from the 1980s onwards. Third, it targets the limbic brain.

   Infectious childhood vaccines are a plausible contender; however, multiple statistical analyses have excluded them as a causal factor in more than around 5% of ASD cases. Organometals and other pollutants are more plausible.

2. **Combination theory**. *No single exposure produces ASD, but a combination of exposures, including heavy metals, endocrine disruptors, and other chemical toxins, combined with biochemical insufficiencies (dietary deficiencies, occult genetic and metabolic deficits), converge to produce the disorder.* Four independent exposures each augmenting ASD risk by a factor of 1.8 will together increase overall risk ten-fold, and possibly rather more if they act synergistically.

Heavy metals are clearly a factor, evidenced by deficits in mercury handling, aggravated body burdens, and porphyrinuria in ASD. The source of the heavy metals is not entirely clear, and remains somewhat of a puzzle. For mercury, prenatal exposure to metal released from maternal dental amalgams is a major source, though organomercury (thimerosal or thiomersal) contained in medications such as Rho immunoglobulin has been identified as a specific risk factor. Childhood vaccinations containing mercurials are without any doubt a further risk factor for ASD development. More generally, however, seafood assumes a greater importance in the postnatal period. While mercury in early breast milk is primarily mercuric ion derived from maternal amalgams, after two or more months the predominant source is methylmercury from maternal seafood consumption.[69,70] Other metals such as tin (Sn), also found in both dental amalgams and in seafood, are likely to contribute to ASD risk. However, given that organometals appear to present a rather greater threat than metal ions, organic derivatives of tin (tributyltin and triethyltin) found widely in seafood afford a major risk factor. A range of other heavy metals are also found at increasing levels in foodstuffs, all with a propensity to cause the same type of brain damage. The finding that ASD development correlates with environmental (predominantly atmospheric) mercury release in the USA[71] could suggest that heavy metal contamination of drinking water (rather than food) is an important route of toxic exposure to mercury and other metals co-released in the same industrial processes.

Alongside heavy metals and mineral deficiencies, chemical pollutants are very likely to be second factors. There is ample evidence for chemical toxin exposure in ASD, though no two cases showed the same combination of toxic agents in excess of norms.[51]

Impairments of mental and motor development correlate statistically with polychlorinated biphenyl (PCB) exposure.[72] There is clear synergy between mercury and PCB toxicity.[46] It is uncertain whether PCB specifically can be blamed, because environmental contamination of foodstuffs is widespread, and individuals exposed to PCB, principally through food, will almost inevitably be exposed to other persistent aromatic compounds such as dioxins[73] as well as heavy metals. However, PCB remains co-suspect.

An environmental warning was issued as early as 1991 regarding the potential long-term detrimental effects of endocrine disruptors (EDs) including PCBs and dioxins,[74] as revisited recently.[75] The warnings focused exclusively on EDs. In the meantime there is evidence that some chemical EDs are slowly but extensively broken down in the environment; the same is not true of heavy metals. Once they enter the biosphere there is no obvious mechanism by which they can be removed. Lead levels in freshly deposited Greenland ice were still elevated 500 years after the collapse of the Roman empire.[76] Ocean floor sedimentation may contribute; the rate of such removal is not known.

If ASD is the result of environmental toxicant exposure exacerbated by singular susceptibility of the limbic brain, then other disorders of limbic function will surely and inevitably rise in our populations.

Concluding remarks

Autism is not a unitary disorder – a wider view encompasses a spectrum of conditions that extends from the pervasive developmental disorders of autism, Asperger, and PDD-NOS to related conditions including ADHD, and further to anxiety, epilepsy, and affective disorders.

There is substantial overlap between all these conditions. ASD individuals have a greatly increased rate of other brain conditions; first-degree relatives of individuals diagnosed as "autistic" display elevated rates of behavioral individualities dubbed "the broader phenotype,"[77,78] including specific deficits such as dyslexia and dyspraxia, and mood disorders including anxiety and depression. These conditions could have a common cause, with local factors guiding progression toward autism or epilepsy, or a different causality. However, it is argued that the common thread linking all these conditions is the involvement of the limbic brain.

The focus on the hippocampus and amygdala is also a simplification, as hypothalamic and brainstem nuclei participate in all the regulatory circuits discussed here, but are much harder to analyze and have been relegated to the periphery of many if not the majority of studies reviewed here. However, the underlying mechanisms (and potential therapies) may be shared between all these regions.

On balance, it is argued that environmental toxins, particularly heavy metals, combined with intestinal infection/inflammation and other physiological perturbations, jointly predispose to neuronal damage in the limbic brain regions. The concept of a specific "autism gene" is put aside, favoring the notion that a wide range of genetic predispositions contribute to the ASD phenotype, exact identity differing between families and indeed populations.

This study reaches the following conclusions:

1. The rising prevalence of ASD (new phase autism) may be ascribed to environmental toxicity, notably including heavy metals in combination with organic endocrine disruptors and other chemical toxins.

2. Physiological dysregulation including but not restricted to gut inflammation contributes to aberrant function of the limbic brain, predisposing to ASD.

3. These insults only maximally exert their impact on subjects with a pre-existing genetic or physiological predisposition – such as a subclinical metabolic deficiency or undiagnosed inflammatory disorders. Biochemical and behavioral therapies are therefore likely to be of major benefit in the management of ASD and related neuropsychiatric conditions.

Looking to the future, it is impossible to say how present-day conditions will evolve, but one must suspect that the consequences of environmental degradation could become progressively more severe, with brain conditions including ASD rising further in our populations. And we care greatly if our child is autistic, or anxious, or delinquent. History sometimes repeats itself. S. Colum Gilfillan,[79] in 1965, put forward a well-argued and compelling case that the fall of the Roman civilization was due to pervasive lead (Pb) exposure of the upper echelons of Roman society. The Romans were wholly unaware of the risk; Pliny gave explicit directions for reducing grapes to sweet syrup – "Leaden and not bronze pots should be used."[79]

Key points

"Genetic" disease can be uncovered by an "environmental" stress.

In humans, early stresses predispose to later brain and behavior problems; pre-existing genetic predispositions are inferred.

Heavy metal toxicity has been associated with ADHD, dyslexia, anxiety, schizophrenia, and Alzheimer. Non-brain disorders include asthma.

ASD children have a high rate of co-disorders including other metal-sensitive behavioral problems and asthma.

The specific susceptibility of the limbic brain requires an explanation. It is suggested that a limbic damage (self-destruct) mechanism links diet and health to social status – fittest individuals taking group decisions confers a population advantage.

A combination of environmental toxins, exacerbated by physiological dysregulation and genetic predisposition, act on the susceptible brain to produce ASD. Toxic environmental influences are likely to be increasing.

References

Chapter 1 Introduction

1. Rapin, I. (2001) "An 8-year-old boy with autism." *J. Am. Med. Assoc. 285*, 1749–1757.
2. Wing, L. (1996) "Autistic spectrum disorders." *Brit. Med. J. 312*, 327–328.
3. Gillberg, C. and Coleman, M. (2000) *The Biology of the Autistic Syndromes.* Cambridge: MacKeith–Cambridge University Press.
4. Asperger, H. (1992) "Autistic psychopathy in childhood – 1944 (translation)." In U.T. Frith (ed) *Autism and Asperger Syndrome.* Cambridge: Cambridge University Press.
5. Hippler, K. and Klicpera, C. (2003) "A retrospective analysis of the clinical case records of 'autistic psychopaths' diagnosed by Hans Asperger and his team at the University Children's Hospital, Vienna." *Philos. Trans. R. Soc. Lond. B. Biol. Sci. 358*, 291–301.
6. Kanner, L. (1943) "Autistic disturbances of affective contact." *Nervous Child 2*, 217–250.
7. Kanner, L. (1971) "Follow-up study of eleven autistic children originally reported in 1943." *J. Autism Child Schizophr. 1*, 119–145.
8. Dancey, T.E. (1957) "Early infantile autism, 1943–1955; discussion of paper presented by Leo Kanner, M.D." *Psychiatr. Res. Rep. Am. Psychiatr. Assoc. 7*, 66–88.
9. Bleuler, E. (1950) *Dementia Praecox or the Group of Schizophrenias 1911.* (Translation J. Zinkin.) New York: International University Press.
10. Ssucharewa, G.E. and Wolff, S. (1996) "The first account of the syndrome Asperger described? Translation of a paper entitled 'Die schizoiden Psychopathien im Kindesalter' by Dr. G.E. Ssucharewa; scientific assistant, which appeared in 1926 in the Monatsschrift für Psychiatrie und Neurologie 60:235–261." *Eur. Child Adolesc. Psychiatry 5*, 119–132.
11. Hauser, S.L., DeLong, G.R. and Rosman, N.P. (1975) "Pneumographic findings in the infantile autism syndrome. A correlation with temporal lobe disease." *Brain 98*, 667–688.
12. Kaufman, B.N. (1995) *Son-Rise: The Miracle Continues.* Tiburon, CA: H.J. Kramer Press.
13. Jarbrink, K. and Knapp, M. (2001) "The economic impact of autism in Britain." *Autism 5*, 7–22.
14. Loynes, F. (2001) *The Impact of Autism.* Report for the All Party Parliamentary Group on Autism. Online at: http://www.nas.org.uk/content/1/c4/28/62/impact.pdf

Chapter 2 Autism and Autism Spectrum Disorders: An Introduction to the Problem of Recognition and Diagnosis

1. Wing, L. and Gould, J. (1979) "Severe impairments of social interaction and associated abnormalities in children: epidemiology and classification." *J. Autism Dev. Disord. 9*, 11–29.
2. Gillberg, C. and Coleman, M. (2000) *The Biology of the Autistic Syndromes.* Cambridge: MacKeith–Cambridge University Press.
3. Wing, L. (1996) "Autistic spectrum disorders." *Brit. Med. J. 312*, 327–328.
4. Tidmarsh, L. and Volkmar, F.R. (2003) "Diagnosis and epidemiology of autism spectrum disorders." *Can. J. Psychiatry 48*, 517–525.
5. Nataf, R., Skorupka, C., Amet, L., Lam, A., Springbett, A. and Lathe, R. (2005) "Porphyrinuria in childhood autistic disorder." Submitted for publication.
6. Fombonne, E. (2003) "The prevalence of autism." *J. Am. Med. Assoc. 289*, 87–89.
7. Fombonne, E. (2003) "Epidemiology of pervasive developmental disorders." *Trends Evidence-Based Neuropsychiatry 5*, 29–36.

8. Fombonne, E. (2003) "Epidemiological surveys of autism and other pervasive developmental disorders: an update." *J. Autism Dev. Disord. 33*, 365–382.

9. Baird, G., Charman, T., Baron-Cohen, S., Cox, A., Swettenham, J., Wheelwright, S. *et al.* (2000) "A screening instrument for autism at 18 months of age: a 6-year follow-up study." *J. Am. Acad. Child Adolesc. Psychiatry 39*, 694–702.

10. World Health Organization (WHO) (1992) *The ICD-10 Classification of Mental and Behavioural Disorders.* Geneva: World Health Organization.

11. American Psychiatric Association (1994) *Diagnostic and Statistical Manual of Mental Disorders (DSM-IV).* Washington, DC: American Psychiatric Association.

12. Kopp, S. and Gillberg, C. (2003) "Swedish child and adolescent psychiatric out-patients – a five-year cohort." *Eur. Child Adolesc. Psychiatry 12*, 30–35.

13. Lotspeich, L.J., Kwon, H., Schumann, C.M., Fryer, S.L., Goodlin-Jones, B.L., Buonocore, M.H. *et al.* (2004) "Investigation of neuroanatomical differences between autism and Asperger syndrome." *Arch. Gen. Psychiatry 61*, 291–298.

14. Mayes, S.D., Calhoun, S.L. and Crites, D.L. (2001) "Does DSM-IV Asperger's disorder exist?" *J. Abnorm. Child Psychol. 29*, 263–271.

15. Hippler, K. and Klicpera, C. (2003) "A retrospective analysis of the clinical case records of 'autistic psychopaths' diagnosed by Hans Asperger and his team at the University Children's Hospital, Vienna." *Philos. Trans. R. Soc. Lond. B. Biol. Sci. 358*, 291–301.

16. Asperger, H. (1991) "Autistic psychopathy in childhood – 1944 (translation)." In U.T. Frith (ed) *Autism and Asperger Syndrome.* pp.37–39. Cambridge: Cambridge University Press.

17. Kanner, L. (1943) "Autistic disturbances of affective contact." *Nervous Child 2*, 217–250.

18. Kanner, L. (1971) "Follow-up study of eleven autistic children originally reported in 1943." *J. Autism Child Schizophr. 1*, 119–145.

19. Dancey, T.E. (1957) "Early infantile autism, 1943–1955; discussion of paper presented by Leo Kanner, M.D." *Psychiatr. Res. Rep. Am. Psychiatr. Assoc.*, 66–88.

20. Gillberg, C. and Billstedt, E. (2000) "Autism and Asperger syndrome: coexistence with other clinical disorders." *Acta Psychiatr. Scand. 102*, 321–330.

21. Ghaziuddin, M., Al Khouri, I. and Ghaziuddin, N. (2002) "Autistic symptoms following herpes encephalitis." *Eur. Child Adolesc. Psychiatry 11*, 142–146.

22. Gillberg, C. (1986) "Onset at age 14 of a typical autistic syndrome. A case report of a girl with herpes simplex encephalitis." *J. Autism Dev. Disord. 16*, 369–375.

23. Gillberg, I.C. (1991) "Autistic syndrome with onset at age 31 years: herpes encephalitis as a possible model for childhood autism." *Dev. Med. Child Neurol. 33*, 920–924.

24. Baird, G., Cass, H. and Slonims, V. (2003) "Diagnosis of autism." *BMJ 327*, 488–493.

25. Filipek, P.A., Accardo, P.J., Ashwal, S., Baranek, G.T., Cook, E.H., Jr., Dawson, G. *et al.* (2000) "Practice parameter: screening and diagnosis of autism: report of the Quality Standards Subcommittee of the American Academy of Neurology and the Child Neurology Society." *Neurology 55*, 468–479.

26. Robins, D.L., Fein, D., Barton, M.L. and Green, J.A. (2001) "The Modified Checklist for Autism in Toddlers: an initial study investigating the early detection of autism and pervasive developmental disorders." *J. Autism Dev. Disord. 31*, 131–144.

27. Dumont-Mathieu, T., Fein, D. and Kleinman, J. (2005) "Screening for autism in young children: the Modified Checklist for Autism in Toddlers (M-CHAT)." *Dev. Behav. Pediatrics Online*: http://www.dbpeds .org/articles/detail.cfm?TextID=377

28. Lord, C., Rutter, M. and Le Couteur, A. (1994) "Autism Diagnostic Interview – Revised: a revised version of a diagnostic interview for caregivers of individuals with possible pervasive developmental disorders." *J. Autism Dev. Disord. 24*, 659–685.

29. Herault, J., Petit, E., Martineau, J., Cherpi, C., Perrot, A., Barthelemy, C. *et al.* (1996) "Serotonin and autism: biochemical and molecular biology features." *Psychiatry Res. 65*, 33–43.

30. Schopler, E., Reichler, R.J., DeVellis, R.F. and Daly, K. (1980) "Toward objective classification of childhood autism: Childhood Autism Rating Scale (CARS)." *J. Autism Dev. Disord. 10*, 91–103.

31. Perry, A., Condillac, R.A., Freeman, N.L., Dunn-Geier, J. and Belair, J. (2006) "Multi-site study of the Childhood Autism Rating Scale (CARS) in five clinical groups of young children." *J. Autism Dev. Disord.*, in press.

32. Croen, L.A., Grether, J.K., Hoogstrate, J. and Selvin, S. (2002) "The changing prevalence of autism in California." *J. Autism Dev. Disord. 32*, 207–215.

33. Newschaffer, C.J., Falb, M.D. and Gurney, J.G. (2005) "National autism prevalence trends from United States special education data." *Pediatrics 115*, e277–e282.

34. Le Couteur, A., Bailey, A., Goode, S., Pickles, A., Robertson, S., Gottesman, I. *et al.* (1996) "A broader phenotype of autism: the clinical spectrum in twins." *J. Child Psychol. Psychiatry 37*, 785–801.

35. Gillberg, C., Gillberg, I.C. and Steffenburg, S. (1992) "Siblings and parents of children with autism: a controlled population-based study." *Dev. Med. Child Neurol. 34*, 389–398.

36. Folstein, S.E., Santangelo, S.L., Gilman, S.E., Piven, J., Landa, R., Lainhart, J. *et al.* (1999) "Predictors of cognitive test patterns in autism families." *J. Child Psychol. Psychiatry 40*, 1117–1128.

37. Lauritsen, M. and Ewald, H. (2001) "The genetics of autism." *Acta Psychiatr. Scand. 103*, 411–427.

38. Spiker, D., Lotspeich, L.J., Dimiceli, S., Myers, R.M. and Risch, N. (2002) "Behavioral phenotypic variation in autism multiplex families: evidence for a continuous severity gradient." *Am. J. Med. Genet. 114*, 129–136.

39. Amaral, D.G. (2003) "Report from the research director." *MIND Institute Newsletter 4*, 1–2.

40. Hrdlicka, M., Dudova, I., Beranova, I., Lisy, J., Belsan, T., Neuwirth, J. *et al.* (2005) "Subtypes of autism by cluster analysis based on structural MRI data." *Eur. Child Adolesc. Psychiatry 14*, 138–144.

41. Miles, J.H., Takahashi, T.N., Bagby, S., Sahota, P.K., Vaslow, D.F., Wang, C.H. *et al.* (2005) "Essential versus complex autism: definition of fundamental prognostic subtypes." *Am. J. Med. Genet. A 135*, 171–180.

Chapter 3 Genetic Contribution to Autistic Spectrum Disorders: Diversity and Insufficiency

1. Folstein, S. and Rutter, M. (1977) "Infantile autism: a genetic study of 21 twin pairs." *J. Child Psychol. Psychiatry 18*, 297–321.

2. Steffenburg, S., Gillberg, C., Hellgren, L., Andersson, L., Gillberg, I.C., Jakobsson, G. *et al.* (1989) "A twin study of autism in Denmark, Finland, Iceland, Norway and Sweden." *J. Child Psychol. Psychiatry 30*, 405–416.

3. Ritvo, E.R., Freeman, B.J., Mason-Brothers, A., Mo, A. and Ritvo, A.M. (1985) "Concordance for the syndrome of autism in 40 pairs of afflicted twins." *Am. J. Psychiatry 142*, 74–77.

4. Bailey, A., Le Couteur, A., Gottesman, I., Bolton, P., Simonoff, E., Yuzda, E. *et al.* (1995) "Autism as a strongly genetic disorder: evidence from a British twin study." *Psychol. Med. 25*, 63–77.

5. Muhle, R., Trentacoste, S.V. and Rapin, I. (2004) "The genetics of autism." *Pediatrics 113*, e472–e486.

6. Gillberg, C., Gillberg, I.C. and Steffenburg, S. (1992) "Siblings and parents of children with autism: a controlled population-based study." *Dev. Med. Child Neurol. 34*, 389–398.

7. Folstein, S.E., Santangelo, S.L., Gilman, S.E., Piven, J., Landa, R., Lainhart, J. *et al.* (1999) "Predictors of cognitive test patterns in autism families." *J. Child Psychol. Psychiatry 40*, 1117–1128.

8. Lauritsen, M. and Ewald, H. (2001) "The genetics of autism." *Acta Psychiatr. Scand. 103*, 411–427.

9. Spiker, D., Lotspeich, L.J., Dimiceli, S., Myers, R.M. and Risch, N. (2002) "Behavioral phenotypic variation in autism multiplex families: evidence for a continuous severity gradient." *Am. J. Med. Genet. 114*, 129–136.

10. Hippler, K. and Klicpera, C. (2003) "A retrospective analysis of the clinical case records of 'autistic psychopaths' diagnosed by Hans Asperger and his team at the University Children's Hospital, Vienna." *Philos. Trans. R. Soc. Lond. B. Biol. Sci. 358*, 291–301.

11. Wing, L. (1981) "Sex ratios in early childhood autism and related conditions." *Psychiatry Res. 5*, 129–137.

12. Ehlers, S. and Gillberg, C. (1993) "The epidemiology of Asperger syndrome. A total population study." *J. Child Psychol. Psychiatry 34*, 1327–1350.

13. Fombonne, E. (2002) "Epidemiological trends in rates of autism." *Mol. Psychiatry 7*, Suppl 2, S4–S6.

14. Lord, C. and Schopler, E. (1985) "Differences in sex ratios in autism as a function of measured intelligence." *J. Autism Dev. Disord. 15*, 185–193.

15. Tsai, L.Y. and Beisler, J.M. (1983) "The development of sex differences in infantile autism." *Br. J. Psychiatry* *142*, 373–378.

16. Kopp, S. and Gillberg, C. (2003) "Swedish child and adolescent psychiatric out-patients – a five-year cohort." *Eur. Child Adolesc. Psychiatry 12*, 30–35.

17. Kendler, K.S. and Aggen, S.H. (2001) "Time, memory and the heritability of major depression." *Psychol. Med. 31*, 923–928.

18. Cardno, A.G., Marshall, E.J., Coid, B., Macdonald, A.M., Ribchester, T.R., Davies, N.J. *et al.* (1999) "Heritability estimates for psychotic disorders: the Maudsley twin psychosis series." *Arch. Gen. Psychiatry 56*, 162–168.

19. Lewis, K.E., Lubetsky, M.J., Wenger, S.L. and Steele, M.W. (1995) "Chromosomal abnormalities in a psychiatric population." *Am. J. Med. Genet. 60*, 53–54.

20. Wassink, T.H., Piven, J. and Patil, S.R. (2001) "Chromosomal abnormalities in a clinic sample of individuals with autistic disorder." *Psychiatr. Genet. 11*, 57–63.

21. Reddy, K.S. (2005) "Cytogenetic abnormalities and fragile-X syndrome in autism spectrum disorder." *BMC Med. Genet. 6*, 3.

22. Yu, C.E., Dawson, G., Munson, J., D'Souza, I., Osterling, J., Estes, A. *et al.* (2002) "Presence of large deletions in kindreds with autism." *Am. J. Hum. Genet. 71*, 100–115.

23. Baker, P., Piven, J., Schwartz, S. and Patil, S. (1994) "Brief report: duplication of chromosome 15q11–13 in two individuals with autistic disorder." *J. Autism Dev. Disord. 24*, 529–535.

24. Brown, W.T., Friedman, E., Jenkins, E.C., Brooks, J., Wisniewski, K., Raguthu, S. *et al.* (1982) "Association of fragile X syndrome with autism." *Lancet 1*, 100.

25. Verkerk, A.J., Pieretti, M., Sutcliffe, J.S., Fu, Y.H., Kuhl, D.P., Pizzuti, A. *et al.* (1991) "Identification of a gene (FMR-1) containing a CGG repeat coincident with a breakpoint cluster region exhibiting length variation in fragile X syndrome." *Cell 65*, 905–914.

26. Castermans, D., Wilquet, V., Steyaert, J., Van de Ven, W., Fryns, J.P. and Devriendt, K. (2004) "Chromosomal anomalies in individuals with autism: a strategy towards the identification of genes involved in autism." *Autism 8*, 141–161.

27. Lamb, J.A., Parr, J.R., Bailey, A.J. and Monaco, A.P. (2002) "Autism: in search of susceptibility genes." *Neuromolecular. Med. 2*, 11–28.

28. Gillberg, C. and Coleman, M. (2000) *The Biology of the Autistic Syndromes.* Cambridge: MacKeith–Cambridge University Press.

29. Kotsopoulos, S. and Kutty, K.M. (1979) "Histidinemia and infantile autism." *J. Autism Dev. Disord. 9*, 55–60.

30. Baieli, S., Pavone, L., Meli, C., Fiumara, A. and Coleman, M. (2003) "Autism and phenylketonuria." *J. Autism Dev. Disord. 33*, 201–204.

31. Cohen, L.H., Vamos, E., Heinrichs, C., Toppet, M., Courtens, W., Kumps, A. *et al.* (1997) "Growth failure, encephalopathy, and endocrine dysfunctions in two siblings, one with 5-oxoprolinase deficiency." *Eur. J. Pediatr. 156*, 935–938.

32. Page, T. and Coleman, M. (2000) "Purine metabolism abnormalities in a hyperuricosuric subclass of autism." *Biochim. Biophys. Acta 1500*, 291–296.

33. Marie, S., Race, V., Nassogne, M.C., Vincent, M.F. and Van den, B.G. (2002) "Mutation of a nuclear respiratory factor 2 binding site in the 5' untranslated region of the ADSL gene in three patients with adenylosuccinate lyase deficiency." *Am. J. Hum. Genet. 71*, 14–21.

34. Zannolli, R., Micheli, V., Mazzei, M.A., Sacco, P., Piomboni, P., Bruni, E. *et al.* (2003) "Hereditary xanthinuria type II associated with mental delay, autism, cortical renal cysts, nephrocalcinosis, osteopenia, and hair and teeth defects." *J. Med. Genet. 40*, e121.

35. Tierney, E., Nwokoro, N.A., Porter, F.D., Freund, L.S., Ghuman, J.K. and Kelley, R.I. (2001) "Behavior phenotype in the RSH/Smith-Lemli-Opitz syndrome." *Am. J. Med. Genet. 98*, 191–200.

36. Fillano, J.J., Goldenthal, M.J., Rhodes, C.H. and Marin-Garcia, J. (2002) "Mitochondrial dysfunction in patients with hypotonia, epilepsy, autism, and developmental delay: HEADD syndrome." *J. Child Neurol. 17*, 435–439.

37. Pons, R., Andreu, A.L., Checcarelli, N., Vila, M.R., Engelstad, K., Sue, C.M. *et al.* (2004) "Mitochondrial DNA abnormalities and autistic spectrum disorders." *J. Pediatr. 144*, 81–85.

38. Gropman, A. (2003) "Vigabatrin and newer interventions in succinic semialdehyde dehydrogenase deficiency." *Ann. Neurol. 54*, Suppl 6, S66–S72.

39. Jamain, S., Quach, H., Betancur, C., Rastam, M., Colineaux, C., Gillberg, I.C. *et al.* (2003) "Mutations of the X-linked genes encoding neuroligins NLGN3 and NLGN4 are associated with autism." *Nat. Genet. 34*, 27–29.

40. Amir, R.E., Van de Veyver, I.B., Wan, M., Tran, C.Q., Francke, U. and Zoghbi, H.Y. (1999) "Rett syndrome is caused by mutations in X-linked MECP2, encoding methyl-CpG-binding protein 2." *Nat. Genet. 23*, 185–188.

41. Brown, W.T., Jenkins, E.C., Cohen, I.L., Fisch, G.S., Wolf-Schein, E.G., Gross, A. *et al.* (1986) "Fragile X and autism: a multicenter survey." *Am. J. Med. Genet. 23*, 341–352.

42. Mansheim, P. (1979) "Tuberous sclerosis and autistic behavior." *J. Clin. Psychiatry 40*, 97–98.

43. Smalley, S.L. (1998) "Autism and tuberous sclerosis." *J. Autism Dev. Disord. 28*, 407–414.

44. Erlandson, A. and Hagberg, B. (2005) "MECP2 abnormality phenotypes: clinicopathologic area with broad variability." *J. Child Neurol. 20*, 727–732.

45. Naidu, S., Bibat, G., Kratz, L., Kelley, R.I., Pevsner, J., Hoffman, E. *et al.* (2003) "Clinical variability in Rett syndrome." *J. Child Neurol. 18*, 662–668.

46. Edery, P., Chabrier, S., Ceballos-Picot, I., Marie, S., Vincent, M.F. and Tardieu, M. (2003) "Intrafamilial variability in the phenotypic expression of adenylosuccinate lyase deficiency: a report on three patients." *Am. J. Med. Genet. 120A*, 185–190.

47. Maestrini, E., Paul, A., Monaco, A.P. and Bailey, A. (2000) "Identifying autism susceptibility genes." *Neuron 28*, 19–24.

48. Page, T. (2000) "Metabolic approaches to the treatment of autism spectrum disorders." *J. Autism Dev. Disord. 30*, 463–469.

49. International HapMap Consortium (2005) "A haplotype map of the human genome." *Nature 437*, 1299–1320.

50. Beaudet, A., Bowcock, A., Buchwald, M., Cavalli-Sforza, L., Farrall, M., King, M.C. *et al.* (1986) "Linkage of cystic fibrosis to two tightly linked DNA markers: joint report from a collaborative study." *Am. J. Hum. Genet. 39*, 681–693.

51. Folstein, S.E. and Rosen-Sheidley, B. (2001) "Genetics of autism: complex aetiology for a heterogeneous disorder." *Nat. Rev. Genet. 2*, 943–955.

52. Yonan, A.L., Palmer, A.A., Smith, K.C., Feldman, I., Lee, H.K., Yonan, J.M. *et al.* (2003) "Bioinformatic analysis of autism positional candidate genes using biological databases and computational gene network prediction." *Genes Brain Behav. 2*, 303–320.

53. McCauley, J.L., Li, C., Jiang, L., Olson, L.M., Crockett, G., Gainer, K. *et al.* (2005) "Genome-wide and ordered-subset linkage analyses provide support for autism loci on 17q and 19p with evidence of phenotypic and interlocus genetic correlates." *BMC Med. Genet. 6*, 1.

54. Buxbaum, J.D., Silverman, J.M., Smith, C.J., Greenberg, D.A., Kilifarski, M., Reichert, J. *et al.* (2002) "Association between a GABRB3 polymorphism and autism." *Mol. Psychiatry 7*, 311–316.

55. Alarcón, M., Yonan, A.L., Gilliam, T.C., Cantor, R.M. and Geschwind, D.H. (2005) "Quantitative genome scan and ordered-subsets analysis of autism endophenotypes support language QTLs." *Mol. Psychiatry 10*, 747–757.

56. Molloy, C.A., Keddache, M. and Martin, L.J. (2005) "Evidence for linkage on 21q and 7q in a subset of autism characterized by developmental regression." *Mol. Psychiatry 10*, 741–746.

57. Shao, Y., Cuccaro, M.L., Hauser, E.R., Raiford, K.L., Menold, M.M., Wolpert, C.M. *et al.* (2003) "Fine mapping of autistic disorder to chromosome 15q11–q13 by use of phenotypic subtypes." *Am. J. Hum. Genet. 72*, 539–548.

58. National Alliance for Autism Research (2004) *What is the NAAR Autism Genome Project?* http://www.tgen.org/downloads/autism/NAAR_Autism_Genome_Project.pdf

59. AGRE (2005) *The AGRE Program.* http://www.agre.org/program/intro.cfm?do=program

60. Cold Spring Harbor Laboratory (2005) *Landmark Autism Initiative at CSHL.* http://www.cshl.edu/public/releases/simons_05.html

61. Dean, J.C., Moore, S.J., Osborne, A., Howe, J. and Turnpenny, P.D. (1999) "Fetal anticonvulsant syndrome and mutation in the maternal MTHFR gene." *Clin. Genet. 56*, 216–220.

62. Stone, J.L., Merriman, B., Cantor, R.M., Yonan, A.L., Gilliam, T.C., Geschwind, D.H. *et al.* (2004) "Evidence for sex-specific risk alleles in autism spectrum disorder." *Am. J. Hum. Genet. 75*, 1117–1123.

63. Oliveira, G., Diogo, L., Grazina, M., Garcia, P., Ataide, A., Marques, C. *et al.* (2005) "Mitochondrial dysfunction in autism spectrum disorders: a population-based study." *Dev. Med. Child Neurol. 47*, 185–189.

64. Trask, B., van den, E.G., Mayall, B. and Gray, J.W. (1989) "Chromosome heteromorphism quantified by high-resolution bivariate flow karyotyping." *Am. J. Hum. Genet. 45*, 739–752.

65. Feuk, L., Macdonald, J.R., Tang, T., Carson, A.R., Li, M., Rao, G. *et al.* (2005) "Discovery of human inversion polymorphisms by comparative analysis of human and chimpanzee DNA sequence assemblies." *PLoS Genet. 1*, e56.

66. Sebat, J., Lakshmi, B., Troge, J., Alexander, J., Young, J., Lundin, P. *et al.* (2004) "Large-scale copy number polymorphism in the human genome." *Science 305*, 525–528.

67. Check, E. (2005) "Human genome: patchwork people." *Nature 437*, 1084–1086.

68. Jaenisch, R. and Bird, A. (2003) "Epigenetic regulation of gene expression: how the genome integrates intrinsic and environmental signals." *Nat. Genet. 33 Suppl*, 245–254.

69. Meehan, R.R. (2003) "DNA methylation in animal development." *Semin. Cell Dev. Biol. 14*, 53–65.

70. Petronis, A. (2000) "The genes for major psychosis: aberrant sequence or regulation?" *Neuropsychopharmacology 23*, 1–12.

71. Petronis, A. (2004) "The origin of schizophrenia: genetic thesis, epigenetic antithesis, and resolving synthesis." *Biol. Psychiatry 55*, 965–970.

72. Hall, J.G. (1996) "Twinning: mechanisms and genetic implications." *Curr. Opin. Genet. Dev. 6*, 343–347.

73. Singh, S.M., Murphy, B. and O'Reilly, R. (2002) "Epigenetic contributors to the discordance of monozygotic twins." *Clin. Genet. 62*, 97–103.

74. Bestor, T.H. (2003) "Imprinting errors and developmental asymmetry." *Philos. Trans. R. Soc. Lond. B. Biol. Sci. 358*, 1411–1415.

75. Weksberg, R., Shuman, C., Caluseriu, O., Smith, A.C., Fei, Y.L., Nishikawa, J. *et al.* (2002) "Discordant KCNQ1OT1 imprinting in sets of monozygotic twins discordant for Beckwith-Wiedemann syndrome." *Hum. Mol. Genet. 11*, 1317–1325.

76. Boklage, C.E. (2005) "The biology of human twinning: a needed change of perspective." In I. Blickstein and G. Keith (eds) *Multiple Pregnancy: Epidemiology, Gestation and Perinatal Outcome*. London: Taylor and Francis; pp.255–264.

77. Golbin, A., Golbin, Y., Keith, L. and Keith, D. (1993) "Mirror imaging in twins: biological polarization – an evolving hypothesis." *Acta Genet. Med. Gemellol. (Roma.) 42*, 237–243.

78. Rutter, M. (2000) "Genetic studies of autism: from the 1970s into the millennium." *J. Abnormal Child Psychol. 28*, 3–14.

Chapter 4 New Phase Autism: Rising Prevalence

1. American Psychiatric Association (1994) *Diagnostic and Statistical Manual of Mental Disorders (DSM-IV)*. Washington, DC: American Psychiatric Association.

2. World Health Organization (WHO) (1992) *The ICD-10 Classification of Mental and Behavioural Disorders*. Geneva: World Health Organization.

3. Volkmar, F.R., Bregman, J., Cohen, D.J. and Cicchetti, D.V. (1988) "DSM-III and DSM-III-R diagnoses of autism." *Am. J. Psychiatry 145*, 1404–1408.

4. Tidmarsh, L. and Volkmar, F.R. (2003) "Diagnosis and epidemiology of autism spectrum disorders." *Can. J. Psychiatry 48*, 517–525.

5. Fombonne, E. (2003) "The prevalence of autism." *J. Am. Med. Assoc. 289*, 87–89.

6. Wing, L. (1996) "Autistic spectrum disorders." *Brit. Med. J. 312*, 327–328.

7. Rutter, M. (2005) "Aetiology of autism: findings and questions." *J. Intellect. Disabil. Res. 49*, 231–238.

8. Ritvo, E.R., Freeman, B.J., Pingree, C., Mason-Brothers, A., Jorde, L., Jenson, W.R. *et al.* (1989) "The UCLA-University of Utah epidemiologic survey of autism: prevalence." *Am. J. Psychiatry 146*, 194–199.

9. Madsen, K.M., Hviid, A., Vestergaard, M., Schendel, D., Wohlfahrt, J., Thorsen, P. *et al.* (2002) "A population-based study of measles, mumps, and rubella vaccination and autism." *N. Engl. J. Med. 347*, 1477–1482.

10. Kaye, J.A., Mar Melero-Montes, M. and Jick, H. (2001) "Mumps, measles, and rubella vaccine and the incidence of autism recorded by general practitioners: a time trend analysis." *Brit. Med. J. 322*, 460–463.

11. Medical Research Council (2001) *MRC Review of Autism Research; Epidemiology and Causes.* http://www.mrc.ac.uk/pdf-autism-report.pdf

12. Barnard, J., Broach, S., Potter, D. and Prior, A. (2002) *Autism in Schools, Crisis or Challenge?* London: National Autistic Society.

13. NHS Health Scotland (2004) *ASD Audit 2004.* http://www.scotland.gov.uk/Topics/Health/care/18950/19650

14. California Dept. Developmental Services (2003) *Autistic Spectrum Disorders: Changes in the California Caseload; An Update: 1999 Through 2002.* www.dds.cahwnet.gov/autism/pdf/AutismReport2003.pdf

15. Yazbak, F.E. (2003) "Autism in the United States: a perspective." *J. Am. Phys. Surg. 8*, 103–107.

16. Newschaffer, C.J., Falb, M.D. and Gurney, J.G. (2005) "National autism prevalence trends from United States special education data." *Pediatrics 115*, e277–e282.

17. Goldman, G.S. and Yazbak, F.E. (2004) "An investigation of the association between MMR vaccination and autism in Denmark." *J. Am. Phys. Surg. 9*, 70–75.

18. Lauritsen, M.B., Pedersen, C.B. and Mortensen, P.B. (2004) "The incidence and prevalence of pervasive developmental disorders: a Danish population-based study." *Psychol. Med. 34*, 1339–1346.

19. Gillberg, C. and Wing, L. (1999) "Autism: not an extremely rare disorder." *Acta Psychiatr. Scand. 99*, 399–406.

20. Fombonne, E., Simmons, H., Ford, T., Meltzer, H. and Goodman, R. (2003) "Prevalence of pervasive developmental disorders in the British nationwide survey of child mental health." *Int. Rev. Psychiatry 15*, 158–165.

21. Wing, L. and Potter, D. (2002) "The epidemiology of autistic spectrum disorders: is the prevalence rising?" *Ment. Retard. Dev. Disabil. Res. Rev. 8*, 151–161.

22. Fombonne, E. (2003) "Epidemiological surveys of autism and other pervasive developmental disorders: an update." *J. Autism Dev. Disord. 33*, 365–382.

23. Blaxill, M.F. (2004) "What's going on? The question of time trends in autism." *Publ. Health Repts. 119*, 536–551.

24. Williams, J.G., Higgins, J.P. and Brayne, C.E. (2006) "Systematic review of prevalence studies of autism spectrum disorders." *Arch. Dis. Child 91*, 8–15.

25. Deb, S. and Prasad, K.B. (1994) "The prevalence of autistic disorder among children with a learning disability." *Br. J. Psychiatry 165*, 395–399.

26. Palmer, R.F., Blanchard, S., Stein, Z., Mandell, D. and Miller, C. (2006) "Environmental mercury release, special education rates, and autism disorder: an ecological study of Texas." *Health & Place 12*, 203–209.

27. Croen, L.A., Grether, J.K., Hoogstrate, J. and Selvin, S. (2002) "The changing prevalence of autism in California." *J. Autism Dev. Disord. 32*, 207–215.

28. Blaxill, M.F., Baskin, D.S. and Spitzer, W.O. (2003) "Commentary: Blaxill, Baskin, and Spitzer on Croen (2002), the changing prevalence of autism in California." *J. Autism Dev. Disord. 33*, 223–226.

29. Croen, L.A. and Grether, J.K. (2003) "A response to Blaxill, Baskin, and Spitzer on Croen *et al.* (2002), the changing prevalence of autism in California." *J. Autism Dev. Disord. 33*, 227–229.

30. Smeeth, L., Cook, C., Fombonne, E., Heavey, L., Rodrigues, L.C., Smith, P.G. *et al.* (2004) "Rate of first recorded diagnosis of autism and other pervasive developmental disorders in United Kingdom general practice, 1988 to 2001." *BMC Medicine 2.* http://www.biomedcentral.com/1741-7015/2/39

31. Barbaresi, W.J., Katusic, S.K., Colligan, R.C., Weaver, A.L. and Jacobsen, S.J. (2005) "The incidence of autism in Olmsted County, Minnesota, 1976–1997: results from a population-based study." *Arch. Pediatr. Adolesc. Med. 159*, 37–44.

32. MIND Institute (2002) *Report to the Legislature on the Principal Findings from the Epidemiology of Autism in California: A Comprehensive Pilot Study.* http://www.dds.cahwnet.gov/autism/pdf/study_final.pdf

33. New Jersey State Department of Education (2001) *Number of Public Students with Disabilities Ages 3–21 By Eligibility Category and Age and Percent of Enrollment.* http://www.state.nj.us/njded/specialed/data/excel/NJT052000.pdf

34. Williams, K., Glasson, E.J., Wray, J., Tuck, M., Helmer, M., Bower, C.I. *et al.* (2005) "Incidence of autism spectrum disorders in children in two Australian states." *Med. J. Aust. 182*, 108–111.

35. Magnusson, P. and Saemundsen, E. (2001) "Prevalence of autism in Iceland." *J. Autism Dev. Disord. 31*, 153–163.

36. Seltzer, M.M., Krauss, M.W., Shattuck, P.T., Orsmond, G., Swe, A. and Lord, C. (2003) "The symptoms of autism spectrum disorders in adolescence and adulthood." *J. Autism Dev. Disord. 33*, 565–581.

37. McGovern, C.W. and Sigman, M. (2005) "Continuity and change from early childhood to adolescence in autism." *J. Child Psychol. Psychiatry 46*, 401–408.

38. Folstein, S. and Rutter, M. (1977) "Infantile autism: a genetic study of 21 twin pairs." *J. Child Psychol. Psychiatry 18*, 297–321.

39. Steffenburg, S., Gillberg, C., Hellgren, L., Andersson, L., Gillberg, I.C., Jakobsson, G. *et al.* (1989) "A twin study of autism in Denmark, Finland, Iceland, Norway and Sweden." *J. Child Psychol. Psychiatry 30*, 405–416.

40. Bailey, A., Le Couteur, A., Gottesman, I., Bolton, P., Simonoff, E., Yuzda, E. *et al.* (1995) "Autism as a strongly genetic disorder: evidence from a British twin study." *Psychol. Med. 25*, 63–77.

41. Muhle, R., Trentacoste, S.V. and Rapin, I. (2004) "The genetics of autism." *Pediatrics 113*, e472–e486.

42. Betancur, C., Leboyer, M. and Gillberg, C. (2002) "Increased rate of twins among affected sibling pairs with autism." *Am. J. Hum. Genet. 70*, 1381–1383.

43. Hallmayer, J., Glasson, E.J., Bower, C., Petterson, B., Croen, L., Grether, J. *et al.* (2002) "On the twin risk in autism." *Am. J. Hum. Genet. 71*, 941–946.

44. Kates, W.R., Burnette, C.P., Eliez, S., Strunge, L.A., Kaplan, D., Landa, R. *et al.* (2004) "Neuroanatomic variation in monozygotic twin pairs discordant for the narrow phenotype for autism." *Am. J. Psychiatry 161*, 539–546.

45. Lamb, J.A., Parr, J.R., Bailey, A.J. and Monaco, A.P. (2002) "Autism: in search of susceptibility genes." *Neuromolecular Med. 2*, 11–28.

46. Laxova, R. (1994) "Fragile X syndrome." *Adv. Pediatr. 41*, 305–342.

47. Brown, W.T., Jenkins, E.C., Cohen, I.L., Fisch, G.S., Wolf-Schein, E.G., Gross, A. *et al.* (1986) "Fragile X and autism: a multicenter survey." *Am. J. Med. Genet. 23*, 341–352.

48. Demark, J.L., Feldman, M.A. and Holden, J.J. (2003) "Behavioral relationship between autism and fragile X syndrome." *Am. J. Ment. Retard. 108*, 314–326.

49. Brown, W.T., Friedman, E., Jenkins, E.C., Brooks, J., Wisniewski, K., Raguthu, S. *et al.* (1982) "Association of fragile X syndrome with autism." *Lancet 1*, 100.

50. McInnes, L.A., Jimenez, G.P., Manghi, E.R., Esquivel, M., Monge, M.S., Fallas, D.M. *et al.* (2005) "A genetic study of autism in Costa Rica: multiple variables affecting IQ scores observed in a preliminary sample of autistic cases." *BMC Psychiatry 5*, 15; http://www.biomedcentral.com/1471-244X/5/15

51. Kosinovsky, B., Hermon, S., Yoran-Hegesh, R., Golomb, A., Senecky, Y., Goez, H. *et al.* (2005) "The yield of laboratory investigations in children with infantile autism." *J. Neural Transm. 112*, 587–596.

52. Nataf, R., Skorupka, C., Amet, L., Lam, A., Springbett, A. and Lathe, R. (2005) "Porphyrinuria in childhood autistic disorder." Submitted for publication.

53. Gillberg, C. and Wahlstrom, J. (1985) "Chromosome abnormalities in infantile autism and other childhood psychoses: a population study of 66 cases." *Dev. Med. Child Neurol. 27*, 293–304.

54. Fisch, G.S., Cohen, I.L., Wolf, E.G., Brown, W.T., Jenkins, E.C. and Gross, A. (1986) "Autism and the fragile X syndrome." *Am. J. Psychiatry 143*, 71–73.

55. Wahlstrom, J., Gillberg, C., Gustavson, K.H. and Holmgren, G. (1986) "Infantile autism and the fragile X. A Swedish multicenter study." *Am. J. Med. Genet. 23*, 403–408.

56. Piven, J., Gayle, J., Landa, R., Wzorek, M. and Folstein, S. (1991) "The prevalence of fragile X in a sample of autistic individuals diagnosed using a standardized interview." *J. Am. Acad. Child Adolesc. Psychiatry 30*, 825–830.

57. Wong, V.C. and Lam, S.T. (1992) "Fragile X positivity in Chinese children with autistic spectrum disorder." *Pediatr. Neurol. 8*, 272–274.

58. Fisch, G.S. (1992) "Is autism associated with the fragile X syndrome?" *Am. J. Med. Genet. 43*, 47–55.

59. Bailey, A., Bolton, P., Butler, L., Le Couteur, A., Murphy, M., Scott, S. *et al.* (1993) "Prevalence of the fragile X anomaly amongst autistic twins and singletons." *J. Child Psychol. Psychiatry 34*, 673–688.

60. Li, S.Y., Chen, Y.C., Lai, T.J., Hsu, C.Y. and Wang, Y.C. (1993) "Molecular and cytogenetic analyses of autism in Taiwan." *Hum. Genet. 92*, 441–445.

61. Kielinen, M., Rantala, H., Timonen, E., Linna, S.L. and Moilanen, I. (2004) "Associated medical disorders and disabilities in children with autistic disorder: a population-based study." *Autism 8*, 49–60.

62. Murray, J., Cuckle, H., Taylor, G. and Hewison, J. (1997) "Screening for fragile X syndrome." *Health Technol. Assess. 1*, 1–71.

63. Fombonne, E., Du, M.C., Cans, C. and Grandjean, H. (1997) "Autism and associated medical disorders in a French epidemiological survey." *J. Am. Acad. Child Adolesc. Psychiatry 36*, 1561–1569.

64. Wassink, T.H., Piven, J. and Patil, S.R. (2001) "Chromosomal abnormalities in a clinic sample of individuals with autistic disorder." *Psychiatr. Genet. 11*, 57–63.

65. Reddy, K.S. (2005) "Cytogenetic abnormalities and fragile-X syndrome in autism spectrum disorder." *BMC Med. Genet. 6*, 3.

66. Turner, G., Webb, T., Wake, S. and Robinson, H. (1996) "Prevalence of fragile X syndrome." *Am. J. Med. Genet. 64*, 196–197.

67. Morton, J.E., Bundey, S., Webb, T.P., MacDonald, F., Rindl, P.M. and Bullock, S. (1997) "Fragile X syndrome is less common than previously estimated." *J. Med. Genet. 34*, 1–5.

68. Song, F.J., Barton, P., Sleightholme, V., Yao, G.L. and Fry-Smith, A. (2003) "Screening for fragile X syndrome: a literature review and modelling study." *Health Technol. Assess. 7*, 1–106.

69. Fombonne, E. (2001) "Is there an epidemic of autism?" *Pediatrics 107*, 411–412.

70. Merrick, J., Kandel, I. and Morad, M. (2004) "Trends in autism." *Int. J. Adolesc. Med. Health 16*, 75–78.

71. Tebruegge, M., Nandini, V. and Ritchie, J. (2004) "Does routine child health surveillance contribute to the early detection of children with pervasive developmental disorders? An epidemiological study in Kent, UK." *BMC Pediatr. 4*, 4.

72. Chakrabarti, S. and Fombonne, E. (2005) "Pervasive developmental disorders in preschool children: confirmation of high prevalence." *Am. J. Psychiatry 162*, 1133–1141.

73. Brown, E.L.R. (2002) "Risk of outbreaks." *The Scotsman*, 16 February.

Chapter 5 Brain Abnormalities: Focus on the Limbic System

1. HOPES: Huntington's Outreach Project for Education, S.U. (2005) *Build a Brain.* http://www.stanford.edu/group/hopes/basics/braintut/ab9.html

2. Structural Informatics Group, U.o.W. (2005) *Digital Anatomist Information System.* http://sig.biostr.washington.edu/projects/da/

3. Johnson, K.A. and Becker, J.A. (2005) *The Whole Brain Atlas.* http://www.med.harvard.edu/AANLIB/

4. Kandel, E., Schwartz, J.H. and Jessel, T.M. (2000) *Principles of Neural Science.* New York: McGraw-Hill.

5. Lathe, R. (2001) "Hormones and the hippocampus." *J. Endocrinol. 169*, 205–231.

6. Angevine, J.B., Jr. (1965) "Time of neuron origin in the hippocampal region." *Exp. Neurol. S2*, 1–70.

7. Redcay, E. and Courchesne, E. (2005) "When is the brain enlarged in autism? A meta-analysis of all brain size reports." *Biol. Psychiatry 58*, 1–9.

8. Palmen, S.J., Hulshoff Pol, H.E., Kemner, C., Schnack, H.G., Durston, S., Lahuis, B.E. *et al.* (2005) "Increased gray-matter volume in medication-naive high-functioning children with autism spectrum disorder." *Psychol. Med. 35*, 561–570.

9. McAlonan, G.M., Cheung, V., Cheung, C., Suckling, J., Lam, G.Y., Tai, K.S. *et al.* (2005) "Mapping the brain in autism. A voxel-based MRI study of volumetric differences and intercorrelations in autism." *Brain 128*, 268–276.

10. Waiter, G.D., Williams, J.H., Murray, A.D., Gilchrist, A., Perrett, D.I. and Whiten, A. (2005) "Structural white matter deficits in high-functioning individuals with autistic spectrum disorder: a voxel-based investigation." *Neuroimage 24*, 455–461.

11. Rice, S.A., Bigler, E.D., Cleavinger, H.B., Tate, D.F., Sayer, J., McMahon, W. *et al.* (2005) "Macrocephaly, corpus callosum morphology, and autism." *J. Child Neurol. 20*, 34–41.

12. Bauman, M. and Kemper, T.L. (1985) "Histoanatomic observations of the brain in early infantile autism." *Neurology 35*, 866–874.

13. Kemper, T.L. and Bauman, M.L. (1993) "The contribution of neuropathologic studies to the understanding of autism." *Neurol. Clin. 11*, 175–187.

14. Maurer, R.G. and Damasio, A.R. (1982) "Childhood autism from the point of view of behavioral neurology." *J. Autism Dev. Disord. 12*, 195–205.

15. Damasio, A.R. and Maurer, R.G. (1978) "A neurological model for childhood autism." *Arch. Neurol. 35*, 777–786.

16. DeLong, G.R. (1992) "Autism, amnesia, hippocampus, and learning." *Neurosci. Biobehav. Rev. 16*, 63–70.

17. Palmen, S.J., Van Engeland, H., Hof, P.R. and Schmitz, C. (2004) "Neuropathological findings in autism." *Brain 127*, 2572–2583.

18. Raymond, G.V., Bauman, M.L. and Kemper, T.L. (1996) "Hippocampus in autism: a Golgi analysis." *Acta Neuropathol. (Berl.) 91*, 117–119.

19. Kemper, T.L. and Bauman, M. (1998) "Neuropathology of infantile autism." *J. Neuropathol. Exp. Neurol. 57*, 645–652.

20. Kemper, T.L. and Bauman, M.L. (2002) "Neuropathology of infantile autism." *Mol. Psychiatry 7 Suppl 2*, S12–S13.

21. Green-Hopkins, I., Kemper, T.L., Bauman, M. and Blatt, G.J. (2004) "Increased density of Nissl-stained hippocampal neurons in autism." *Soc. Neurosci. Abs. 1028.15.*

22. Lawrence, Y.A., Kemper, T.L., Bauman, M. and Blatt, G.J. (2004) "Increased density of parvalbumin-labelled hippocampal interneurons in autism." *Soc. Neurosci. Abs. 1028.14.*

23. Aylward, E.H., Minshew, N.J., Goldstein, G., Honeycutt, N.A., Augustine, A.M., Yates, K.O. *et al.* (1999) "MRI volumes of amygdala and hippocampus in non-mentally retarded autistic adolescents and adults." *Neurology 53*, 2145–2150.

24. Sparks, B.F., Friedman, S.D., Shaw, D.W., Aylward, E.H., Echelard, D., Artru, A.A. *et al.* (2002) "Brain structural abnormalities in young children with autism spectrum disorder." *Neurology 59*, 184–192.

25. Schumann, C.M., Hamstra, J., Goodlin-Jones, B.L., Lotspeich, L.J., Kwon, H., Buonocore, M.H. *et al.* (2004) "The amygdala is enlarged in children but not adolescents with autism; the hippocampus is enlarged at all ages." *J. Neurosci. 24*, 6392–6401.

26. Saitoh, O., Karns, C.M. and Courchesne, E. (2001) "Development of the hippocampal formation from 2 to 42 years: MRI evidence of smaller area dentata in autism." *Brain 124*, 1317–1324.

27. Salmond, C.H., Ashburner, J., Connelly, A., Friston, K.J., Gadian, D.G. and Vargha-Khadem, F. (2005) "The role of the medial temporal lobe in autistic spectrum disorders." *Eur. J. Neurosci. 22*, 764–772.

28. Piven, J., Bailey, J., Ranson, B.J. and Arndt, S. (1998) "No difference in hippocampus volume detected on magnetic resonance imaging in autistic individuals." *J. Autism Dev. Disord. 28*, 105–110.

29. Howard, M.A., Cowell, P.E., Boucher, J., Broks, P., Mayes, A., Farrant, A. *et al.* (2000) "Convergent neuroanatomical and behavioural evidence of an amygdala hypothesis of autism." *Neuroreport 11*, 2931–2935.

30. Boddaert, N., Chabane, N., Gervais, H., Good, C.D., Bourgeois, M., Plumet, M.H. *et al.* (2004) "Superior temporal sulcus anatomical abnormalities in childhood autism: a voxel-based morphometry MRI study." *Neuroimage 23*, 364–369.

31. Boddaert, N. and Zilbovicius, M. (2002) "Functional neuroimaging and childhood autism." *Pediatr. Radiol. 32*, 1–7.

32. Welchew, D.E., Ashwin, C., Berkouk, K., Salvador, R., Suckling, J., Baron-Cohen, S. *et al.* (2005) "Functional disconnectivity of the medial temporal lobe in Asperger's syndrome." *Biol. Psychiatry 57*, 991–998.

33. Zilbovicius, M., Boddaert, N., Belin, P., Poline, J.B., Remy, P., Mangin, J.F. *et al.* (2000) "Temporal lobe dysfunction in childhood autism: a PET study. Positron emission tomography." *Am. J. Psychiatry 157*, 1988–1993.

34. Otsuka, H., Harada, M., Mori, K., Hisaoka, S. and Nishitani, H. (1999) "Brain metabolites in the hippocampus-amygdala region and cerebellum in autism: an 1H-MR spectroscopy study." *Neuroradiology 41*, 517–519.

35. Ito, H., Mori, K., Hashimoto, T., Miyazaki, M., Hori, A., Kagami, S. *et al.* (2005) "Findings of brain 99mTc-ECD SPECT in high-functioning autism – 3-dimensional stereotactic ROI template analysis of brain SPECT." *J. Med. Invest. 52*, 49–56.

36. Gendry Meresse, I., Zilbovicius, M., Boddaert, N., Robel, L., Philippe, A., Sfaello, I. *et al.* (2005) "Autism severity and temporal lobe functional abnormalities." *Ann. Neurol. 58*, 466–469.

37. Vargas, D.L., Nascimbene, C., Krishnan, C., Zimmerman, A.W. and Pardo, C.A. (2005) "Neuroglial activation and neuroinflammation in the brain of patients with autism." *Ann. Neurol. 57*, 67–81.

38. Courchesne, E. (1991) "Neuroanatomic imaging in autism." *Pediatrics 87*, 781–790.

39. Courchesne, E., Townsend, J. and Saitoh, O. (1994) "The brain in infantile autism: posterior fossa structures are abnormal." *Neurology 44*, 214–223.

40. Hardan, A.Y., Minshew, N.J., Harenski, K. and Keshavan, M.S. (2001) "Posterior fossa magnetic resonance imaging in autism." *J. Am. Acad. Child Adolesc. Psychiatry 40*, 666–672.

41. Courchesne, E. (2002) "Abnormal early brain development in autism." *Mol. Psychiatry 7*, Suppl 2, S21–S23.

42. Holttum, J.R., Minshew, N.J., Sanders, R.S. and Phillips, N.E. (1992) "Magnetic resonance imaging of the posterior fossa in autism." *Biol. Psychiatry 32*, 1091–1101.

43. Ryu, Y.H., Lee, J.D., Yoon, P.H., Kim, D.I., Lee, H.B. and Shin, Y.J. (1999) "Perfusion impairments in infantile autism on technetium-99m ethyl cysteinate dimer brain single-photon emission tomography: comparison with findings on magnetic resonance imaging." *Eur. J. Nucl. Med. 26*, 253–259.

44. Allen, G., Muller, R.A. and Courchesne, E. (2004) "Cerebellar function in autism: functional magnetic resonance image activation during a simple motor task." *Biol. Psychiatry 56*, 269–278.

45. Minshew, N.J., Sung, K., Jones, B.L. and Furman, J.M. (2004) "Underdevelopment of the postural control system in autism." *Neurology 63*, 2056–2061.

46. Ahsgren, I., Baldwin, I., Goetzinger-Falk, C., Erikson, A., Flodmark, O. and Gillberg, C. (2005) "Ataxia, autism, and the cerebellum: a clinical study of 32 individuals with congenital ataxia." *Dev. Med. Child Neurol. 47*, 193–198.

47. Mostofsky, S.H., Bunoski, R., Morton, S.M., Goldberg, M.C. and Bastian, A.J. (2004) "Children with autism adapt normally during a catching task requiring the cerebellum." *Neurocase 10*, 60–64.

48. Heath, R.G., Dempesy, C.W., Fontana, C.J. and Fitzjarrell, A.T. (1980) "Feedback loop between cerebellum and septal-hippocampal sites: its role in emotion and epilepsy." *Biol. Psychiatry 15*, 541–556.

49. Schmahmann, J.D. (1994) "The cerebellum in autism; clinical and anatomic perspectives." In M. Bauman and T.L. Kemper (eds) *The Neurobiology of Autism.* Baltimore: Johns Hopkins University Press; pp.195–226.

50. Carper, R.A. and Courchesne, E. (2005) "Localized enlargement of the frontal cortex in early autism." *Biol. Psychiatry 57*, 126–133.

51. Casanova, M.F., Buxhoeveden, D.P., Switala, A.E. and Roy, E. (2002) "Minicolumnar pathology in autism." *Neurology 58*, 428–432.

52. Casanova, M.F., Buxhoeveden, D.P., Switala, A.E. and Roy, E. (2002) "Neuronal density and architecture (Gray Level Index) in the brains of autistic patients." *J. Child Neurol. 17*, 515–521.

53. Bailey, A., Luthert, P., Dean, A., Harding, B., Janota, I., Montgomery, M. *et al.* (1998) "A clinicopathological study of autism." *Brain 121*, Pt 5, 889–905.

54. Lotspeich, L.J., Kwon, H., Schumann, C.M., Fryer, S.L., Goodlin-Jones, B.L., Buonocore, M.H. *et al.* (2004) "Investigation of neuroanatomical differences between autism and Asperger syndrome." *Arch. Gen. Psychiatry 61*, 291–298.

55. Hrdlicka, M., Dudova, I., Beranova, I., Lisy, J., Belsan, T., Neuwirth, J. *et al.* (2005) "Subtypes of autism by cluster analysis based on structural MRI data." *Eur. Child Adolesc. Psychiatry 14*, 138–144.

56. Cody, H., Pelphrey, K. and Piven, J. (2002) "Structural and functional magnetic resonance imaging of autism." *Int. J. Dev. Neurosci. 20*, 421.

57. Dawson, G., Webb, S., Schellenberg, G.D., Dager, S., Friedman, S., Aylward, E. *et al.* (2002) "Defining the broader phenotype of autism: genetic, brain, and behavioral perspectives." *Dev. Psychopathol. 14*, 581–611.

58. Kates, W.R., Mostofsky, S.H., Zimmerman, A.W., Mazzocco, M.M., Landa, R., Warsofsky, I.S. *et al.* (1998) "Neuroanatomical and neurocognitive differences in a pair of monozygous twins discordant for strictly defined autism." *Ann. Neurol. 43*, 782–791.

59. Corkin, S., Amaral, D.G., Gonzalez, R.G., Johnson, K.A. and Hyman, B.T. (1997) "HM's medial temporal lobe lesion: findings from magnetic resonance imaging." *J. Neurosci. 17*, 3964–3979.

60. Aitken, K. (1991) "Examining the evidence for a common structural basis to autism." *Dev. Med. Child Neurol. 33*, 930–934.

Chapter 6 Limbic Dysfunction Correlates with the Autistic Phenotype

1. Corkin, S., Amaral, D.G., Gonzalez, R.G., Johnson, K.A. and Hyman, B.T. (1997) "HM's medial temporal lobe lesion: findings from magnetic resonance imaging." *J. Neurosci. 17,* 3964–3979.

2. Corkin, S. (2002) "What's new with the amnesic patient HM?" *Nat. Rev. Neurosci. 3,* 153–160.

3. Scoville, W.B. and Milner, B. (1957) "Loss of recent memory after bilateral hippocampal lesions." *J. Neurol. Neurosurg. Psychiat. 20,* 11–21.

4. Cohen, N.J. and Eichenbaum, H. (1993) *Memory, Amnesia and the Hippocampal System.* Cambridge, MA: MIT.

5. Milner, B., Corkin, S. and Teuber, H.-L. (1968) "Further analysis of the hippocampal amnesic syndrome: 14-year follow-up study of HM." *Neuropsychologia 215,* 234.

6. Zola-Morgan, S., Squire, L.R. and Amaral, D.G. (1986) "Human amnesia and the medial temporal region: enduring memory impairment following a bilateral lesion limited to field CA1 of the hippocampus." *J. Neurosci. 6,* 2950–2967.

7. Stefanacci, L., Buffalo, E.A., Schmolck, H. and Squire, L.R. (2000) "Profound amnesia after damage to the medial temporal lobe: a neuroanatomical and neuropsychological profile of patient EP." *J. Neurosci. 20,* 7024–7036.

8. Isaacson, R.L. (2002) "Unsolved mysteries: the hippocampus." *Behav. Cogn. Neurosci. Rev. 1,* 87–107.

9. Zola-Morgan, S. and Squire, L.R. (1985) "Medial temporal lesions in monkeys impair memory on a variety of tasks sensitive to human amnesia." *Behav. Neurosci. 99,* 22–34.

10. Zola-Morgan, S., Squire, L.R. and Amaral, D.G. (1989) "Lesions of the amygdala that spare adjacent cortical regions do not impair memory or exacerbate the impairment following lesions of the hippocampal formation." *J. Neurosci. 9,* 1922–1936.

11. Zola-Morgan, S., Squire, L.R., Amaral, D.G. and Suzuki, W.A. (1989) "Lesions of perirhinal and parahippocampal cortex that spare the amygdala and hippocampal formation produce severe memory impairment." *J. Neurosci. 9,* 4355–4370.

12. Boucher, J. and Warrington, E.K. (1976) "Memory deficits in early infantile autism: some similarities to the amnesic syndrome." *Br. J. Psychol. 67,* 73–87.

13. Boucher, J. (1981) "Memory for recent events in autistic children." *J. Autism Dev. Disord. 11,* 293–301.

14. Boucher, J. (1981) "Immediate free recall in early childhood autism: another point of behavioural similarity with the amnesic syndrome." *Br. J. Psychol. 72,* 211–215.

15. Killiany, R.J. and Moss, M.B. (1994) "Memory function in autism." In M. Bauman and T.L. Kemper (eds) *The Neurobiology of Autism.* Baltimore: Johns Hopkins University Press; pp.170–194.

16. Burack, J.A. (1994) "Selective attention deficits in persons with autism: preliminary evidence of an inefficient attentional lens." *J. Abnorm. Psychol. 103,* 535–543.

17. Dunn, M. (1994) "Neurophysiologic observations in autism and their implications for neurologic dysfunction." In M. Bauman and T.L. Kemper (eds) *The Neurobiology of Autism.* Baltimore: Johns Hopkins University Press; pp.45–65.

18. Goldstein, G., Johnson, C.R. and Minshew, N.J. (2001) "Attentional processes in autism." *J. Autism Dev. Disord. 31,* 433–440.

19. Belmonte, M.K. and Yurgelun-Todd, D.A. (2003) "Functional anatomy of impaired selective attention and compensatory processing in autism." *Brain Res. Cogn. Brain Res. 17,* 651–664.

20. Grastyan, E. and Buzsaki, G. (1979) "The orienting-exploratory response hypothesis of discriminative conditioning." *Acta Neurobiol. Exp. (Wars.) 39,* 491–501.

21. Shors, T.J. and Matzel, L.D. (1997) "Long-term potentiation: what's learning got to do with it?" *Behav. Brain Sci. 20,* 597–614.

22. Minshew, N.J. and Goldstein, G. (2001) "The pattern of intact and impaired memory functions in autism." *J. Child Psychol. Psychiatry 42,* 1095–1101.

23. Williams, D.L., Goldstein, G. and Minshew, N.J. (2005) "Impaired memory for faces and social scenes in autism: clinical implications of memory dysfunction." *Arch. Clin. Neuropsychol. 20,* 1–15.

24. Salmond, C.H., Ashburner, J., Connelly, A., Friston, K.J., Gadian, D.G. and Vargha-Khadem, F. (2005) "The role of the medial temporal lobe in autistic spectrum disorders." *Eur. J. Neurosci. 22,* 764–772.

25. Morris, R.G.M. and Frey, U. (1997) "Hippocampal synaptic plasticity: role in spatial learning or the automatic recording of attended experience?" *Phil. Trans. R. Soc. Lond. 352*, 1489–1503.

26. Morris, R.G. (2001) "Episodic-like memory in animals: psychological criteria, neural mechanisms and the value of episodic-like tasks to investigate animal models of neurodegenerative disease." *Philos. Trans. R. Soc. Lond. B. Biol. Sci. 356*, 1453–1465.

27. Chen, G., Chen, K.S., Knox, J., Inglis, J., Bernard, A., Martin, S.J. *et al.* (2000) "A learning deficit related to age and beta-amyloid plaques in a mouse model of Alzheimer's disease." *Nature 408*, 975–979.

28. Lidsky, T.I. and Schneider, J.S. (2005) "Autism and autistic symptoms associated with childhood lead poisoning." *J. Appl. Res. 5*, 80–87.

29. Lainhart, J.E. and Folstein, S.E. (1994) "Affective disorders in people with autism: a review of published cases." *J. Autism Dev. Disord. 24*, 587–601.

30. Gillberg, C. and Billstedt, E. (2000) "Autism and Asperger syndrome: coexistence with other clinical disorders." *Acta Psychiatr. Scand. 102*, 321–330.

31. Muris, P., Steerneman, P., Merckelbach, H., Holdrinet, I. and Meesters, C. (1998) "Comorbid anxiety symptoms in children with pervasive developmental disorders." *J. Anxiety Disord. 12*, 387–393.

32. Weisbrot, D.M., Gadow, K.D., DeVincent, C.J. and Pomeroy, J. (2005) "The presentation of anxiety in children with pervasive developmental disorders." *J. Child Adolesc. Psychopharmacol. 15*, 477–496.

33. Gray, J.A. (1982) *The Neuropsychology of Anxiety: An Enquiry into the Functions of the Septo-Hippocampal System.* Oxford: Oxford University Press.

34. Gray, J.A. and McNaughton, N. (2000) *The Neuropsychology of Anxiety: An Enquiry into the Functions of the Septo-Hippocampal System.* Oxford: Oxford University Press.

35. Jackson, W.J. (1984) "Regional hippocampal lesions alter matching by monkeys: an anorexiant effect." *Physiol. Behav. 32*, 593–601.

36. Davidson, R.J., Pizzagalli, D., Nitschke, J.B. and Putnam, K. (2002) "Depression: perspectives from affective neuroscience." *Annu. Rev. Psychol. 53*, 545–574.

37. Ploghaus, A., Narain, C., Beckmann, C.F., Clare, S., Bantick, S., Wise, R. *et al.* (2001) "Exacerbation of pain by anxiety is associated with activity in a hippocampal network." *J. Neurosci. 21*, 9896–9903.

38. Prather, M.D., Lavenex, P., Mauldin-Jourdain, M.L., Mason, W.A., Capitanio, J.P., Mendoza, S.P. *et al.* (2001) "Increased social fear and decreased fear of objects in monkeys with neonatal amygdala lesions." *Neuroscience 106*, 653–658.

39. Kalin, N.H., Shelton, S.E. and Davidson, R.J. (2004) "The role of the central nucleus of the amygdala in mediating fear and anxiety in the primate." *J. Neurosci. 24*, 5506–5515.

40. Kanner, L. (1943) "Autistic disturbances of affective contact." *Nervous Child 2*, 217–250.

41. Rutter, M. (1978) "Diagnosis and definition of childhood autism." *J. Autism Child Schizophr. 8*, 139–161.

42. Klüver, H. (1965) "Neurobiology of normal and abnormal perception." In P.C. Hoch and J. Zubin (eds) *Psychopathology of Perception.* pp.1–40. New York: Grune and Stratton.

43. Douglas, R.J. and Isaacson, R.L. (1964) "Hippocampal lesions and activity." *Psychonomic Sci. 1*, 187–188.

44. Vinogradova, O.S. (1975) "Functional organization of the limbic system in the process of registration of information: facts and hypotheses." In R.L. Isaacson and K.H. Pribram (eds) *The Hippocampus, Vol. 2: Neurophysiology and Behavior.* New York: Plenum; pp.3–69.

45. Davis, M. (1992) "The role of the amygdala in fear-potentiated startle: implications for animal models of anxiety." *Trends Pharmacol. Sci. 13*, 35–41.

46. Pribram, K.H. (1971) *Languages of the Brain: Experimental Paradoxes and Principles in Neuropsychology.* New Jersey: Prentice-Hall.

47. Kaufman, B.N. (1995) *Son-Rise: The Miracle Continues.* Tiburon, CA: H.J. Kramer Press.

48. Hobson, R.P. (1986) "The autistic child's appraisal of expressions of emotion: a further study." *J. Child Psychol. Psychiatry 27*, 671–680.

49. Hobson, R.P., Ouston, J. and Lee, A. (1988) "What's in a face? The case of autism." *Br. J. Psychol. 79*, Pt 4, 441–453.

50. Blair, R.J. (2003) "Facial expressions, their communicatory functions and neuro-cognitive substrates." *Philos. Trans. R. Soc. Lond. B. Biol. Sci. 358*, 561–572.

51. Zola-Morgan, S., Squire, L.R., Rempel, N.L., Clower, R.P. and Amaral, D.G. (1992) "Enduring memory impairment in monkeys after ischemic damage to the hippocampus." *J. Neurosci. 12*, 2582–2596.

52. Keane, J., Calder, A.J., Hodges, J.R. and Young, A.W. (2002) "Face and emotion processing in frontal variant frontotemporal dementia." *Neuropsychologia 40,* 655–665.

53. Rosen, H.J., Perry, R.J., Murphy, J., Kramer, J.H., Mychack, P., Schuff, N. *et al.* (2002) "Emotion comprehension in the temporal variant of frontotemporal dementia." *Brain 125,* 2286–2295.

54. Rosen, H.J., Pace-Savitsky, K., Perry, R.J., Kramer, J.H., Miller, B.L. and Levenson, R.W. (2004) "Recognition of emotion in the frontal and temporal variants of frontotemporal dementia." *Dement. Geriatr. Cogn. Disord. 17,* 277–281.

55. Frisoni, G.B., Beltramello, A., Geroldi, C., Weiss, C., Bianchetti, A. and Trabucchi, M. (1996) "Brain atrophy in frontotemporal dementia." *J. Neurol. Neurosurg. Psychiatry 61,* 157–165.

56. Laakso, M.P., Frisoni, G.B., Kononen, M., Mikkonen, M., Beltramello, A., Geroldi, C. *et al.* (2000) "Hippocampus and entorhinal cortex in frontotemporal dementia and Alzheimer's disease: a morphometric MRI study." *Biol. Psychiatry 47,* 1056–1063.

57. Hatanpaa, K.J., Blass, D.M., Pletnikova, O., Crain, B.J., Bigio, E.H., Hedreen, J.C. *et al.* (2004) "Most cases of dementia with hippocampal sclerosis may represent frontotemporal dementia." *Neurology 63,* 538–542.

58. Hall, J., Harris, J.M., Sprengelmeyer, R., Sprengelmeyer, A., Young, A.W., Santos, I.M. *et al.* (2004) "Social cognition and face processing in schizophrenia." *Br. J. Psychiatry 185,* 169–170.

59. Harrison, P.J. (2004) "The hippocampus in schizophrenia: a review of the neuropathological evidence and its pathophysiological implications." *Psychopharmacology (Berl.) 174,* 151–162.

60. Schmajuk, N.A. (2001) "Hippocampal dysfunction in schizophrenia." *Hippocampus 11,* 599–613.

61. Lawrie, S.M., Whalley, H.C., Job, D.E. and Johnstone, E.C. (2003) "Structural and functional abnormalities of the amygdala in schizophrenia." *Ann. NY Acad. Sci. 985,* 445–460.

62. Voeller, K.K. (1995) "Clinical neurologic aspects of the right-hemisphere deficit syndrome." *J. Child Neurol. 10,* Suppl 1, S16–S22.

63. Emery, N.J. (2000) "The eyes have it: the neuroethology, function and evolution of social gaze." *Neurosci. Biobehav. Rev. 24,* 581–604.

64. Klin, A., Jones, W., Schultz, R., Volkmar, F. and Cohen, D. (2002) "Defining and quantifying the social phenotype in autism." *Am. J. Psychiatry 159,* 895–908.

65. Adolphs, R., Tranel, D. and Damasio, A.R. (1998) "The human amygdala in social judgment." *Nature 393,* 470–474.

66. Kimble, D.P. (1963) "The effects of bilateral hippocampal lesions in rats." *J. Comp. Physiol. Psychol. 56,* 273–283.

67. Maaswinkel, H., Baars, A.M., Gispen, W.H. and Spruijt, B.M. (1996) "Roles of the basolateral amygdala and hippocampus in social recognition in rats." *Physiol. Behav. 60,* 55–63.

68. Sams-Dodd, F., Lipska, B.K. and Weinberger, D.R. (1997) "Neonatal lesions of the rat ventral hippocampus result in hyperlocomotion and deficits in social behaviour in adulthood." *Psychopharmacology (Berl.) 132,* 303–310.

69. Becker, A., Grecksch, G., Bernstein, H.G., Hollt, V. and Bogerts, B. (1999) "Social behaviour in rats lesioned with ibotenic acid in the hippocampus: quantitative and qualitative analysis." *Psychopharmacology (Berl.) 144,* 333–338.

70. Bannerman, D.M., Lemaire, M., Beggs, S., Rawlins, J.N. and Iversen, S.D. (2001) "Cytotoxic lesions of the hippocampus increase social investigation but do not impair social-recognition memory." *Exp. Brain Res. 138,* 100–109.

71. Beauregard, M., Malkova, L. and Bachevalier, J. (1995) "Stereotypies and loss of social affiliation after early hippocampectomy in primates." *Neuroreport 6,* 2521–2526.

72. Wolterink, G., Daenen, L.E., Dubbeldam, S., Gerrits, M.A., van Rijn, R., Kruse, C.G. *et al.* (2001) "Early amygdala damage in the rat as a model for neurodevelopmental psychopathological disorders." *Eur. Neuropsychopharmacol. 11,* 51–59.

73. Beauregard, M. and Bachevalier, J. (1996) "Neonatal insult to the hippocampal region and schizophrenia: a review and a putative animal model." *Can. J. Psychiatry 41,* 446–456.

74. Amaral, D.G. (2002) "The primate amygdala and the neurobiology of social behavior: implications for understanding social anxiety." *Biol. Psychiatry 51,* 11–17.

75. Bachevalier, J. (1994) "Medial temporal lobe structures and autism: a review of clinical and experimental findings." *Neuropsychologia 32,* 627–648.

76. Bachevalier, J. (1996) "Brief report: medial temporal lobe and autism: a putative animal model in primates." *J. Autism Dev. Disord. 26*, 217–220.

77. Hippler, K. and Klicpera, C. (2003) "A retrospective analysis of the clinical case records of 'autistic psychopaths' diagnosed by Hans Asperger and his team at the University Children's Hospital, Vienna." *Philos. Trans. R. Soc. Lond. B. Biol. Sci. 358*, 291–301.

78. Dlugos, D.J., Moss, E.M., Duhaime, A.C. and Brooks-Kayal, A.R. (1999) "Language-related cognitive declines after left temporal lobectomy in children." *Pediatr. Neurol. 21*, 444–449.

79. Lord, C., Cook, E.H., Leventhal, B.L. and Amaral, D.G. (2000) "Autism spectrum disorders." *Neuron 28*, 355–363.

80. Schmolck, H., Stefanacci, L. and Squire, L.R. (2000) "Detection and explanation of sentence ambiguity are unaffected by hippocampal lesions but are impaired by larger temporal lobe lesions." *Hippocampus 10*, 759–770.

81. Schmolck, H., Kensinger, E.A., Corkin, S. and Squire, L.R. (2002) "Semantic knowledge in patient HM and other patients with bilateral medial and lateral temporal lobe lesions." *Hippocampus 12*, 520–533.

82. Bartha, L., Trinka, E., Ortler, M., Donnemiller, E., Felber, S., Bauer, G. *et al.* (2004) "Linguistic deficits following left selective amygdalohippocampectomy: a prospective study." *Epilepsy Behav. 5*, 348–357.

83. Dawson, G., Webb, S., Schellenberg, G.D., Dager, S., Friedman, S., Aylward, E. *et al.* (2002) "Defining the broader phenotype of autism: genetic, brain, and behavioral perspectives." *Dev. Psychopathol. 14*, 581–611.

84. Tuchman, R. and Rapin, I. (2002) "Epilepsy in autism." *Lancet Neurol. 1*, 352–358.

85. Kielinen, M., Rantala, H., Timonen, E., Linna, S.L. and Moilanen, I. (2004) "Associated medical disorders and disabilities in children with autistic disorder: a population-based study." *Autism 8*, 49–60.

86. Canitano, R., Luchetti, A. and Zappella, M. (2005) "Epilepsy, electroencephalographic abnormalities, and regression in children with autism." *J. Child Neurol. 20*, 27–31.

87. Hughes, J.R. and Melyn, M. (2005) "EEG and seizures in autistic children and adolescents: further findings with therapeutic implications." *Clin. EEG Neurosci. 36*, 15–20.

88. Small, J.G. (1975) "EEG and neurophysiological studies of early infantile autism." *Biol. Psychiatry 10*, 385–397.

89. Rossi, P.G., Parmeggiani, A., Bach, V., Santucci, M. and Visconti, P. (1995) "EEG features and epilepsy in patients with autism." *Brain Dev. 17*, 169–174.

90. Kawasaki, Y., Yokota, K., Shinomiya, M., Shimizu, Y. and Niwa, S. (1997) "Brief report: electroencephalographic paroxysmal activities in the frontal area emerged in middle childhood and during adolescence in a follow-up study of autism." *J. Autism Dev. Disord. 27*, 605–620.

91. Ballaban-Gil, K. and Tuchman, R. (2000) "Epilepsy and epileptiform EEG: association with autism and language disorders." *Ment. Retard. Dev. Disabil. Res. Rev. 6*, 300–308.

92. Tuchman, R.F. and Rapin, I. (1997) "Regression in pervasive developmental disorders: seizures and epileptiform electroencephalogram correlates." *Pediatrics 99*, 560–566.

93. McDermott, S., Moran, R., Platt, T., Wood, H., Isaac, T. and Dasari, S. (2005) "Prevalence of epilepsy in adults with mental retardation and related disabilities in primary care." *Am. J. Ment. Retard. 110*, 48–56.

94. Danielsson, S., Gillberg, I.C., Billstedt, E., Gillberg, C. and Olsson, I. (2005) "Epilepsy in young adults with autism: a prospective population-based follow-up study of 120 individuals diagnosed in childhood." *Epilepsia 46*, 918–923.

95. Gastaut, H. (1970) "Clinical and electroencephalographical classification of epileptic seizures." *Epilepsia 11*, 102–113.

96. Fried, I. (1993) "Anatomic temporal lobe resections for temporal lobe epilepsy." *Neurosurg. Clin. N. Am. 4*, 233–242.

97. Lothman, E.W., Stringer, J.L. and Bertram, E.H. (1992) "The dentate gyrus as a control point for seizures in the hippocampus and beyond." *Epilepsy Res. Suppl. 7*, 301–313.

98. Carvill, S. (2001) "Sensory impairments, intellectual disability and psychiatry." *J. Intellect. Disabil. Res. 45*, 467–483.

99. Novick, B., Vaughan, H.G., Jr., Kurtzberg, D. and Simson, R. (1980) "An electrophysiologic indication of auditory processing defects in autism." *Psychiatry Res. 3*, 107–114.

100. Khalfa, S., Bruneau, N., Roge, B., Georgieff, N., Veuillet, E., Adrien, J.L. *et al.* (2004) "Increased perception of loudness in autism." *Hear. Res. 198*, 87–92.

101. Tordjman, S., Antoine, C., Cohen, D.J., Gauvain-Piquard, A., Carlier, M., Roubertoux, P. *et al.* (1999) "Study of the relationships between self-injurious behavior and pain reactivity in infantile autism." *Encephale 25*, 122–134.

102. Hauser, S.L., DeLong, G.R. and Rosman, N.P. (1975) "Pneumographic findings in the infantile autism syndrome. A correlation with temporal lobe disease." *Brain 98*, 667–688.

103. Klüver, H. and Bucy, P.C. (1939) "Preliminary analysis of functions of the temporal lobe in monkeys." *Arch. Neurol. Psychiatry 42*, 979–1000.

104. Hebben, N., Corkin, S., Eichenbaum, H. and Shedlack, K. (1985) "Diminished ability to interpret and report internal states after bilateral medial temporal resection: case HM." *Behav. Neurosci. 99*, 1031–1039.

105. Clifton, P.G., Vickers, S.P. and Somerville, E.M. (1998) "Little and often: ingestive behaviour patterns following hippocampal lesions in rats." *Behav. Neurosci. 112*, 502–511.

106. Osborne, B. and Dodek, A.B. (1986) "Disrupted patterns of consummatory behavior in rats with fornix transections." *Behav. Neural Biol. 45*, 212–222.

107. Osborne, B. and Flashman, L.A. (1986) "Meal patterns following changes in procurement cost for rats with fornix transection." *Behav. Neural Biol. 46*, 123–136.

108. Terzian, H. and Dalle Ore, G. (1955) "Syndrome of Klüver and Bucy reproduced in man by bilateral removal of the temporal lobes." *Neurology 5*, 373–380.

109. Overman, W.H. (1991) "Performance on traditional match-to-sample and non-match to sample, and object recognition tasks, by 12- and 32-month old children: a developmental progression." In A. Diamond (ed) *Developmental and Neural Basis of Higher Cognitive Function.* New York: New York Academy of Sciences; pp.365–393.

110. Fitzgerald, J.M. (1991) "A developmental account of early childhood amnesia." *J. Genet. Psychol. 152*, 159–171.

111. Douglas, R.J. (1975) "The development of hippocampal function: implications for theory and for therapy." In R.L. Isaacson and K.H. Pribram (eds) *The Hippocampus, Vol. 2, Neurophysiology and Behavior.* New York: Plenum; pp.327–361.

112. Wen, X., Fuhrman, S., Michaels, G.S., Carr, D.B., Smith, S., Barker, J.L. *et al.* (1998) "Large-scale temporal gene expression mapping of central nervous system development." *Proc. Natl. Acad. Sci. USA 95*, 334–339.

113. Wakefield, A.J., Murch, S.H., Anthony, A., Linnell, J., Casson, D.M., Malik, M. *et al.* (1998) "Ileal-lymphoid-nodular hyperplasia, non-specific colitis, and pervasive developmental disorder in children." *Lancet 351*, 637–641.

114. Amaral, D.G., Bauman, M.D. and Schumann, C.M. (2003) "The amygdala and autism: implications from non-human primate studies." *Genes Brain Behav. 2*, 295–302.

115. DeLong, G.R. and Heinz, E.R. (1997) "The clinical syndrome of early-life bilateral hippocampal sclerosis." *Ann. Neurol. 42*, 11–17.

116. Lathe, R. (2001) "Hormones and the hippocampus." *J. Endocrinol. 169*, 205–231.

117. Kates, W.R., Mostofsky, S.H., Zimmerman, A.W., Mazzocco, M.M., Landa, R., Warsofsky, I.S. *et al.* (1998) "Neuroanatomical and neurocognitive differences in a pair of monozygous twins discordant for strictly defined autism." *Ann. Neurol. 43*, 782–791.

118. Gendry, M.I., Zilbovicius, M., Boddaert, N., Robel, L., Philippe, A., Sfaello, I. *et al.* (2005) "Autism severity and temporal lobe functional abnormalities." *Ann. Neurol. 58*, 466–469.

119. Bolton, P.F. and Griffiths, P.D. (1997) "Association of tuberous sclerosis of temporal lobes with autism and atypical autism." *Lancet 349*, 392–395.

120. Chugani, H.T., Da Silva, E. and Chugani, D.C. (1996) "Infantile spasms: III. Prognostic implications of bitemporal hypometabolism on positron emission tomography." *Ann. Neurol. 39*, 643–649.

121. Bachevalier, J. and Merjanian, P.M. (1994) "The contribution of medial temporal lobe structures in infantile autism: a neurobehavioral study in primates." In M. Bauman and T.L. Kemper (eds) *The Neurobiology of Autism.* Baltimore: Johns Hopkins University Press; pp.146–169.

122. Tulving, D. (1972) "Episodic and semantic memory." In E. Tulving and W. Donaldson (eds) *The Organization of Memory.* pp.381–403. New York: Academic Press.

123. Benton, A. (2000) *Exploring the History of Neuropsychology.* Oxford: Oxford University Press.

124. Kertesz, A. and Munoz, D.G. (1997) "Primary progressive aphasia." *Clin. Neurosci. 4*, 95–102.

125. Assal, F. and Cummings, J.L. (2002) "Neuropsychiatric symptoms in the dementias." *Curr. Opin. Neurol. 15*, 445–450.

126. Lavenu, I., Pasquier, F., Lebert, F., Petit, H. and Van der, L.M. (1999) "Perception of emotion in frontotemporal dementia and Alzheimer disease." *Alzheimer Dis. Assoc. Disord. 13*, 96–101.

127. Armstrong, R.A., Cairns, N.J. and Lantos, P.L. (1999) "Quantification of pathological lesions in the frontal and temporal lobe of ten patients diagnosed with Pick's disease." *Acta Neuropathol. (Berl.) 97*, 456–462.

128. Dickson, D.W. (1998) "Pick's disease: a modern approach." *Brain Pathol. 8*, 339–354.

129. Alzheimer's Association (1999) *Understanding Early-stage Alzheimer's Disease: A Guide for Health Care Professionals.* Chicago, IL: Alzheimer's Association.

130. Grossman, M. (2002) "Progressive aphasic syndromes: clinical and theoretical advances." *Curr. Opin. Neurol. 15*, 409–413.

131. Davidson, P.W., Willoughby, R.H., O'Tuama, L.A., Swisher, C.N. and Benjamins, D. (1978) "Neurological and intellectual sequelae of Reye's syndrome." *Am. J. Ment. Defic. 82*, 535–541.

132. DeLong, G.R., Bean, S.C. and Brown, F.R., III (1981) "Acquired reversible autistic syndrome in acute encephalopathic illness in children." *Arch. Neurol. 38*, 191–194.

133. Quart, E.J., Buchtel, H.A. and Sarnaik, A.P. (1988) "Long-lasting memory deficits in children recovered from Reye's syndrome." *J. Clin. Exp. Neuropsychol. 10*, 409–420.

134. Pearl, P.L., Carrazana, E.J. and Holmes, G.L. (2001) "The Landau-Kleffner Syndrome." *Epilepsy Curr. 1*, 39–45.

135. Glasgow, J.F. and Middleton, B. (2001) "Reye syndrome – insights on causation and prognosis." *Arch. Dis. Child 85*, 351–353.

136. Blass, D.M., Hatanpaa, K.J., Brandt, J., Rao, V., Steinberg, M., Troncoso, J.C. *et al.* (2004) "Dementia in hippocampal sclerosis resembles frontotemporal dementia more than Alzheimer disease." *Neurology 63*, 492–497.

137. Lanska, D.J. and Lanska, M.J. (1994) "Klüver-Bucy syndrome in juvenile neuronal ceroid lipofuscinosis." *J. Child Neurol. 9*, 67–69.

Chapter 7 Environmental Factors, Heavy Metals, and Brain Function

1. Deb, S. and Prasad, K.B. (1994) "The prevalence of autistic disorder among children with a learning disability." *Br. J. Psychiatry 165*, 395–399.

2. Palmer, R.F., Blanchard, S., Stein, Z., Mandell, D. and Miller, C. (2006) "Environmental mercury release, special education rates, and autism disorder: an ecological study of Texas." *Health & Place 12*, 203–209.

3. Gillberg, C. (1980) "Maternal age and infantile autism." *J. Autism Dev. Disord. 10*, 293–297.

4. Hultman, C.M., Sparen, P. and Cnattingius, S. (2002) "Perinatal risk factors for infantile autism." *Epidemiology 13*, 417–423.

5. Stromland, K., Nordin, V., Miller, M., Akerstrom, B. and Gillberg, C. (1994) "Autism in thalidomide embryopathy: a population study." *Dev. Med. Child Neurol. 36*, 351–356.

6. Nanson, J.L. (1992) "Autism in fetal alcohol syndrome: a report of six cases." *Alcohol Clin. Exp. Res. 16*, 558–565.

7. Harris, S.R., MacKay, L.L. and Osborn, J.A. (1995) "Autistic behaviors in offspring of mothers abusing alcohol and other drugs: a series of case reports." *Alcohol Clin. Exp. Res. 19*, 660–665.

8. Fombonne, E. (2002) "Is exposure to alcohol during pregnancy a risk factor for autism?" *J. Autism Dev. Disord. 32*, 243.

9. Davis, E., Fennoy, I., Laraque, D., Kanem, N., Brown, G. and Mitchell, J. (1992) "Autism and developmental abnormalities in children with perinatal cocaine exposure." *J. Natl. Med. Assoc. 84*, 315–319.

10. Moore, S.J., Turnpenny, P., Quinn, A., Glover, S., Lloyd, D.J., Montgomery, T. *et al.* (2000) "A clinical study of 57 children with fetal anticonvulsant syndromes." *J. Med. Genet. 37*, 489–497.

11. Schneider, T. and Przewlocki, R. (2005) "Behavioral alterations in rats prenatally exposed to valproic acid: animal model of autism." *Neuropsychopharmacology 30*, 80–89.

12. Hightower, J.M. and Moore, D. (2003) "Mercury levels in high-end consumers of fish." *Environ. Health Perspect. 111*, 604–608.

13. Carlsen, E., Giwercman, A., Keiding, N. and Skakkebaek, N.E. (1992) "Evidence for decreasing quality of semen during past 50 years." *Brit. Med. J. 305*, 609–613.

14. Swan, S.H., Elkin, E.P. and Fenster, L. (2000) "The question of declining sperm density revisited: an analysis of 101 studies published 1934–1996." *Environ. Health Perspect. 108*, 961–966.

15. Telisman, S., Cvitkovic, P., Jurasovic, J., Pizent, A., Gavella, M. and Rocic, B. (2000) "Semen quality and reproductive endocrine function in relation to biomarkers of lead, cadmium, zinc, and copper in men." *Environ. Health Perspect. 108*, 45–53.

16. Cohen, D.J., Johnson, W.T. and Caparulo, B.K. (1976) "Pica and elevated blood lead level in autistic and atypical children." *Am. J. Dis. Child. 130*, 47–48.

17. Cohen, D.J., Paul, R., Anderson, G.M. and Harcherik, D.F. (1982) "Blood lead in autistic children." *Lancet 2*, 94–95.

18. Shearer, T.R., Larson, K., Neuschwander, J. and Gedney, B. (1982) "Minerals in the hair and nutrient intake of autistic children." *J. Autism Dev. Disord. 12*, 25–34.

19. Bithoney, W.G. (1986) "Elevated lead levels in children with nonorganic failure to thrive." *Pediatrics 78*, 891–895.

20. Accardo, P., Whitman, B., Caul, J. and Rolfe, U. (1988) "Autism and plumbism. A possible association." *Clin. Pediatr. (Phila.) 27*, 41–44.

21. Shannon, M.W. and Graef, J.W. (1992) "Lead intoxication in infancy." *Pediatrics 89*, 87–90.

22. Shannon, M. and Graef, J.W. (1996) "Lead intoxication in children with pervasive developmental disorders." *J. Toxicol. Clin. Toxicol. 34*, 177–181.

23. Eppright, T.D., Sanfacon, J.A. and Horwitz, E.A. (1996) "Attention deficit hyperactivity disorder, infantile autism, and elevated blood-lead: a possible relationship." *Missouri Med. 93*, 136–138.

24. Kumar, A., Dey, P.K., Singla, P.N., Ambasht, R.S. and Upadhyay, S.K. (1998) "Blood lead levels in children with neurological disorders." *J. Trop. Pediatr. 44*, 320–322.

25. Coltman, C.A., Jr. (1969) "Pagophagia and iron lack." *J. Am. Med. Assoc. 207*, 513–516.

26. Denton, D. (1982) *The Hunger for Salt.* Berlin: Springer.

27. Baldwin, D.R. and Marshall, W.J. (1999) "Heavy metal poisoning and its laboratory investigation." *Ann. Clin. Biochem. 36 (Pt 3)*, 267–300.

28. Lidsky, T.I. and Schneider, J.S. (2005) "Autism and autistic symptoms associated with childhood lead poisoning." *J. Appl. Res. 5*, 80–87.

29. Hallaway, N. and Strauts, Z. (1995) *Turning Lead into Gold: How Heavy Metal Poisoning Can Affect Your Child and How to Prevent and Treat It.* Vancouver: New Start.

30. Bernard, S., Enayati, A., Redwood, L., Roger, H. and Binstock, T. (2001) "Autism: a novel form of mercury poisoning." *Med. Hypotheses 56*, 462–471.

31. Farris, F.F., Dedrick, R.L., Allen, P.V. and Smith, J.C. (1993) "Physiological model for the pharmacokinetics of methyl mercury in the growing rat." *Toxicol. Appl. Pharmacol. 119*, 74–90.

32. Suzuki, T., Hongo, T., Yoshinaga, J., Imai, H., Nakazawa, M., Matsuo, N. *et al.* (1993) "The hair–organ relationship in mercury concentration in contemporary Japanese." *Arch. Environ. Health 48*, 221–229.

33. Wecker, L., Miller, S.B., Cochran, S.R., Dugger, D.L. and Johnson, W.D. (1985) "Trace element concentrations in hair from autistic children." *J. Ment. Defic. Res. 29 (Pt 1)*, 15–22.

34. Ip, P., Wong, V., Ho, M., Lee, J. and Wong, W. (2004) "Mercury exposure in children with autistic spectrum disorder: case-control study." *J. Child Neurol. 19*, 431–434.

35. Fido, A. and Al Saad, S. (2005) "Toxic trace elements in the hair of children with autism." *Autism 9*, 290–298.

36. Audhya, T. (2004) "Nutritional intervention in autism." *Proc. Autism 1. Conf. June 28.* Online at: http://www.fltwood.com/onsite/autism/2004/03.shtml

37. Adams, J.B., Romdalvik, J., Ramanujam, V.M.S. and Legator, M. (2003) "Research programs: current projects. Baby tooth study." *Autism/Asperger's Research Program at Arizona State University.* http://www.eas.asu.edu/~autism/Research/Current.html

38. Gonzalez-Ramirez, D., Maiorino, R.M., Zuniga-Charles, M., Xu, Z., Hurlbut, K.M., Junco-Munoz, P. *et al.* (1995) "Sodium 2,3-dimercaptopropane-1-sulfonate challenge test for mercury in humans: II. Urinary

mercury, porphyrins and neurobehavioral changes of dental workers in Monterrey, Mexico." *J. Pharmacol. Exp. Ther. 272,* 264–274.

39. Woods, J.S., Martin, M.D., Naleway, C.A. and Echeverria, D. (1993) "Urinary porphyrin profiles as a biomarker of mercury exposure: studies on dentists with occupational exposure to mercury vapor." *J. Toxicol. Environ. Health 40,* 235–246.

40. Pingree, S.D., Simmonds, P.L., Rummel, K.T. and Woods, J.S. (2001) "Quantitative evaluation of urinary porphyrins as a measure of kidney mercury content and mercury body burden during prolonged methylmercury exposure in rats." *Toxicol. Sci. 61,* 234–240.

41. Rosen, J.F. and Markowitz, M.E. (1993) "Trends in the management of childhood lead poisonings." *Neurotoxicology 14,* 211–217.

42. Nataf, R., Skorupka, C., Amet, L., Lam, A., Springbett, A. and Lathe, R. (2005) "Porphyrinuria in child-hood autistic disorder." Submitted for publication.

43. Woods, J.S. (1996) "Altered porphyrin metabolism as a biomarker of mercury exposure and toxicity." *Can. J. Physiol. Pharmacol. 74,* 210–215.

44. Wang, J.P., Qi, L., Zheng, B., Liu, F., Moore, M.R. and Ng, J.C. (2002) "Porphyrins as early biomarkers for arsenic exposure in animals and humans." *Cell Mol. Biol. (Noisy.-le-grand) 48,* 835–843.

45. Marks, G.S., Zelt, D.T. and Cole, S.P. (1982) "Alterations in the heme biosynthetic pathway as an index of exposure to toxins." *Can. J. Physiol. Pharmacol. 60,* 1017–1026.

46. Hill, R.H. (1985) "Effects of polyhalogenated aromatic compounds on porphyrin metabolism." *Environ. Health Perspect. 60,* 139–143.

47. Holmes, A.S., Blaxill, M.F. and Haley, B.E. (2003) "Reduced levels of mercury in first baby haircuts of autistic children." *Int. J. Toxicol. 22,* 277–285.

48. Juul-Dam, N., Townsend, J. and Courchesne, E. (2001) "Prenatal, perinatal, and neonatal factors in autism, pervasive developmental disorder-not otherwise specified, and the general population." *Pediatrics 107,* E63.

49. Lonsdale, D., Shamberger, R.J. and Audhya, T. (2002) "Treatment of autism spectrum children with thiamine tetrahydrofurfuryl disulfide: a pilot study." *Neuroendocrinol. Lett. 23,* 303–308.

50. Bradstreet, J. (2003) "A case control study of mercury burden in children with autistic spectrum disor-ders." *J. Am. Phys. Surg. 8,* 76–79.

51. Holmes, A.S. (2003) *Chelation of Mercury for the Treatment of Autism.* http://www.healing-arts.org /children/holmes.htm

52. Myers, G.J., Davidson, P.W., Palumbo, D., Shamlaye, C., Cox, C., Cernichiari, E. *et al.* (2000) "Secondary analysis from the Seychelles Child Development Study: the child behavior checklist." *Environ. Res. 84,* 12–19.

53. Grandjean, P., Weihe, P. and White, R.F. (1995) "Milestone development in infants exposed to methylmercury from human milk." *Neurotoxicology 16,* 27–33.

54. Steuerwald, U., Weihe, P., Jorgensen, P.J., Bjerve, K., Brock, J., Heinzow, B. *et al.* (2000) "Maternal seafood diet, methylmercury exposure, and neonatal neurologic function." *J. Pediatr. 136,* 599–605.

55. Hu, L.-W., Bernard, J.A. and Che, J. (2003) "Neutron activation analysis of hair samples for the identifica-tion of autism." *Trans. Am. Nuclear Soc. 89,* 16–20.

56. Adams, J.B. and Romdalvik, J. (2004) *Arizona State University: Autism Baby Hair Study.* http://www .bridges4kids.org/articles/8-04/AZ7-04.html

57. Adams, J.B. (2004) "A review of the autism–mercury connection." Conference presentation, *Proc. Ann. Meeting Autism Soc. America.*

58. Grandjean, P., Jorgensen, P.J. and Weihe, P. (1994) "Human milk as a source of methylmercury exposure in infants." *Environ. Health Perspect. 102,* 74–77.

59. Brouwer, O.F., Onkenhout, W., Edelbroek, P.M., de Kom, J.F., de Wolff, F.A. and Peters, A.C. (1992) "Increased neurotoxicity of arsenic in methylenetetrahydrofolate reductase deficiency." *Clin. Neurol. Neurosurg. 94,* 307–310.

60. Kang, S.S., Zhou, J., Wong, P.W., Kowalisyn, J. and Strokosch, G. (1988) "Intermediate homocysteinemia: a thermolabile variant of methylenetetrahydrofolate reductase." *Am. J. Hum. Genet. 43,* 414–421.

61. Frosst, P., Blom, H.J., Milos, R., Goyette, P., Sheppard, C.A., Matthews, R.G. *et al.* (1995) "A candidate genetic risk factor for vascular disease: a common mutation in methylenetetrahydrofolate reductase." *Nat. Genet. 10,* 111–113.

62. Rozen, R. (1996) "Molecular genetics of methylenetetrahydrofolate reductase deficiency." *J. Inherit. Metab. Dis. 19*, 589–594.

63. Dean, J.C., Moore, S.J., Osborne, A., Howe, J. and Turnpenny, P.D. (1999) "Fetal anticonvulsant syndrome and mutation in the maternal MTHFR gene." *Clin. Genet. 56*, 216–220.

64. Boris, M., Goldblatt, A., Galanko, J. and James, S.J. (2004) "Association of MTHFR gene variants with autism." *J. Am. Phys. Surg. 9*, 106–108.

65. Walsh, T.J., Usman, A. and Tarpey, J. (2001) "Disordered metal metabolism in a large autism population." *Proc. Am. Psychol. Assoc. Conf. New Orleans.* http://www.hriptc.org/metal_autism.html

66. Serajee, F.J., Nabi, R., Zhong, H. and Huq, M. (2004) "Polymorphisms in xenobiotic metabolism genes and autism." *J. Child Neurol. 19*, 413–417.

67. Woods, J.S., Echeverria, D., Heyer, N.J., Simmonds, P.L., Wilkerson, J. and Farin, F.M. (2005) "The association between genetic polymorphisms of coproporphyrinogen oxidase and an atypical porphyrinogenic response to mercury exposure in humans." *Toxicol. Appl. Pharmacol. 206*, 113–120.

68. Brown, A.W., Aldridge, W.N., Street, B.W. and Verschoyle, R.D. (1979) "The behavioral and neuropathologic sequelae of intoxication by trimethyltin compounds in the rat." *Am. J. Pathol. 97*, 59–82.

69. Kutscher, C.L. (1992) "A morphometric analysis of trimethyltin-induced change in rat brain using the Timm technique." *Brain Res. Bull. 28*, 519–527.

70. Dyer, R.S., Deshields, T.L. and Wonderlin, W.F. (1982) "Trimethyltin-induced changes in gross morphology of the hippocampus." *Neurobehav. Toxicol. Teratol. 4*, 141–147.

71. Chang, L.W., Tiemeyer, T.M., Wenger, G.R. and McMillan, D.E. (1982) "Neuropathology of mouse hippocampus in acute trimethyltin intoxication." *Neurobehav. Toxicol. Teratol. 4*, 149–156.

72. Ruppert, P.H., Walsh, T.J., Reiter, L.W. and Dyer, R.S. (1982) "Trimethyltin-induced hyperactivity: time course and pattern." *Neurobehav. Toxicol. Teratol. 4*, 135–139.

73. Miller, D.B. and O'Callaghan, J.P. (1984) "Biochemical, functional and morphological indicators of neurotoxicity: effects of acute administration of trimethyltin to the developing rat." *J. Pharmacol. Exp. Ther. 231*, 744–751.

74. Paule, M.G., Reuhl, K., Chen, J.J., Ali, S.F. and Slikker, W., Jr. (1986) "Developmental toxicology of trimethyltin in the rat." *Toxicol. Appl. Pharmacol. 84*, 412–417.

75. Robertson, D.G., Gray, R.H. and de la Iglesia, F.A. (1987) "Quantitative assessment of trimethyltin induced pathology of the hippocampus." *Toxicol. Pathol. 15*, 7–17.

76. Ishida, N., Akaike, M., Tsutsumi, S., Kanai, H., Masui, A., Sadamatsu, M. *et al.* (1997) "Trimethyltin syndrome as a hippocampal degeneration model: temporal changes and neurochemical features of seizure susceptibility and learning impairment." *Neuroscience 81*, 1183–1191.

77. Tsunashima, K., Sadamatsu, M., Takahashi, Y., Kato, N. and Sperk, G. (1998) "Trimethyltin intoxication induces marked changes in neuropeptide expression in the rat hippocampus." *Synapse 29*, 333–342.

78. Fiedorowicz, A., Figiel, I., Kaminska, B., Zaremba, M., Wilk, S. and Oderfeld-Nowak, B. (2001) "Dentate granule neuron apoptosis and glia activation in murine hippocampus induced by trimethyltin exposure." *Brain Res. 912*, 116–127.

79. Bruccoleri, A., Pennypacker, K.R. and Harry, G.J. (1999) "Effect of dexamethasone on elevated cytokine mRNA levels in chemical-induced hippocampal injury." *J. Neurosci. Res. 57*, 916–926.

80. Bruccoleri, A., Brown, H. and Harry, G.J. (1998) "Cellular localization and temporal elevation of tumor necrosis factor-alpha, interleukin-1 alpha, and transforming growth factor-beta 1 mRNA in hippocampal injury response induced by trimethyltin." *J. Neurochem. 71*, 1577–1587.

81. Brown, A.W., Verschoyle, R.D., Street, B.W., Aldridge, W.N. and Grindley, H. (1984) "The neurotoxicity of trimethyltin chloride in hamsters, gerbils and marmosets." *J. Appl. Toxicol. 4*, 12–21.

82. Gozzo, S., Perretta, G., Monaco, V., Andreozzi, U. and Rossiello, E. (1993) "The neuropathology of trimethyltin in the marmoset (*Callithrix jacchus*) hippocampal formation." *Ecotoxicol. Environ. Saf. 26*, 293–301.

83. Rey, C., Reinecke, H.J. and Besser, R. (1984) "Methyltin intoxication in six men; toxicologic and clinical aspects." *Vet. Hum. Toxicol. 26*, 121–122.

84. Besser, R., Kramer, G., Thumler, R., Bohl, J., Gutmann, L. and Hopf, H.C. (1987) "Acute trimethyltin limbic-cerebellar syndrome." *Neurology 37*, 945–950.

85. van Heijst, A.N.P. (1993) "Trimethyltin compounds." *Int. Prog. Chem. Safety Group: Poisons Information Monograph G019.* http://www.inchem.org/documents/pims/chemical/pimg019.htm

86. Kreyberg, S., Torvik, A., Bjorneboe, A., Wiik-Larsen, W. and Jacobsen, D. (1992) "Trimethyltin poisoning: report of a case with postmortem examination." *Clin. Neuropathol. 11*, 256–259.

87. Aschner, M. and Aschner, J.L. (1992) "Cellular and molecular effects of trimethyltin and triethyltin: relevance to organotin neurotoxicity." *Neurosci. Biobehav. Rev. 16*, 427–435.

88. Thompson, T.A., Lewis, J.M., Dejneka, N.S., Severs, W.B., Polavarapu, R. and Billingsley, M.L. (1996) "Induction of apoptosis by organotin compounds in vitro: neuronal protection with antisense oligonucleotides directed against stannin." *J. Pharmacol. Exp. Ther. 276*, 1201–1216.

89. Doctor, S.V., Costa, L.G. and Murphy, S.D. (1982) "Effect of trimethyltin on chemically-induced seizures." *Toxicol. Lett. 13*, 217–223.

90. Wenger, G.R., McMillan, D.E. and Chang, L.W. (1984) "Behavioral effects of trimethyltin in two strains of mice. I. Spontaneous motor activity." *Toxicol. Appl. Pharmacol. 73*, 78–88.

91. Isaacson, R.L. (2002) "Unsolved mysteries: the hippocampus." *Behav. Cogn. Neurosci. Rev. 1*, 87–107.

92. Ishido, M., Masuo, Y., Oka, S., Kunimoto, M. and Morita, M. (2002) "Application of supermex system to screen behavioral traits produced by tributyltin in the rat." *J. Health Sci. 48*, 451–454.

93. Reiter, L.W. and Ruppert, P.H. (1984) "Behavioral toxicity of trialkyltin compounds: a review." *Neurotoxicology 5*, 177–186.

94. Reuhl, K.R. and Cranmer, J.M. (1984) "Developmental neuropathology of organotin compounds." *Neurotoxicology 5*, 187–204.

95. Chang, L.W. (1990) "The neurotoxicology and pathology of organomercury, organolead, and organotin." *J. Toxicol. Sci. 15*, Suppl 4, 125–151.

96. Koczyk, D. (1996) "How does trimethyltin affect the brain? Facts and hypotheses." *Acta Neurobiol. Exp. (Wars.) 56*, 587–596.

97. Swartzwelder, H.S., Holahan, W. and Myers, R.D. (1983) "Antagonism by d-amphetamine of trimethyltin-induced hyperactivity evidence toward an animal model of hyperkinetic behavior." *Neuropharmacology 22*, 1049–1054.

98. Young, J.S. and Fechter, L.D. (1986) "Trimethyltin exposure produces an unusual form of toxic auditory damage in rats." *Toxicol. Appl. Pharmacol. 82*, 87–93.

99. Eastman, C.L., Young, J.S. and Fechter, L.D. (1987) "Trimethyltin ototoxicity in albino rats." *Neurotoxicol. Teratol. 9*, 329–332.

100. Hoeffding, V. and Fechter, L.D. (1991) "Trimethyltin disrupts auditory function and cochlear morphology in pigmented rats." *Neurotoxicol. Teratol. 13*, 135–145.

101. Tang, X.J., Lai, G.C., Huang, J.X., Li, L.Y., Deng, Y.Y., Yue, F. *et al.* (2002) "Studies on hypokalemia induced by trimethyltin chloride." *Biomed. Environ. Sci. 15*, 16–24.

102. Chang, L.W. (1984) "Hippocampal lesions induced by trimethyltin in the neonatal rat brain." *Neurotoxicology 5*, 205–215.

103. Swartzwelder, H.S., Dyer, R.S., Holahan, W. and Myers, R.D. (1981) "Activity changes in rats following acute trimethyltin exposure." *Neurotoxicology 2*, 589–593.

104. Miller, D.B., Eckerman, D.A., Krigman, M.R. and Grant, L.D. (1982) "Chronic neonatal organotin exposure alters radial-arm maze performance in adult rats." *Neurobehav. Toxicol. Teratol. 4*, 185–190.

105. Walsh, T.J., Gallagher, M., Bostock, E. and Dyer, R.S. (1982) "Trimethyltin impairs retention of a passive avoidance task." *Neurobehav. Toxicol. Teratol. 4*, 163–167.

106. Messing, R.B., Bollweg, G., Chen, Q. and Sparber, S.B. (1988) "Dose-specific effects of trimethyltin poisoning on learning and hippocampal corticosterone binding." *Neurotoxicology 9*, 491–502.

107. Walsh, T.J., McLamb, R.L. and Tilson, H.A. (1984) "Organometal-induced antinociception: a time- and dose-response comparison of triethyl and trimethyl lead and tin." *Toxicol. Appl. Pharmacol. 73*, 295–299.

108. Dyer, R.S., Wonderlin, W.F. and Walsh, T.J. (1982) "Increased seizure susceptibility following trimethyltin administration in rats." *Neurobehav. Toxicol. Teratol. 4*, 203–208.

109. Sloviter, R.S., von Knebel, D.C., Walsh, T.J. and Dempster, D.W. (1986) "On the role of seizure activity in the hippocampal damage produced by trimethyltin." *Brain Res. 367*, 169–182.

110. Johnson, C.T., Dunn, A.R. and Swartzwelder, H.S. (1984) "Disruption of learned and spontaneous alternation in the rat by trimethyltin: chronic effects." *Neurobehav. Toxicol. Teratol. 6*, 337–340.

111. Stanton, M.E., Jensen, K.F. and Pickens, C.V. (1991) "Neonatal exposure to trimethyltin disrupts spatial delayed alternation learning in preweanling rats." *Neurotoxicol. Teratol. 13*, 525–530.

112. Dyer, R.S., Howell, W.E. and Wonderlin, W.F. (1982) "Visual system dysfunction following acute trimethyltin exposure in rats." *Neurobehav. Toxicol. Teratol. 4,* 191–195.

113. Yanofsky, N.N., Nierenberg, D. and Turco, J.H. (1991) "Acute short-term memory loss from trimethyltin exposure." *J. Emerg. Med. 9,* 137–139.

114. Gale, N.L., Adams, C.D., Wixson, B.G., Loftin, K.A. and Huang, Y.W. (2002) "Lead concentrations in fish and river sediments in the old lead belt of Missouri." *Environ. Sci. Technol. 36,* 4262–4268.

115. Petit, T.L., Alfano, D.P. and LeBoutillier, J.C. (1983) "Early lead exposure and the hippocampus: a review and recent advances." *Neurotoxicology 4,* 79–94.

116. Munoz, C., Garbe, K., Lilienthal, H. and Winneke, G. (1988) "Significance of hippocampal dysfunction in low level lead exposure of rats." *Neurotoxicol. Teratol. 10,* 245–253.

117. Lorenzo, A.V., Gewirtz, M. and Averill, D. (1978) "CNS lead toxicity in rabbit offspring." *Environ. Res. 17,* 131–150.

118. Bondy, S.C., Hong, J.S., Tilson, H.A. and Walsh, T.J. (1985) "Effects of triethyl lead on hot-plate responsiveness and biochemical properties of hippocampus." *Pharmacol. Biochem. Behav. 22,* 1007–1011.

119. Moreira, E.G., Vassilieff, I. and Vassilieff, V.S. (2001) "Developmental lead exposure: behavioral alterations in the short and long term." *Neurotoxicol. Teratol. 23,* 489–495.

120. Stiles, K.M. and Bellinger, D.C. (1993) "Neuropsychological correlates of low-level lead exposure in school-age children: a prospective study." *Neurotoxicol. Teratol. 15,* 27–35.

121. IARC (1987) "Fluorides (inorganic) used in drinking water." *International Agency for Research on Cancer (IARC) Monographs Programme on the Evaluation of Carcinogenic Risks to Humans. Supplement 7,* 208. http://www-cie.iarc.fr/htdocs/monographs/suppl7/fluorides.html

122. Wilkinson, R.R. (1984) "Technoeconomic and environmental assessment of industrial organotin compounds." *Neurotoxicology 5,* 141–158.

123. Hoch, M. (2001) "Organotin compounds in the environment – an overview." *Appl. Geochem. 16,* 719–743.

124. Borghi, V. and Porte, C. (2002) "Organotin pollution in deep-sea fish from the northwestern Mediterranean." *Environ. Sci. Technol. 36,* 4224–4228.

125. Goldman, L.R. and Shannon, M.W. (2001) "Technical report: mercury in the environment: implications for pediatricians." *Pediatrics 108,* 197–205.

126. Falter, R. and Scholer, H.F. (1994) "Determination of methyl-, ethyl-, phenyl and total mercury in Neckar River fish." *Chemosphere 29,* 1333–1338.

127. Burger, J. and Campbell, K.R. (2004) "Species differences in contaminants in fish on and adjacent to the Oak Ridge Reservation, Tennessee." *Environ. Res. 96,* 145–155.

128. Johnsson, C., Sallsten, G., Schutz, A., Sjors, A. and Barregard, L. (2004) "Hair mercury levels versus freshwater fish consumption in household members of Swedish angling societies." *Environ. Res. 96,* 257–263.

129. United Nations Environment Program (2003) *Global Mercury Assessment Report; Mercury Levels in Fish/ Shellfish in Different Regions of the World.* Online at http://www.chem.unep.ch/mercury/Report/GMA-report-TOC.htm, Chapter 4, Table 0.5.

130. Geier, D.A. and Geier, M.R. (2004) "A comparative evaluation of the effects of MMR immunization and mercury doses from thimerosal-containing childhood vaccines on the population prevalence of autism." *Med. Sci. Monit. 10,* 133–139.

131. Verstraeten, T., Davis, R.L., DeStefano, F., Lieu, T.A., Rhodes, P.H., Black, S.B. *et al.* (2003) "Safety of thimerosal-containing vaccines: a two-phased study of computerized health maintenance organization databases." *Pediatrics 112,* 1039–1048.

132. Mulder, E.J., Anderson, G.M., Kema, I.P., de Bildt, A., van Lang, N.D., den Boer, J.A. *et al.* (2004) "Platelet serotonin levels in pervasive developmental disorders and mental retardation: diagnostic group differences, within-group distribution, and behavioral correlates." *J. Am. Acad. Child Adolesc. Psychiatry 43,* 491–499.

133. Grandjean, P., White, R.F., Weihe, P. and Jorgensen, P.J. (2003) "Neurotoxic risk caused by stable and variable exposure to methylmercury from seafood." *Ambul. Pediatr. 3,* 18–23.

134. Murata, K., Weihe, P., Budtz-Jorgensen, E., Jorgensen, P.J. and Grandjean, P. (2004) "Delayed brainstem auditory evoked potential latencies in 14-year-old children exposed to methylmercury." *J. Pediatr. 144,* 177–183.

135. Marsh, D.O., Clarkson, T.W., Cox, C., Myers, G.J., Amin-Zaki, L. and Al Tikriti, S. (1987) "Fetal methylmercury poisoning. Relationship between concentration in single strands of maternal hair and child effects." *Arch. Neurol. 44*, 1017–1022.

136. Harada, M. (1995) "Minamata disease: methylmercury poisoning in Japan caused by environmental pollution." *Crit. Rev. Toxicol. 25*, 1–24.

137. Iesato, K., Wakashin, M., Wakashin, Y. and Tojo, S. (1977) "Renal tubular dysfunction in Minamata disease. Detection of renal tubular antigen and beta-2-microglobin in the urine." *Ann. Intern. Med. 86*, 731–737.

138. Chrysochoou, C., Rutishauser, C., Rauber-Luthy, C., Neuhaus, T., Boltshauser, E. and Superti-Furga, A. (2003) "An 11-month-old boy with psychomotor regression and auto-aggressive behaviour." *Eur. J. Pediatr. 162*, 559–561.

139. Korogi, Y., Takahashi, M., Sumi, M., Hirai, T., Okuda, T., Shinzato, J. *et al.* (1994) "MR imaging of Minamata disease: qualitative and quantitative analysis." *Radiat. Med. 12*, 249–253.

140. Korogi, Y., Takahashi, M., Okajima, T. and Eto, K. (1998) "MR findings of Minamata disease – organic mercury poisoning." *J. Magn. Reson. Imaging 8*, 308–316.

141. Moller-Madsen, B. and Danscher, G. (1991) "Localization of mercury in CNS of the rat. IV. The effect of selenium on orally administered organic and inorganic mercury." *Toxicol. Appl. Pharmacol. 108*, 457–473.

142. Sakamoto, M., Kakita, A., Wakabayashi, K., Takahashi, H., Nakano, A. and Akagi, H. (2002) "Evaluation of changes in methylmercury accumulation in the developing rat brain and its effects: a study with consecutive and moderate dose exposure throughout gestation and lactation periods." *Brain Res. 949*, 51–59.

143. Cicmanec, J.L. (1996) "Comparison of four human studies of perinatal exposure to methylmercury for use in risk assessment." *Toxicology 111*, 157–162.

144. Shenker, B.J., Guo, T.L. and Shapiro, I.M. (2000) "Mercury-induced apoptosis in human lymphoid cells: evidence that the apoptotic pathway is mercurial species dependent." *Environ. Res. 84*, 89–99.

145. Magos, L., Brown, A.W., Sparrow, S., Bailey, E., Snowden, R.T. and Skipp, W.R. (1985) "The comparative toxicology of ethyl- and methylmercury." *Arch. Toxicol. 57*, 260–267.

146. Lehotzky, K., Szeberenyi, J.M., Ungvary, G. and Kiss, A. (1988) "Behavioral effects of prenatal methoxy-ethyl-mercury chloride exposure in rat pups." *Neurotoxicol. Teratol. 10*, 471–474.

147. Pichichero, M.E., Cernichiari, E., Lopreiato, J. and Treanor, J. (2002) "Mercury concentrations and metabolism in infants receiving vaccines containing thiomersal: a descriptive study." *Lancet 360*, 1737–1741.

148. Ueha-Ishibashi, T., Oyama, Y., Nakao, H., Umebayashi, C., Nishizaki, Y., Tatsuishi, T. *et al.* (2004) "Effect of thimerosal, a preservative in vaccines, on intracellular Ca2+ concentration of rat cerebellar neurons." *Toxicology 195*, 77–84.

149. Burbacher, T.M., Shen, D.D., Liberato, N., Grant, K.S., Cernichiari, E. and Clarkson, T. (2005) "Comparison of blood and brain mercury levels in infant monkeys exposed to methylmercury or vaccines containing thimerosal." *Environ. Health Perspect. 113*, 1015–1021.

150. Havarinasab, S., Haggqvist, B., Bjorn, E., Pollard, K.M. and Hultman, P. (2005) "Immunosuppressive and autoimmune effects of thimerosal in mice." *Toxicol. Appl. Pharmacol. 204*, 109–121.

151. Haggqvist, B., Havarinasab, S., Bjorn, E. and Hultman, P. (2005) "The immunosuppressive effect of methylmercury does not preclude development of autoimmunity in genetically susceptible mice." *Toxicology 208*, 149–164.

152. Hornig, M., Chian, D. and Lipkin, W.I. (2004) "Neurotoxic effects of postnatal thimerosal are mouse strain dependent." *Mol. Psychiatry 9*, 833–845.

153. Miu, A.C., Andreescu, C.E., Vasiu, R. and Olteanu, A.I. (2003) "A behavioral and histological study of the effects of long-term exposure of adult rats to aluminum." *Int. J. Neurosci. 113*, 1197–1211.

154. Offit, P.A. and Jew, R.K. (2003) "Addressing parents' concerns: do vaccines contain harmful preservatives, adjuvants, additives, or residuals?" *Pediatrics 112*, 1394–1397.

155. Golub, M.S. and Germann, S.L. (2001) "Long-term consequences of developmental exposure to aluminum in a suboptimal diet for growth and behavior of Swiss Webster mice." *Neurotoxicol. Teratol. 23*, 365–372.

156. Golub, M.S., Gershwin, M.E., Donald, J.M., Negri, S. and Keen, C.L. (1987) "Maternal and developmental toxicity of chronic aluminum exposure in mice." *Fundam. Appl. Toxicol. 8*, 346–357.

157. Ministry of Agriculture, F.a.F.U. (1999) "The 1997 total diet study: aluminium, arsenic, cadmium, chromium, copper, lead, mercury, nickel, selenium, tin and zinc." *Food Surveillance Information Sheet 191.*

158. Petit, T.L. and LeBoutillier, J.C. (1986) "Zinc deficiency in the postnatal rat: implications for lead toxicity." *Neurotoxicology 7*, 237–246.

159. Hunt, C.D. and Idso, J.P. (1995) "Moderate copper deprivation during gestation and lactation affects dentate gyrus and hippocampal maturation in immature male rats." *J. Nutr. 125*, 2700–2710.

160. Latif, A., Heinz, P. and Cook, R. (2002) "Iron deficiency in autism and Asperger syndrome." *Autism 6*, 103–114.

161. Rao, R., de Ungria, M., Sullivan, D., Wu, P., Wobken, J.D., Nelson, C.A. *et al.* (1999) "Perinatal brain iron deficiency increases the vulnerability of rat hippocampus to hypoxic ischemic insult." *J. Nutr. 129*, 199–206.

162. Bradman, A., Eskenazi, B., Sutton, P., Athanasoulis, M. and Goldman, L.R. (2001) "Iron deficiency associated with higher blood lead in children living in contaminated environments." *Environ. Health Perspect. 109*, 1079–1084.

163. Rayman, M.P. (2000) "The importance of selenium to human health." *Lancet 356*, 233–241.

164. Whanger, P.D. (2001) "Selenium and the brain: a review." *Nutr. Neurosci. 4*, 81–97.

165. Kryukov, G.V., Castellano, S., Novoselov, S.V., Lobanov, A.V., Zehtab, O., Guigo, R. *et al.* (2003) "Characterization of mammalian selenoproteomes." *Science 300*, 1439–1443.

166. Arthur, J.R. (2000) "The glutathione peroxidases." *Cell Mol. Life Sci. 57*, 1825–1835.

167. Schomburg, L., Schweizer, U., Holtmann, B., Flohe, L., Sendtner, M. and Kohrle, J. (2003) "Gene disruption discloses role of selenoprotein P in selenium delivery to target tissues." *Biochem. J. 370*, 397–402.

168. Sasakura, C. and Suzuki, K.T. (1998) "Biological interaction between transition metals (Ag, Cd and Hg), selenide/sulfide and selenoprotein P." *J. Inorg. Biochem. 71*, 159–162.

169. Hill, K.E., Zhou, J., McMahan, W.J., Motley, A.K. and Burk, R.F. (2004) "Neurological dysfunction occurs in mice with targeted deletion of the selenoprotein P gene." *J. Nutr. 134*, 157–161.

170. Morimoto, K., Iijima, S. and Koizumi, A. (1982) "Selenite prevents the induction of sister-chromatid exchanges by methyl mercury and mercuric chloride in human whole-blood cultures." *Mutat. Res. 102*, 183–192.

171. Frisk, P., Wester, K., Yaqob, A. and Lindh, U. (2003) "Selenium protection against mercury-induced apoptosis and growth inhibition in cultured K-562 cells." *Biol. Trace Elem. Res. 92*, 105–114.

172. Satoh, H., Yasuda, N. and Shimai, S. (1985) "Development of reflexes in neonatal mice prenatally exposed to methylmercury and selenite." *Toxicol. Lett. 25*, 199–203.

173. Watanabe, C., Yin, K., Kasanuma, Y. and Satoh, H. (1999) "In utero exposure to methylmercury and Se deficiency converge on the neurobehavioral outcome in mice." *Neurotoxicol. Teratol. 21*, 83–88.

174. James, S.J., Slikker, W., III, Melnyk, S., New, E., Pogribna, M. and Jernigan, S. (2005) "Thimerosal neurotoxicity is associated with glutathione depletion: protection with glutathione precursors." *Neurotoxicology 26*, 1–8.

175. Yorbik, O., Sayal, A., Akay, C., Akbiyik, D.I. and Sohmen, T. (2002) "Investigation of antioxidant enzymes in children with autistic disorder." *Prostaglandins Leukot. Essent. Fatty Acids 67*, 341–343.

176. Weber, G.F., Maertens, P., Meng, X.Z. and Pippenger, C.E. (1991) "Glutathione peroxidase deficiency and childhood seizures." *Lancet 337*, 1443–1444.

177. Ramaekers, V.T., Calomme, M., Vanden Berghe, D. and Makropoulos, W. (1994) "Selenium deficiency triggering intractable seizures." *Neuropediatrics 25*, 217–223.

178. Esworthy, R.S., Binder, S.W., Doroshow, J.H. and Chu, F.F. (2003) "Microflora trigger colitis in mice deficient in selenium-dependent glutathione peroxidase and induce Gpx2 gene expression." *Biol. Chem. 384*, 597–607.

179. Chu, F.F., Esworthy, R.S., Chu, P.G., Longmate, J.A., Huycke, M.M., Wilczynski, S. *et al.* (2004) "Bacteria-induced intestinal cancer in mice with disrupted Gpx1 and Gpx2 genes." *Cancer Res. 64*, 962–968.

180. Adams, J.B., Holloway, C.E., George, F. and Quig, D. (2003) "Toxic metals and essential metals in the hair of children with autism and their mothers." *DAN! Conference*, 3–5 October. Online at: http://www.autismwebsite.com/ari/dan/adams1.htm

181. Donnelly, S., Loscher, C.E., Lynch, M.A. and Mills, K.H. (2001) "Whole-cell but not acellular pertussis vaccines induce convulsive activity in mice: evidence of a role for toxin-induced interleukin-1beta in a new murine model for analysis of neuronal side effects of vaccination." *Infect. Immun. 69*, 4217–4223.

182. Braun, J.S., Sublett, J.E., Freyer, D., Mitchell, T.J., Cleveland, J.L., Tuomanen, E.I. *et al.* (2002) "Pneumococcal pneumolysin and H(2)O(2) mediate brain cell apoptosis during meningitis." *J. Clin. Invest. 109,* 19–27.

183. Visser, P.J., Krabbendam, L., Verhey, F.R., Hofman, P.A., Verhoeven, W.M., Tuinier, S. *et al.* (1999) "Brain correlates of memory dysfunction in alcoholic Korsakoff's syndrome." *J. Neurol. Neurosurg. Psychiatry 67,* 774–778.

184. Martin, P.R., Singleton, C.K. and Hiller-Sturmhofel, S. (2003) "The role of thiamine deficiency in alcoholic brain disease." *Alcohol Res. Health 27,* 134–142.

185. Kurth, C., Wegerer, V., Reulbach, U., Lewczuk, P., Kornhuber, J., Steinhoff, B.J. *et al.* (2004) "Analysis of hippocampal atrophy in alcoholic patients by a Kohonen feature map." *Neuroreport 15,* 367–371.

186. den Heijer, T., Vermeer, S.E., Clarke, R., Oudkerk, M., Koudstaal, P.J., Hofman, A. *et al.* (2003) "Homocysteine and brain atrophy on MRI of non-demented elderly." *Brain 126,* 170–175.

187. Watanabe, A. (1998) "Cerebral changes in hepatic encephalopathy." *J. Gastroenterol. Hepatol. 13,* 752–760.

188. Shapre, L.G., Olney, J.W., Ohlendorf, C., Lyss, A., Zimmerman, M. and Gale, B. (1975) "Brain damage and associated behavioral deficits following the administration of L-cysteine to infant rats." *Pharmacol. Biochem. Behav. 3,* 291–298.

189. Streck, E.L., Bavaresco, C.S., Netto, C.A. and Wyse, A.T. (2004) "Chronic hyperhomocysteinemia provokes a memory deficit in rats in the Morris water maze task." *Behav. Brain Res. 153,* 377–381.

190. Kubova, H., Folbergrova, J. and Mares, P. (1995) "Seizures induced by homocysteine in rats during ontogenesis." *Epilepsia 36,* 750–756.

191. Stoltenburg-Didinger, G. (1994) "Neuropathology of the hippocampus and its susceptibility to neurotoxic insult." *Neurotoxicology 15,* 445–450.

192. Zola-Morgan, S., Squire, L.R., Rempel, N.L., Clower, R.P. and Amaral, D.G. (1992) "Enduring memory impairment in monkeys after ischemic damage to the hippocampus." *J. Neurosci. 12,* 2582–2596.

193. DeLong, G.R. and Heinz, E.R. (1997) "The clinical syndrome of early-life bilateral hippocampal sclerosis." *Ann. Neurol. 42,* 11–17.

194. Takeda, A. (2000) "Movement of zinc and its functional significance in the brain." *Brain Res. Rev. 34,* 137–148.

195. Scheuhammer, A.M. and Cherian, M.G. (1982) "The regional distribution of lead in normal rat brain." *Neurotoxicology 3,* 85–92.

196. Pellmar, T.C., Fuciarelli, A.F., Ejnik, J.W., Hamilton, M., Hogan, J., Strocko, S. *et al.* (1999) "Distribution of uranium in rats implanted with depleted uranium pellets." *Toxicol. Sci. 49,* 29–39.

197. Feng, W., Wang, M., Li, B., Liu, J., Chai, Z., Zhao, J. *et al.* (2004) "Mercury and trace element distribution in organic tissues and regional brain of fetal rat after in utero and weaning exposure to low dose of inorganic mercury." *Toxicol. Lett. 152,* 223–234.

198. Cook, L.L., Stine, K.E. and Reiter, L.W. (1984) "Tin distribution in adult rat tissues after exposure to trimethyltin and triethyltin." *Toxicol. Appl. Pharmacol. 76,* 344–348.

199. Naeve, G.S., Vana, A.M., Eggold, J.R., Kelner, G.S., Maki, R., Desouza, E.B. *et al.* (1999) "Expression profile of the copper homeostasis gene, rAtox1, in the rat brain." *Neuroscience 93,* 1179–1187.

200. Kobayashi, M., Takamatsu, K., Saitoh, S., Miura, M. and Noguchi, T. (1992) "Molecular cloning of hippocalcin, a novel calcium-binding protein of the recovering family exclusively expressed in hippocampus." *Biochem. Biophys. Res. Commun. 189,* 511–517.

201. Masters, B.A., Quaife, C.J., Erickson, J.C., Kelly, E.J., Froelick, G.J., Zambrowicz, B.P. *et al.* (1994) "Metallothionein III is expressed in neurons that sequester zinc in synaptic vesicles." *J. Neurosci. 14,* 5844–5857.

202. Palumaa, P., Eriste, E., Njunkova, O., Pokras, L., Jornvall, H. and Sillard, R. (2002) "Brain-specific metallothionein-3 has higher metal-binding capacity than ubiquitous metallothioneins and binds metals noncooperatively." *Biochemistry 41,* 6158–6163.

203. Toggas, S.M., Krady, J.K. and Billingsley, M.L. (1992) "Molecular neurotoxicology of trimethyltin: identification of stannin, a novel protein expressed in trimethyltin-sensitive cells." *Mol. Pharmacol. 42,* 44–56.

204. Dejneka, N.S., Patanow, C.M., Polavarapu, R., Toggas, S.M., Krady, J.K. and Billingsley, M.L. (1997) "Localization and characterization of stannin: relationship to cellular sensitivity to organotin compounds." *Neurochem. Int. 31,* 801–815.

205. Pullen, R.G., Candy, J.M., Morris, C.M., Taylor, G., Keith, A.B. and Edwardson, J.A. (1990) "Gallium-67 as a potential marker for aluminium transport in rat brain: implications for Alzheimer's disease." *J. Neurochem.* 55, 251–259.

206. Morris, C.M., Candy, J.M., Kerwin, J.M. and Edwardson, J.A. (1994) "Transferrin receptors in the normal human hippocampus and in Alzheimer's disease." *Neuropathol. Appl. Neurobiol.* 20, 473–477.

207. Wenzel, H.J., Cole, T.B., Born, D.E., Schwartzkroin, P.A. and Palmiter, R.D. (1997) "Ultrastructural localization of zinc transporter-3 (ZnT-3) to synaptic vesicle membranes within mossy fiber boutons in the hippocampus of mouse and monkey." *Proc. Natl. Acad. Sci. USA* 94, 12676–12681.

208. Davidson, C.E., Reese, B.E., Billingsley, M.L. and Yun, J.K. (2004) "Stannin, a protein that localizes to the mitochondria and sensitizes NIH-3T3 cells to trimethyltin and dimethyltin toxicity." *Mol. Pharmacol.* 66, 855–863.

209. Buck, B., Mascioni, A., Que, L., Jr. and Veglia, G. (2003) "Dealkylation of organotin compounds by biological dithiols: toward the chemistry of organotin toxicity." *J. Am. Chem. Soc.* 125, 13316–13317.

210. Buck, B., Mascioni, A., Cramer, C.J. and Veglia, G. (2004) "Interaction of alkyltin salts with biological dithiols: dealkylation and induction of a regular beta-turn structure in peptides." *J. Am. Chem. Soc.* 126, 14400–14410.

211. DeSilva, T.M., Veglia, G., Porcelli, F., Prantner, A.M. and Opella, S.J. (2002) "Selectivity in heavy metal-binding to peptides and proteins." *Biopolymers* 64, 189–197.

212. Dejneka, N.S., Polavarapu, R., Deng, X., Martin-DeLeon, P.A. and Billingsley, M.L. (1998) "Chromosomal localization and characterization of the stannin (Snn) gene." *Mamm. Genome* 9, 556–564.

213. Gould, E., Reeves, A.J., Fallah, M., Tanapat, P., Gross, C.G. and Fuchs, E. (1999) "Hippocampal neurogenesis in adult Old World primates." *Proc. Natl. Acad. Sci. USA* 96, 5263–5267.

214. Kornack, D.R. and Rakic, P. (1999) "Continuation of neurogenesis in the hippocampus of the adult macaque monkey." *Proc. Natl. Acad. Sci. USA* 96, 5768–5773.

215. Eriksson, P.S., Perfilieva, E., Bjork-Eriksson, T., Alborn, A.M., Nordborg, C., Peterson, D.A. *et al.* (1998) "Neurogenesis in the adult human hippocampus." *Nat. Med.* 4, 1313–1317.

216. Bernier, P.J., Bedard, A., Vinet, J., Levesque, M. and Parent, A. (2002) "Newly generated neurons in the amygdala and adjoining cortex of adult primates." *Proc. Natl. Acad. Sci. USA* 99, 11464–11469.

217. Yamaguchi, M., Saito, H., Suzuki, M. and Mori, K. (2000) "Visualization of neurogenesis in the central nervous system using nesting promoter-GFP transgenic mice." *Neuroreport* 11, 1991–1996.

218. Kornack, D.R. and Rakic, P. (2001) "Cell proliferation without neurogenesis in adult primate neocortex." *Science* 294, 2127–2130.

219. Rogers, S.J., Hepburn, S. and Wehner, E. (2003) "Parent reports of sensory symptoms in toddlers with autism and those with other developmental disorders." *J. Autism Dev. Disord.* 33, 631–642.

220. Boulikas, T. and Vougiouka, M. (2003) "Cisplatin and platinum drugs at the molecular level (Review)." *Oncol. Rep.* 10, 1663–1682.

221. Tulub, A.A. and Stefanov, V.E. (2001) "Cisplatin stops tubulin assembly into microtubules. A new insight into the mechanism of antitumor activity of platinum complexes." *Int. J. Biol. Macromol.* 28, 191–198.

222. Fujii, T. (1997) "Transgenerational effects of maternal exposure to chemicals on the functional development of the brain in the offspring." *Cancer Causes Control* 8, 524–528.

223. Schneider, J.S., Anderson, D.W., Wade, T.V., Smith, M.G., Leibrandt, P., Zuck, L. *et al.* (2005) "Inhibition of progenitor cell proliferation in the dentate gyrus of rats following post-weaning lead exposure." *Neurotoxicology* 26, 141–145.

224. Keates, R.A. and Yott, B. (1984) "Inhibition of microtubule polymerization by micromolar concentrations of mercury (II)." *Can. J. Biochem. Cell Biol.* 62, 814–818.

225. Imura, N., Miura, K., Inokawa, M. and Nakada, S. (1980) "Mechanism of methylmercury cytotoxicity: by biochemical and morphological experiments using cultured cells." *Toxicology* 17, 241–254.

226. Kaufmann, W.E. and Moser, H.W. (2000) "Dendritic anomalies in disorders associated with mental retardation." *Cereb. Cortex* 10, 981–991.

227. Vogel, D.G., Margolis, R.L. and Mottet, N.K. (1985) "The effects of methyl mercury binding to microtubules." *Toxicol. Appl. Pharmacol.* 80, 473–486.

228. Brown, D.L., Reuhl, K.R., Bormann, S. and Little, J.E. (1988) "Effects of methyl mercury on the microtubule system of mouse lymphocytes." *Toxicol. Appl. Pharmacol.* 94, 66–75.

229. Leong, C.C., Syed, N.I. and Lorscheider, F.L. (2001) "Retrograde degeneration of neurite membrane structural integrity of nerve growth cones following in vitro exposure to mercury." *Neuroreport 12*, 733–737.

230. Nyka, W.M. (1976) "Cerebral lesions of mature newborn due to perinatal hypoxia. I. Placental and umbilical cord pathology." *Z. Geburtshilfe Perinatol. 180*, 290–294.

231. Tasker, R.C. (2001) "Hippocampal selective regional vulnerability and development." *Dev. Med. Child Neurol. Suppl. 86*, 6–7.

232. Back, T., Hemmen, T. and Schuler, O.G. (2004) "Lesion evolution in cerebral ischemia." *J. Neurol. 251*, 388–397.

233. Henke, K., Kroll, N.E., Behniea, H., Amaral, D.G., Miller, M.B., Rafal, R. *et al.* (1999) "Memory lost and regained following bilateral hippocampal damage." *J. Cogn. Neurosci. 11*, 682–697.

234. Lathe, R. (2001) "Hormones and the hippocampus." *J. Endocrinol. 169*, 205–231.

235. Tracy, A.L., Jarrard, L.E. and Davidson, T.L. (2001) "The hippocampus and motivation revisited: appetite and activity." *Behav. Brain Res. 127*, 13–23.

236. Garcia-Morales, P., Saceda, M., Kenney, N., Kim, N., Salomon, D.S., Gottardis, M.M. *et al.* (1994) "Effect of cadmium on estrogen receptor levels and estrogen-induced responses in human breast cancer cells." *J. Biol. Chem. 269*, 16896–16901.

237. Stoica, A., Katzenellenbogen, B.S. and Martin, M.B. (2000) "Activation of estrogen receptor-alpha by the heavy metal cadmium." *Mol. Endocrinol. 14*, 545–553.

238. Martin, M.B., Reiter, R., Pham, T., Avellanet, Y.R., Camara, J., Lahm, M. *et al.* (2003) "Estrogen-like activity of metals in MCF-7 breast cancer cells." *Endocrinology 144*, 2425–2436.

239. Johnson, M.D., Kenney, N., Stoica, A., Hilakivi-Clarke, L., Singh, B., Chepko, G. *et al.* (2003) "Cadmium mimics the in vivo effects of estrogen in the uterus and mammary gland." *Nat. Med. 9*, 1081–1084.

240. Martin, M.B., Voeller, H.J., Gelmann, E.P., Lu, J., Stoica, E.G., Hebert, E.J. *et al.* (2002) "Role of cadmium in the regulation of AR gene expression and activity." *Endocrinology 143*, 263–275.

241. Stapleton, G., Steel, M., Richardson, M., Mason, J.O., Rose, K.A., Morris, R.G. *et al.* (1995) "A novel cytochrome P450 expressed primarily in brain." *J. Biol. Chem. 270*, 29739–29745.

242. Lathe, R. (2002) "Steroid and sterol 7-hydroxylation: ancient pathways." *Steroids 67*, 967–977.

243. Weihua, Z., Lathe, R., Warner, M. and Gustafsson, J.-A. (2002) "A novel endocrine pathway in the prostate, ERbeta, AR, 5alpha-androstane-3beta,17beta-diol, and CYP7B, regulates prostate growth." *Proc. Natl. Acad. Sci. USA 99*, 13589–13594.

244. Omoto, Y., Lathe, R., Warner, M. and Gustafsson, J.-A. (2005) "Early onset of puberty and early ovarian failure in CYP7B knockout mice." *Proc. Natl. Acad. Sci. USA, 102*, 2814–2819.

245. Daston, G.P., Cook, J.C. and Kavlock, R.J. (2003) "Uncertainties for endocrine disrupters: our view on progress." *Toxicol. Sci. 74*, 245–252.

246. Witorsch, R.J. (2002) "Low-dose in utero effects of xenoestrogens in mice and their relevance to humans: an analytical review of the literature." *Food Chem. Toxicol. 40*, 905–912.

247. Le, T.N. and Johansson, A. (2001) "Impact of chemical warfare with agent orange on women's reproductive lives in Vietnam: a pilot study." *Reprod. Health Matters 9*, 156–164.

248. Krstevska-Konstantinova, M., Charlier, C., Craen, M., Du, C.M., Heinrichs, C., de Beaufort, C. *et al.* (2001) "Sexual precocity after immigration from developing countries to Belgium: evidence of previous exposure to organochlorine pesticides." *Hum. Reprod. 16*, 1020–1026.

249. Bibbo, M., Gill, W.B., Azizi, F., Blough, R., Fang, V.S., Rosenfield, R.L. *et al.* (1977) "Follow-up study of male and female offspring of DES-exposed mothers." *Obstet. Gynecol. 49*, 1–8.

250. Gill, W.B., Schumacher, G.F. and Bibbo, M. (1977) "Pathological semen and anatomical abnormalities of the genital tract in human male subjects exposed to diethylstilbestrol in utero." *J. Urol. 117*, 477–480.

251. Palanza, P., Morellini, F., Parmigiani, S. and vom Saal, F.S. (1999) "Prenatal exposure to endocrine disrupting chemicals: effects on behavioral development." *Neurosci. Biobehav. Rev. 23*, 1011–1027.

252. Farabollini, F., Porrini, S. and Dessi-Fulgheri, F. (1999) "Perinatal exposure to the estrogenic pollutant bisphenol A affects behavior in male and female rats." *Pharmacol. Biochem. Behav. 64*, 687–694.

253. Weiss, B. (2002) "Sexually dimorphic nonreproductive behaviors as indicators of endocrine disruption." *Environ. Health Perspect. 110*, Suppl 3, 387–391.

254. Levy, C.J. (1988) "Agent Orange exposure and posttraumatic stress disorder." *J. Nerv. Ment. Dis. 176*, 242–245.

255. Food Standards Agency (2004) *Fish Consumption, Benefits and Risks, Part 3*. Online at: http://www .food.gov.uk/multimedia/pdfs/fishreport200403.pdf

256. Kainu, T., Gustafsson, J.A. and Pelto-Huikko, M. (1995) "The dioxin receptor and its nuclear translocator (Arnt) in the rat brain." *Neuroreport 6*, 2557–2560.

257. Hassoun, E.A., Al Ghafri, M. and Abushaban, A. (2003) "The role of antioxidant enzymes in TCDD-induced oxidative stress in various brain regions of rats after subchronic exposure." *Free Radic. Biol. Med. 35*, 1028–1036.

258. Powers, B.E., Lin, T.M., Vanka, A., Peterson, R.E., Juraska, J.M. and Schantz, S.L. (2005) "Tetrachlorodibenzo-p-dioxin exposure alters radial arm maze performance and hippocampal morphology in female AhR mice." *Genes Brain Behav. 4*, 51–59.

259. Edelson, S.B. and Cantor, D.S. (1998) "Autism: xenobiotic influences." *Toxicol. Ind. Health 14*, 553–563.

260. Stubbs, E.G. (1978) "Autistic symptoms in a child with congenital cytomegalovirus infection." *J. Autism Child Schizophr. 8*, 37–43.

261. Stubbs, E.G., Ash, E. and Williams, C.P. (1984) "Autism and congenital cytomegalovirus." *J. Autism Dev. Disord. 14*, 183–189.

262. Ivarsson, S.A., Bjerre, I., Vegfors, P. and Ahlfors, K. (1990) "Autism as one of several disabilities in two children with congenital cytomegalovirus infection." *Neuropediatrics 21*, 102–103.

263. Yamashita, Y., Fujimoto, C., Nakajima, E., Isagai, T. and Matsuishi, T. (2003) "Possible association between congenital cytomegalovirus infection and autistic disorder." *J. Autism Dev. Disord. 33*, 455–459.

264. Sweeten, T.L., Posey, D.J. and McDougle, C.J. (2004) "Brief report: autistic disorder in three children with cytomegalovirus infection." *J. Autism Dev. Disord. 34*, 583–586.

265. Chess, S. (1977) "Follow-up report on autism in congenital rubella." *J. Autism Child Schizophr. 7*, 69–81.

266. Chess, S., Fernandez, P. and Korn, S. (1978) "Behavioral consequences of congenital rubella." *J. Pediatr. 93*, 699–703.

267. Domachowske, J.B., Cunningham, C.K., Cummings, D.L., Crosley, C.J., Hannan, W.P. and Weiner, L.B. (1996) "Acute manifestations and neurologic sequelae of Epstein-Barr virus encephalitis in children." *Pediatr. Infect. Dis. J. 15*, 871–875.

268. DeLong, G.R., Bean, S.C. and Brown, F.R., III (1981) "Acquired reversible autistic syndrome in acute encephalopathic illness in children." *Arch. Neurol. 38*, 191–194.

269. Gillberg, C. (1986) "Onset at age 14 of a typical autistic syndrome. A case report of a girl with herpes simplex encephalitis." *J. Autism Dev. Disord. 16*, 369–375.

270. Ghaziuddin, M., Al Khouri, I. and Ghaziuddin, N. (2002) "Autistic symptoms following herpes encephalitis." *Eur. Child Adolesc. Psychiatry 11*, 142–146.

271. Gillberg, I.C. (1991) "Autistic syndrome with onset at age 31 years: herpes encephalitis as a possible model for childhood autism." *Dev. Med. Child Neurol. 33*, 920–924.

272. Reitman, M.A., Casper, J., Coplan, J., Weiner, L.B., Kellman, R.M. and Kanter, R.K. (1984) "Motor disorders of voice and speech in Reye's syndrome survivors." *Am. J. Dis. Child 138*, 1129–1131.

273. Quart, E.J., Buchtel, H.A. and Sarnaik, A.P. (1988) "Long-lasting memory deficits in children recovered from Reye's syndrome." *J. Clin. Exp. Neuropsychol. 10*, 409–420.

274. Cornford, M.E. and McCormick, G.F. (1997) "Adult-onset temporal lobe epilepsy associated with smoldering herpes simplex 2 infection." *Neurology 48*, 425–430.

275. Stefanacci, L., Buffalo, E.A., Schmolck, H. and Squire, L.R. (2000) "Profound amnesia after damage to the medial temporal lobe: a neuroanatomical and neuropsychological profile of patient EP." *J. Neurosci. 20*, 7024–7036.

276. Shoji, H., Azuma, K., Nishimura, Y., Fujimoto, H., Sugita, Y. and Eizuru, Y. (2002) "Acute viral encephalitis: the recent progress." *Intern. Med. 41*, 420–428.

277. Asaoka, K., Shoji, H., Nishizaka, S., Ayabe, M., Abe, T., Ohori, N. *et al.* (2004) "Non-herpetic acute limbic encephalitis: cerebrospinal fluid cytokines and magnetic resonance imaging findings." *Intern. Med. 43*, 42–48.

278. Rubin, S.A., Sylves, P., Vogel, M., Pletnikov, M., Moran, T.H., Schwartz, G.J. *et al.* (1999) "Borna disease virus-induced hippocampal dentate gyrus damage is associated with spatial learning and memory deficits." *Brain Res. Bull. 48*, 23–30.

279. Gosztonyi, G. and Ludwig, H. (1995) "Borna disease – neuropathology and pathogenesis." *Curr. Top. Microbiol. Immunol. 190*, 39–73.

280. Pletnikov, M.V., Moran, T.H. and Carbone, K.M. (2002) "Borna disease virus infection of the neonatal rat: developmental brain injury model of autism spectrum disorders." *Front Biosci. 7*, d593–d607.

281. Hornig, M., Weissenbock, H., Horscroft, N. and Lipkin, W.I. (1999) "An infection-based model of neurodevelopmental damage." *Proc. Natl. Acad. Sci. USA 96*, 12102–12107.

282. Gianinazzi, C., Grandgirard, D., Imboden, H., Egger, L., Meli, D.N., Bifrare, Y.D. *et al.* (2003) "Caspase-3 mediates hippocampal apoptosis in pneumococcal meningitis." *Acta Neuropathol. (Berl.) 105*, 499–507.

283. Nau, R., Soto, A. and Bruck, W. (1999) "Apoptosis of neurons in the dentate gyrus in humans suffering from bacterial meningitis." *J. Neuropathol. Exp. Neurol. 58*, 265–274.

284. Goldman, G.S. and Yazbak, F.E. (2004) "An investigation of the association between MMR vaccination and autism in Denmark." *J. Am. Phys. Surg. 9*, 70–75.

285. Dyken, P.R. (2004) "Some aspects about the clinical and pathogenetics characteristics of the presumed persistent measles infections: SSPE and MINE." *J. Pediatr. Neurol. 2*, 121–124.

286. Honda, H., Shimizu, Y. and Rutter, M. (2005) "No effect of MMR withdrawal on the incidence of autism: a total population study." *J. Child Psychol. Psychiatry 46*, 572–579.

287. Lingam, R., Simmons, A., Andrews, N., Miller, E., Stowe, J. and Taylor, B. (2003) "Prevalence of autism and parentally reported triggers in a north east London population." *Arch. Dis. Child 88*, 666–670.

288. Taylor, B., Miller, E., Lingam, R., Andrews, N., Simmons, A. and Stowe, J. (2002) "Measles, mumps, and rubella vaccination and bowel problems or developmental regression in children with autism: population study." *Brit. Med. J. 324*, 393–396.

289. Smeeth, L., Cook, C., Fombonne, E., Heavey, L., Rodrigues, L.C., Smith, P.G. *et al.* (2004) "Rate of first recorded diagnosis of autism and other pervasive developmental disorders in United Kingdom general practice, 1988 to 2001." *BMC Medicine 2*. http://www.biomedcentral.com/1741-7015/2/39

290. Carpenter, D.O., Hussain, R.J., Berger, D.F., Lombardo, J.P. and Park, H.Y. (2002) "Electrophysiologic and behavioral effects of perinatal and acute exposure of rats to lead and polychlorinated biphenyls." *Environ. Health Perspect. 110*, Suppl 3, 377–386.

291. Rajapakse, N., Silva, E. and Kortenkamp, A. (2002) "Combining xenoestrogens at levels below individual no-observed-effect concentrations dramatically enhances steroid hormone action." *Environ. Health Perspect. 110*, 917–921.

292. Rutter, M. (2000) "Genetic studies of autism: from the 1970s into the millennium." *J. Abnormal. Child Psychol. 28*, 3–14.

Chapter 8 Gut, Hormones, Immunity: Physiological Dysregulation in Autism

1. Ader, R., Felten, D.L. and Cohen, N. (1991) *Psychoneuroimmunology, Second Edition.* San Diego: Academic Press.

2. Landin, K., Blennow, K., Wallin, A. and Gottfries, C.G. (1993) "Low blood pressure and blood glucose levels in Alzheimer's disease: evidence for a hypometabolic disorder?" *J. Intern. Med. 233*, 357–363.

3. Vanhanen, M. and Soininen, H. (1998) "Glucose intolerance, cognitive impairment and Alzheimer's disease." *Curr. Opin. Neurol. 11*, 673–677.

4. Dunn, A.J. (1988) "Nervous system–immune system interactions: an overview." *J. Recept. Res. 8*, 589–607.

5. Webster, J.I., Tonelli, L. and Sternberg, E.M. (2002) "Neuroendocrine regulation of immunity." *Annu. Rev. Immunol. 20*, 125–163.

6. Lathe, R. (2001) "Hormones and the hippocampus." *J. Endocrinol. 169*, 205–231.

7. Muris, P., Steerneman, P., Merckelbach, H., Holdrinet, I. and Meesters, C. (1998) "Comorbid anxiety symptoms in children with pervasive developmental disorders." *J. Anxiety Disord. 12*, 387–393.

8. Harter, M.C., Conway, K.P. and Merikangas, K.R. (2003) "Associations between anxiety disorders and physical illness." *Eur. Arch. Psychiatry Clin. Neurosci. 253*, 313–320.

9. Shanahan, F. (1999) "Brain-gut axis and mucosal immunity: a perspective on mucosal psycho-neuroimmunology." *Semin. Gastrointest. Dis. 10*, 8–13.

10. Felten, D.L., Felten, S.Y., Carlson, S.L., Olschowka, J.A. and Livnat, S. (1985) "Noradrenergic and peptidergic innervation of lymphoid tissue." *J. Immunol. 135*, 755s–765s.

11. Cassileth, B.R. and Drossman, D.A. (1993) "Psychosocial factors in gastrointestinal illness." *Psychother. Psychosom. 59*, 131–143.

12. Glavin, G.B., Pare, W.P., Sandbak, T., Bakke, H.K. and Murison, R. (1994) "Restraint stress in biomedical research: an update." *Neurosci. Biobehav. Rev. 18*, 223–249.

13. Lewin, J. and Lewis, S. (1995) "Organic and psychosocial risk factors for duodenal ulcer." *J. Psychosom. Res. 39*, 531–548.

14. Hart, A. and Kamm, M.A. (2002) "Review article: mechanisms of initiation and perpetuation of gut inflammation by stress." *Aliment. Pharmacol. Ther. 16*, 2017–2028.

15. Clouse, R.E. (1988) "Anxiety and gastrointestinal illness." *Psychiatr. Clin. North Am. 11*, 399–417.

16. Kim, C., Choi, H., Kim, J.K., Kim, M.S. and Park, H.J. (1976) "Influence of hippocampectomy on gastric ulcer in rats." *Brain Res. 109*, 245–254.

17. Murphy, H.M., Wideman, C.H. and Brown, T.S. (1979) "Plasma corticosterone levels and ulcer formation in rats with hippocampal lesions." *Neuroendocrinology 28*, 123–130.

18. Henke, P.G. (1990) "Hippocampal pathway to the amygdala and stress ulcer development." *Brain Res. Bull. 25*, 691–695.

19. Henke, P.G., Ray, A. and Sullivan, R.M. (1991) "The amygdala. Emotions and gut functions." *Dig. Dis. Sci. 36*, 1633–1643.

20. Henke, P.G. (1992) "Naloxone-sensitive potentiation at granule cell synapses in the ventral dentate gyrus and stress ulcers." *Physiol. Behav. 51*, 823–826.

21. Hernandez, D.E., Salaiz, A.B., Morin, P. and Moreira, M.A. (1990) "Administration of thyrotropin-releasing hormone into the central nucleus of the amygdala induces gastric lesions in rats." *Brain Res. Bull. 24*, 697–699.

22. Uno, H., Tarara, R., Else, J.G., Suleman, M.A. and Sapolsky, R.M. (1989) "Hippocampal damage associated with prolonged and fatal stress in primates." *J. Neurosci. 9*, 1705–1711.

23. Schallert, T., Whishaw, I.Q. and Flannigan, K.P. (1977) "Gastric pathology and feeding deficits induced by hypothalamic damage in rats: effects of lesion type, size, and placement." *J. Comp. Physiol. Psychol. 91*, 598–610.

24. van Gent, T., Heijnen, C.J. and Treffers, P.D. (1997) "Autism and the immune system." *J. Child Psychol. Psychiatry 38*, 337–349.

25. Cohen, D.J. and Johnson, W.T. (1977) "Cardiovascular correlates of attention in normal and psychiatrically disturbed children. Blood pressure, peripheral blood flow, and peripheral vascular resistance." *Arch. Gen. Psychiatry 34*, 561–567.

26. Hutt, C., Forrest, S.J. and Richer, J. (1975) "Cardiac arrhythmia and behaviour in autistic children." *Acta Psychiatr. Scand. 51*, 361–372.

27. Vancassel, S., Durand, G., Barthelemy, C., Lejeune, B., Martineau, J., Guilloteau, D. *et al.* (2001) "Plasma fatty acid levels in autistic children." *Prostaglandins Leukot. Essent. Fatty Acids 65*, 1–7.

28. Ming, X., Stein, T.P., Brimacombe, M., Johnson, W.G., Lambert, G.H. and Wagner, G.C. (2005) "Increased excretion of a lipid peroxidation biomarker in autism." *Prostaglandins Leukot. Essent. Fatty Acids 73*, 379–384.

29. Edelson, S.B. and Cantor, D.S. (1998) "Autism: xenobiotic influences." *Toxicol. Ind. Health 14*, 553–563.

30. Tordjman, S., Ferrari, P., Sulmont, V., Duyme, M. and Roubertoux, P. (1997) "Androgenic activity in autism." *Am. J. Psychiatry 154*, 1626–1627.

31. Horvath, K. and Perman, J.A. (2002) "Autism and gastrointestinal symptoms." *Curr. Gastroenterol. Rep. 4*, 251–258.

32. White, J.F. (2003) "Intestinal pathophysiology in autism." *Exp. Biol. Med. (Maywood.) 228*, 639–649.

33. Wakefield, A.J., Murch, S.H., Anthony, A., Linnell, J., Casson, D.M., Malik, M. *et al.* (1998) "Ileal-lymphoid-nodular hyperplasia, non-specific colitis, and pervasive developmental disorder in children." *Lancet 351*, 637–641.

34. Wakefield, A.J., Anthony, A., Murch, S.H., Thomson, M., Montgomery, S.M., Davies, S. *et al.* (2000) "Enterocolitis in children with developmental disorders." *Am. J. Gastroenterol. 95*, 2285–2295.

35. Krigsman, A. (2002) *Evidence to the Committee on Government Reform, US House of Representatives.* Online at http://www.altcorp.com/DentalInformation/krigsman.htm

36. Finegold, S.M., Molitoris, D., Song, Y., Liu, C., Vaisanen, M.L., Bolte, E. *et al.* (2002) "Gastrointestinal microflora studies in late-onset autism." *Clin. Infect. Dis. 35*, S6–S16.

37. Weihe, E. and Eiden, L.E. (2000) "Chemical neuroanatomy of the vesicular amine transporters." *FASEB J. 14*, 2435–2449.

38. Baumgart, D.C. and Dignass, A.U. (2002) "Intestinal barrier function." *Curr. Opin. Clin. Nutr. Metab. Care 5*, 685–694.

39. D'Eufemia, P., Celli, M., Finocchiaro, R., Pacifico, L., Viozzi, L., Zaccagnini, M. *et al.* (1996) "Abnormal intestinal permeability in children with autism." *Acta Paediatr. 85*, 1076–1079.

40. Jyonouchi, H., Geng, L., Ruby, A., Reddy, C. and Zimmerman-Bier, B. (2005) "Evaluation of an association between gastrointestinal symptoms and cytokine production against common dietary proteins in children with autism spectrum disorders." *J. Pediatr. 146*, 605–610.

41. Horvath, K., Papadimitriou, J.C., Rabsztyn, A., Drachenberg, C. and Tildon, J.T. (1999) "Gastrointestinal abnormalities in children with autistic disorder." *J. Pediatr. 135*, 559–563.

42. Parracho, H.M., Bingham, M.O., Gibson, G.R. and McCartney, A.L. (2005) "Differences between the gut microflora of children with autistic spectrum disorders and that of healthy children." *J. Med. Microbiol. 54*, 987–991.

43. Furlano, R.I., Anthony, A., Day, R., Brown, A., McGarvey, L., Thomson, M.A. *et al.* (2001) "Colonic CD8 and gamma delta T-cell infiltration with epithelial damage in children with autism." *J. Pediatr. 138*, 366–372.

44. Torrente, F., Ashwood, P., Day, R., Machado, N., Furlano, R.I., Anthony, A. *et al.* (2002) "Small intestinal enteropathy with epithelial IgG and complement deposition in children with regressive autism." *Mol. Psychiatry 7*, 375–382, 334.

45. Ashwood, P., Anthony, A., Pellicer, A.A., Torrente, F., Walker-Smith, J.A. and Wakefield, A.J. (2003) "Intestinal lymphocyte populations in children with regressive autism: evidence for extensive mucosal immunopathology." *J. Clin. Immunol. 23*, 504–517.

46. Ashwood, P., Anthony, A., Torrente, F. and Wakefield, A.J. (2004) "Spontaneous mucosal lymphocyte cytokine profiles in children with autism and gastrointestinal symptoms: mucosal immune activation and reduced counter regulatory interleukin-10." *J. Clin. Immunol. 24*, 664–673.

47. Lucarelli, S., Frediani, T., Zingoni, A.M., Ferruzzi, F., Giardini, O., Quintieri, F. *et al.* (1995) "Food allergy and infantile autism." *Panminerva Med. 37*, 137–141.

48. Knivsberg, A.M., Reichelt, K.L. and Nodland, M. (2001) "Reports on dietary intervention in autistic disorders." *Nutr. Neurosci. 4*, 25–37.

49. Knivsberg, A.M., Reichelt, K.L., Hoien, T. and Nodland, M. (2002) "A randomised, controlled study of dietary intervention in autistic syndromes." *Nutr. Neurosci. 5*, 251–261.

50. Alberti, A., Pirrone, P., Elia, M., Waring, R.H. and Romano, C. (1999) "Sulphation deficit in 'low-functioning' autistic children: a pilot study." *Biol. Psychiatry 46*, 420–424.

51. Afzal, N., Murch, S., Thirrupathy, K., Berger, L., Fagbemi, A. and Heuschkel, R. (2003) "Constipation with acquired megarectum in children with autism." *Pediatrics 112*, 939–942.

52. Molloy, C.A. and Manning-Courtney, P. (2003) "Prevalence of chronic gastrointestinal symptoms in children with autism and autistic spectrum disorders." *Autism 7*, 165–171.

53. Valicenti-McDermott, M.R., McVicar, K., Cohen, H., Wershil, B., Rapin, I. and Shinnar, S. (2005) "Frequency of gastrointestinal disorders and family history of autoimmune disease in children with autistic spectrum disorders and controls." *Proc. E. Soc. Pediatric Res. Conf. March 4.* http://www.aps-spr.org/Regional_Societies/ESPR/2005/Program.htm

54. Song, Y., Liu, C. and Finegold, S.M. (2004) "Real-time PCR quantitation of clostridia in feces of autistic children." *Appl. Environ. Microbiol. 70*, 6459–6465.

55. Croonenberghs, J., Bosmans, E., Deboutte, D., Kenis, G. and Maes, M. (2002) "Activation of the inflammatory response system in autism." *Neuropsychobiology 45*, 1–6.

56. DeFelice, M.L., Ruchelli, E.D., Markowitz, J.E., Strogatz, M., Reddy, K.P., Kadivar, K. *et al.* (2003) "Intestinal cytokines in children with pervasive developmental disorders." *Am. J. Gastroenterol. 98*, 1777–1782.

57. Kuddo, T. and Nelson, K.B. (2003) "How common are gastrointestinal disorders in children with autism?" *Curr. Opin. Pediatr. 15,* 339–343.

58. Black, C., Kaye, J.A. and Jick, H. (2002) "Relation of childhood gastrointestinal disorders to autism: nested case-control study using data from the UK General Practice Research Database." *Brit. Med. J. 325,* 419–421.

59. Taylor, B., Miller, E., Lingam, R., Andrews, N., Simmons, A. and Stowe, J. (2002) "Measles, mumps, and rubella vaccination and bowel problems or developmental regression in children with autism: population study." *Brit. Med. J. 324,* 393–396.

60. Melmed, R., Schneider, C., Fabes, R., Phillips, J. and Reichelt, K. (2000) "Metabolic markers and gastrointestinal symptoms in children with autism and related disorders." *J. Pediatr. Gastroenterol. Nutr. 31,* S31–S32.

61. Whiteley, P. (2004) "Developmental, behavioural and somatic factors in pervasive developmental disorders: preliminary analysis." *Child Care Health Dev. 30,* 5–11.

62. Forbes, G.M., Glaser, M.E., Cullen, D.J., Warren, J.R., Christiansen, K.J., Marshall, B.J. *et al.* (1994) "Duodenal ulcer treated with *Helicobacter pylori* eradication: seven-year follow-up." *Lancet 343,* 258–260.

63. Enserink, M. (2005) "Physiology or medicine: triumph of the ulcer-bug theory." *Science 310,* 34a–35a.

64. Stubbs, E.G. (1976) "Autistic children exhibit undetectable hemagglutination-inhibition antibody titers despite previous rubella vaccination." *J. Autism Child Schizophr. 6,* 269–274.

65. Singh, V.K. and Jensen, R.L. (2003) "Elevated levels of measles antibodies in children with autism." *Pediatr. Neurol. 28,* 292–294.

66. Jass, J.R. (2005) "The intestinal lesion of autistic spectrum disorder." *Eur. J. Gastroenterol. Hepatol. 17,* 821–822.

67. Kostial, K., Kargacin, B. and Landeka, M. (1989) "Gut retention of metals in rats." *Biol. Trace Elem. Res. 21,* 213–218.

68. McGinnis, W.R. (2001) "Mercury and autistic gut disease." *Environ. Health Perspect. 109,* A303–A304.

69. Esworthy, R.S., Binder, S.W., Doroshow, J.H. and Chu, F.F. (2003) "Microflora trigger colitis in mice deficient in selenium-dependent glutathione peroxidase and induce Gpx2 gene expression." *Biol. Chem. 384,* 597–607.

70. Chu, F.F., Esworthy, R.S., Chu, P.G., Longmate, J.A., Huycke, M.M., Wilczynski, S. *et al.* (2004) "Bacteria-induced intestinal cancer in mice with disrupted Gpx1 and Gpx2 genes." *Cancer Res. 64,* 962–968.

71. James, S.J., Cutler, P., Melnyk, S., Jernigan, S., Janak, L., Gaylor, D.W. *et al.* (2004) "Metabolic biomarkers of increased oxidative stress and impaired methylation capacity in children with autism." *Am. J. Clin. Nutr. 80,* 1611–1617.

72. Anderson, G.M., Freedman, D.X., Cohen, D.J., Volkmar, F.R., Hoder, E.L., McPhedran, P. *et al.* (1987) "Whole blood serotonin in autistic and normal subjects." *J. Child Psychol. Psychiatry 28,* 885–900.

73. Naffah-Mazzacoratti, M.G., Rosenberg, R., Fernandes, M.J., Draque, C.M., Silvestrini, W., Calderazzo, L. *et al.* (1993) "Serum serotonin levels of normal and autistic children." *Braz. J. Med. Biol. Res. 26,* 309–317.

74. Colombi, A., Maroni, M., Antonini, C., Fait, A., Zocchetti, C. and Foa, V. (1983) "Influence of sex, age, and smoking habits on the urinary excretion of D-glucaric acid." *Clin. Chim. Acta 128,* 349–358.

75. Murch, S.H., MacDonald, T.T., Walker-Smith, J.A., Levin, M., Lionetti, P. and Klein, N.J. (1993) "Disruption of sulphated glycosaminoglycans in intestinal inflammation." *Lancet 341,* 711–714.

76. Wilkinson, L.J. and Waring, R.H. (2002) "Cysteine dioxygenase: modulation of expression in human cell lines by cytokines and control of sulphate production." *Toxicol. In Vitro 16,* 481–483.

77. Kim, M.S., Shigenaga, J., Moser, A., Grunfeld, C. and Feingold, K.R. (2004) "Suppression of DHEA sulfotransferase (Sult2A1) during the acute phase response." *Am. J. Physiol. Endocrinol. Metab. 287,* E731–E738.

78. Strott, C.A. (2002) "Sulfonation and molecular action." *Endocr. Rev. 23,* 703–732.

79. Markovich, D. (2001) "Physiological roles and regulation of mammalian sulfate transporters." *Physiol. Rev. 81,* 1499–1533.

80. Markovich, D. and James, K.M. (1999) "Heavy metals mercury, cadmium, and chromium inhibit the activity of the mammalian liver and kidney sulfate transporter sat-1." *Toxicol. Appl. Pharmacol. 154,* 181–187.

81. Lenz, E.M., Bright, J., Knight, R., Wilson, I.D. and Major, H. (2004) "A metabonomic investigation of the biochemical effects of mercuric chloride in the rat using 1H NMR and HPLC-TOF/MS: time dependent changes in the urinary profile of endogenous metabolites as a result of nephrotoxicity." *Analyst 129*, 535–541.

82. Waly, M., Olteanu, H., Banerjee, R., Choi, S.W., Mason, J.B., Parker, B.S. *et al.* (2004) "Activation of methionine synthase by insulin-like growth factor-1 and dopamine: a target for neurodevelopmental toxins and thimerosal." *Mol. Psychiatry 9*, 358–370.

83. Hanley, H.G., Stahl, S.M. and Freedman, D.X. (1977) "Hyperserotonemia and amine metabolites in autistic and retarded children." *Arch. Gen. Psychiatry 34*, 521–531.

84. Kuperman, S., Beeghly, J., Burns, T. and Tsai, L. (1987) "Association of serotonin concentration to behavior and IQ in autistic children." *J. Autism Dev. Disord. 17*, 133–140.

85. Herault, J., Petit, E., Martineau, J., Cherpi, C., Perrot, A., Barthelemy, C. *et al.* (1996) "Serotonin and autism: biochemical and molecular biology features." *Psychiatry Res. 65*, 33–43.

86. Stone, T.W. (2001) "Kynurenines in the CNS: from endogenous obscurity to therapeutic importance." *Prog. Neurobiol. 64*, 185–218.

87. Pietraszek, M.H., Takada, Y., Yan, D., Urano, T., Serizawa, K. and Takada, A. (1992) "Relationship between serotonergic measures in periphery and the brain of mouse." *Life Sci. 51*, 75–82.

88. Westerink, B.H. and De Vries, J.B. (1991) "Effect of precursor loading on the synthesis rate and release of dopamine and serotonin in the striatum: a microdialysis study in conscious rats." *J. Neurochem. 56*, 228–233.

89. Prichard, B.N. and Smith, C.C. (1990) "Serotonin: receptors and antagonists – summary of symposium." *Clin. Physiol. Biochem. 8*, Suppl 3, 120–128.

90. Hansen, M.B. and Skadhauge, E. (1997) "Signal transduction pathways for serotonin as an intestinal secretagogue." *Comp. Biochem. Physiol. A. Physiol. 118*, 283–290.

91. Ormsbee, H.S., III and Fondacaro, J.D. (1985) "Action of serotonin on the gastrointestinal tract." *Proc. Soc. Exp. Biol. Med. 178*, 333–338.

92. Read, N.W. and Gwee, K.A. (1994) "The importance of 5-hydroxytryptamine receptors in the gut." *Pharmacol. Ther. 62*, 159–173.

93. Hansen, M.B. (2003) "Neurohumoral control of gastrointestinal motility." *Physiol. Res. 52*, 1–30.

94. Hopkinson, G.B., Hinsdale, J. and Jaffe, B.M. (1989) "Contraction of canine stomach and small bowel by intravenous administration of serotonin. A physiologic response?" *Scand. J. Gastroenterol. 24*, 923–932.

95. Nakajima, M., Shiihara, Y., Shiba, Y., Sano, I., Sakai, T., Mizumoto, A. *et al.* (1997) "Effect of 5-hydroxytryptamine on gastrointestinal motility in conscious guinea-pigs." *Neurogastroenterol. Motil. 9*, 205–214.

96. Gronstad, K., Dahlstrom, A., Florence, L., Zinner, M.J., Ahlman, J. and Jaffe, B.M. (1987) "Regulatory mechanisms in endoluminal release of serotonin and substance P from feline jejunum." *Dig. Dis. Sci. 32*, 393–400.

97. Oosterbosch, L., von der, O.M., Valdovinos, M.A., Kost, L.J., Phillips, S.F. and Camilleri, M. (1993) "Effects of serotonin on rat ileocolonic transit and fluid transfer in vivo: possible mechanisms of action." *Gut 34*, 794–798.

98. Anderson, G.M., Feibel, F.C. and Cohen, D.J. (1987) "Determination of serotonin in whole blood, platelet-rich plasma, platelet-poor plasma and plasma ultrafiltrate." *Life Sci. 40*, 1063–1070.

99. Pletscher, A. (1987) "The 5-hydroxytryptamine system of blood platelets: physiology and patho-physiology." *Int. J. Cardiol. 14*, 177–188.

100. Ortiz, J., Artigas, F. and Gelpi, E. (1988) "Serotonergic status in human blood." *Life Sci. 43*, 983–990.

101. Ritvo, E.R., Yuwiler, A., Geller, E., Ornitz, E.M., Saeger, K. and Plotkin, S. (1970) "Increased blood serotonin and platelets in early infantile autism." *Arch. Gen. Psychiatry 23*, 566–572.

102. Takahashi, S., Kanai, H. and Miyamoto, Y. (1976) "Reassessment of elevated serotonin levels in blood platelets in early infantile autism." *J. Autism Child Schizophr. 6*, 317–326.

103. Hoshino, Y., Yamamoto, T., Kaneko, M., Tachibana, R., Watanabe, M., Ono, Y. *et al.* (1984) "Blood serotonin and free tryptophan concentration in autistic children." *Neuropsychobiology 11*, 22–27.

104. Minderaa, R.B., Anderson, G.M., Volkmar, F.R., Akkerhuis, G.W. and Cohen, D.J. (1987) "Urinary 5-hydroxyindoleacetic acid and whole blood serotonin and tryptophan in autistic and normal subjects." *Biol. Psychiatry 22*, 933–940.

105. De Villard, R., Flachaire, E., Laujin, A., Maillet, J., Revol, O., Charles, S. *et al.* (1991) "Platelet serotonin concentration in children under 5 years of age." *Pediatrie. 46*, 813–816.

106. Badcock, N.R., Spence, J.G. and Stern, L.M. (1987) "Blood serotonin levels in adults, autistic and non-autistic children – with a comparison of different methodologies." *Ann. Clin. Biochem. 24*, 625–634.

107. Spivak, B., Golubchik, P., Mozes, T., Vered, Y., Nechmad, A., Weizman, A. *et al.* (2004) "Low platelet-poor plasma levels of serotonin in adult autistic patients." *Neuropsychobiology 50*, 157–160.

108. Vered, Y., Golubchik, P., Mozes, T., Strous, R., Nechmad, A., Mester, R. *et al.* (2003) "The platelet-poor plasma 5-HT response to carbohydrate rich meal administration in adult autistic patients compared with normal controls." *Hum. Psychopharmacol. 18*, 395–399.

109. De Villard, R., Flachaire, E., Thoulon, J.M., Dalery, J., Maillet, J., Chauvin, C. *et al.* (1986) "Platelet serotonin concentrations in autistic children and members of their families." *Encephale 12*, 139–142.

110. Rolf, L.H., Haarmann, F.Y., Grotemeyer, K.H. and Kehrer, H. (1993) "Serotonin and amino acid content in platelets of autistic children." *Acta Psychiatr. Scand. 87*, 312–316.

111. McBride, P.A., Anderson, G.M., Hertzig, M.E., Snow, M.E., Thompson, S.M., Khait, V.D. *et al.* (1998) "Effects of diagnosis, race, and puberty on platelet serotonin levels in autism and mental retardation." *J. Am. Acad. Child Adolesc. Psychiatry 37*, 767–776.

112. Mulder, E.J., Anderson, G.M., Kema, I.P., de Bildt, A., van Lang, N.D., den Boer, J.A. *et al.* (2004) "Platelet serotonin levels in pervasive developmental disorders and mental retardation: diagnostic group differences, within-group distribution, and behavioral correlates." *J. Am. Acad. Child Adolesc. Psychiatry 43*, 491–499.

113. Bolte, A.C., van Geijn, H.P. and Dekker, G.A. (2001) "Pathophysiology of preeclampsia and the role of serotonin." *Eur. J. Obstet. Gynecol. Reprod. Biol. 95*, 12–21.

114. Narayan, M., Srinath, S., Anderson, G.M. and Meundi, D.B. (1993) "Cerebrospinal fluid levels of homovanillic acid and 5-hydroxyindoleacetic acid in autism." *Biol. Psychiatry 33*, 630–635.

115. Piven, J., Tsai, G.C., Nehme, E., Coyle, J.T., Chase, G.A. and Folstein, S.E. (1991) "Platelet serotonin, a possible marker for familial autism." *J. Autism Dev. Disord. 21*, 51–59.

116. Leventhal, B.L., Cook, E.H., Jr., Morford, M., Ravitz, A. and Freedman, D.X. (1990) "Relationships of whole blood serotonin and plasma norepinephrine within families." *J. Autism Dev. Disord. 20*, 499–511.

117. Leboyer, M., Philippe, A., Bouvard, M., Guilloud-Bataille, M., Bondoux, D., Tabuteau, F. *et al.* (1999) "Whole blood serotonin and plasma beta-endorphin in autistic probands and their first-degree relatives." *Biol. Psychiatry 45*, 158–163.

118. Cook, E.H., Leventhal, B.L., Heller, W., Metz, J., Wainwright, M. and Freedman, D.X. (1990) "Autistic children and their first-degree relatives: relationships between serotonin and norepinephrine levels and intelligence." *J. Neuropsychiatry Clin. Neurosci. 2*, 268–274.

119. Sole, M.J., Madapallimattam, A. and Baines, A.D. (1986) "An active pathway for serotonin synthesis by renal proximal tubules." *Kidney Int. 29*, 689–694.

120. Hafdi, Z., Couette, S., Comoy, E., Prie, D., Amiel, C. and Friedlander, G. (1996) "Locally formed 5-hydroxytryptamine stimulates phosphate transport in cultured opossum kidney cells and in rat kidney." *Biochem. J. 320* (Pt 2), 615–621.

121. Sebekova, K., Raucinova, M. and Dzurik, R. (1989) "Serotonin metabolism in patients with decreased renal function." *Nephron 53*, 229–232.

122. Sebekova, K., Spustova, V., Opatrny, K., Jr. and Dzurik, R. (2001) "Serotonin and 5-hydroxyindole-acetic acid." *Bratisl. Lek. Listy 102*, 351–356.

123. Van Vleet, T.R. and Schnellmann, R.G. (2003) "Toxic nephropathy: environmental chemicals." *Semin. Nephrol. 23*, 500–508.

124. Rao, M.L., Stefan, H. and Bauer, J. (1989) "Epileptic but not psychogenic seizures are accompanied by simultaneous elevation of serum pituitary hormones and cortisol levels." *Neuroendocrinology 49*, 33–39.

125. Houghton, L.A., Atkinson, W., Whitaker, R.P., Whorwell, P.J. and Rimmer, M.J. (2003) "Increased platelet depleted plasma 5-hydroxytryptamine concentration following meal ingestion in symptomatic female subjects with diarrhoea predominant irritable bowel syndrome." *Gut 52*, 663–670.

126. Sharma, R. and Schumacher, U. (1996) "The diet and gut microflora influence the distribution of enteroendocrine cells in the rat intestine." *Experientia 52*, 664–670.

127. Farthing, M.J. (2000) "Enterotoxins and the enteric nervous system – a fatal attraction." *Int. J. Med. Microbiol. 290*, 491–496.

128. Oudar, P., Caillard, L. and Fillion, G. (1989) "In vitro effect of organic and inorganic mercury on the serotonergic system." *Pharmacol. Toxicol. 65*, 245–248.

129. Elferink, J.G. (1999) "Thimerosal: a versatile sulfhydryl reagent, calcium mobilizer, and cell function-modulating agent." *Gen. Pharmacol. 33*, 1–6.

130. Lang, I.M. (1999) "Noxious stimulation of emesis." *Dig. Dis. Sci. 44*, 58S–63S.

131. Croonenberghs, J., Verkerk, R., Scharpe, S., Deboutte, D. and Maes, M. (2005) "Serotonergic disturbances in autistic disorder: L-5-hydroxytryptophan administration to autistic youngsters increases the blood concentrations of serotonin in patients but not in controls." *Life Sci. 76*, 2171–2183.

132. Sanger, G.J. (1996) "5-hydroxytryptamine and functional bowel disorders." *Neurogastroenterol. Motil. 8*, 319–331.

133. Mach, T. (2004) "The brain-gut axis in irritable bowel syndrome – clinical aspects." *Med. Sci. Monit. 10*, RA125–RA131.

134. Gershon, M.D. (2004) "Review article: serotonin receptors and transporters – roles in normal and abnormal gastrointestinal motility." *Aliment. Pharmacol. Ther. 20*, Suppl 7, 3–14.

135. Spiller, R.C. (2003) "Postinfectious irritable bowel syndrome." *Gastroenterology 124*, 1662–1671.

136. Singh, R.K., Pandey, H.P. and Singh, R.H. (2003) "Correlation of serotonin and monoamine oxidase levels with anxiety level in diarrhea-predominant irritable bowel syndrome." *Indian J. Gastroenterol. 22*, 88–90.

137. Bearcroft, C.P., Perrett, D. and Farthing, M.J. (1998) "Postprandial plasma 5-hydroxytryptamine in diarrhoea predominant irritable bowel syndrome: a pilot study." *Gut 42*, 42–46.

138. Coutinho, A.M., Oliveira, G., Morgadinho, T., Fesel, C., Macedo, T.R., Bento, C. *et al.* (2004) "Variants of the serotonin transporter gene (SLC6A4) significantly contribute to hyperserotonemia in autism." *Mol. Psychiatry 9*, 264–271.

139. Baron-Cohen, S. (2002) "The extreme male brain theory of autism." *Trends Cogn. Sci. 6*, 248–254.

140. Beuschlein, F., Fassnacht, M., Klink, A., Allolio, B. and Reincke, M. (2001) "ACTH-receptor expression, regulation and role in adrenocortical tumor formation." *Eur. J. Endocrinol. 144*, 199–206.

141. Pritchard, L.E., Turnbull, A.V. and White, A. (2002) "Pro-opiomelanocortin processing in the hypothalamus: impact on melanocortin signalling and obesity." *J. Endocrinol. 172*, 411–421.

142. Wybran, J. (1985) "Enkephalins and endorphins: activation molecules for the immune system and natural killer activity?" *Neuropeptides 5*, 371–374.

143. Carr, D.J. and Klimpel, G.R. (1986) "Enhancement of the generation of cytotoxic T cells by endogenous opiates." *J. Neuroimmunol. 12*, 75–87.

144. Masera, R.G., Staurenghi, A., Sartori, M.L. and Angeli, A. (1999) "Natural killer cell activity in the peripheral blood of patients with Cushing's syndrome." *Eur. J. Endocrinol. 140*, 299–306.

145. Buckley, T.M. and Schatzberg, A.F. (2005) "On the interactions of the hypothalamic-pituitary-adrenal (HPA) axis and sleep: normal HPA axis activity and circadian rhythm, exemplary sleep disorders." *J. Clin. Endocrinol. Metab. 90*, 3106–3114.

146. Malow, B.A. (2004) "Sleep disorders, epilepsy, and autism." *Ment. Retard. Dev. Disabil. Res. Rev. 10*, 122–125.

147. Ivanenko, A., Crabtree, V.M. and Gozal, D. (2004) "Sleep in children with psychiatric disorders." *Pediatr. Clin. North Am. 51*, 51–68.

148. Herman, J.P., Schafer, M.K.H., Young, E.A., Thompson, R., Douglass, J., Akil, H. *et al.* (1989) "Evidence for hippocampal regulation of neuroendocrine neurons of the hypothalamo-pituitary-adrenocortical axis." *J. Neurosci. 9*, 3072–3082.

149. Jansen, L.M., Gispen-de Wied, C.C., Van der Gaag, R.J., ten Hove, F., Willemsen-Swinkels, S.W., Harteveld, E. *et al.* (2000) "Unresponsiveness to psychosocial stress in a subgroup of autistic-like children, multiple complex developmental disorder." *Psychoneuroendocrinology 25*, 753–764.

150. Jansen, L.M., Gispen-de Wied, C.C., Van der Gaag, R.J. and Van Engeland, H. (2003) "Differentiation between autism and multiple complex developmental disorder in response to psychosocial stress." *Neuropsychopharmacology 28*, 582–590.

151. Richdale, A.L. and Prior, M.R. (1992) "Urinary cortisol circadian rhythm in a group of high-functioning children with autism." *J. Autism Dev. Disord. 22*, 433–447.

152. Maher, K.R., Harper, J.F., Macleay, A. and King, M.G. (1975) "Peculiarities in the endocrine response to insulin stress in early infantile autism." *J. Nerv. Ment. Dis. 161*, 180–184.

153. Aihara, R. and Hashimoto, T. (1989) "Neuroendocrinologic studies on autism." *Brain and Development (No To Hattatsu) 21*, 154–162.

154. Curin, J.M., Terzic, J., Petkovic, Z.B., Zekan, L., Terzic, I.M. and Susnjara, I.M. (2003) "Lower cortisol and higher ACTH levels in individuals with autism." *J. Autism Dev. Disord. 33*, 443–448.

155. Corbett, B.A., Mendoza, S., Abdullah, M., Wegelin, J.A. and Levine, S. (2005) "Cortisol circadian rhythms and response to stress in children with autism." *Psychoneuroendocrinology 31*, 59–68.

156. Hoshino, Y., Ohno, Y., Murata, S., Yokoyama, F., Kaneko, M. and Kumashiro, H. (1984) "Dexamethasone suppression test in autistic children." *Folia Psychiatr. Neurol. Jpn. 38*, 445–449.

157. Green, L., Fein, D., Modahl, C., Feinstein, C., Waterhouse, L. and Morris, M. (2001) "Oxytocin and autistic disorder: alterations in peptide forms." *Biol. Psychiatry 50*, 609–613.

158. Tordjman, S., Anderson, G.M., McBride, P.A., Hertzig, M.E., Snow, M.E., Hall, L.M. *et al.* (1997) "Plasma beta-endorphin, adrenocorticotropin hormone, and cortisol in autism." *J. Child Psychol. Psychiatry 38*, 705–715.

159. Tani, P., Lindberg, N., Matto, V., Appelberg, B., Nieminen-von Wendt, T., von Wendt, L. *et al.* (2005) "Higher plasma ACTH levels in adults with Asperger syndrome." *J. Psychosom. Res. 58*, 533–536.

160. Leboyer, M., Bouvard, M.P., Recasens, C., Philippe, A., Guilloud-Bataille, M., Bondoux, D. *et al.* (1994) "Difference between plasma N- and C-terminally directed beta-endorphin immunoreactivity in infantile autism." *Am. J. Psychiatry 151*, 1797–1801.

161. Bouvard, M.P., Leboyer, M., Launay, J.M., Recasens, C., Plumet, M.H., Waller-Perotte, D. *et al.* (1995) "Low-dose naltrexone effects on plasma chemistries and clinical symptoms in autism: a double-blind, placebo-controlled study." *Psychiatry Res. 58*, 191–201.

162. Abbott, R.J., Browning, M.C. and Davidson, D.L. (1980) "Serum prolactin and cortisol concentrations after grand mal seizures." *J. Neurol. Neurosurg. Psychiatry 43*, 163–167.

163. Pritchard, P.B., III (1991) "The effect of seizures on hormones." *Epilepsia 32*, Suppl 6, S46–S50.

164. Swartz, C.M. (1997) "Neuroendocrine effects of electroconvulsive therapy (ECT)." *Psychopharmacol. Bull. 33*, 265–271.

165. Fan, X., Olson, S.J. and Johnson, M.D. (2001) "Immunohistochemical localization and comparison of carboxypeptidases D, E, and Z, alpha-MSH, ACTH, and MIB-1 between human anterior and corticotroph cell 'basophil invasion' of the posterior pituitary." *J. Histochem. Cytochem. 49*, 783–790.

166. Buitelaar, J.K., Van Engeland, H., de Kogel, K., de Vries, H., van Hooff, J. and van Ree, J. (1992) "The adrenocorticotrophic hormone (4–9) analog ORG 2766 benefits autistic children: report on a second controlled clinical trial." *J. Am. Acad. Child Adolesc. Psychiatry 31*, 1149–1156.

167. Matarazzo, E.B. (2002) "Treatment of late onset autism as a consequence of probable autommune processes related to chronic bacterial infection." *World J. Biol. Psychiatry 3*, 162–166.

168. Orentreich, N., Brind, J.L., Vogelman, J.H., Andres, R. and Baldwin, H. (1992) "Long-term longitudinal measurements of plasma dehydroepiandrosterone sulfate in normal men." *J. Clin. Endocrinol. Metab. 75*, 1002–1004.

169. Sapolsky, R.M., Vogelman, J.H., Orentreich, N. and Altmann, J. (1993) "Senescent decline in serum dehydroepiandrosterone sulfate concentrations in a population of wild baboons." *J. Gerontol. 48*, B196–200.

170. Kalimi, M., Shafagoj, Y., Loria, R., Padgett, D. and Regelson, W. (1994) "Anti-glucocorticoid effects of dehydroepiandrosterone (DHEA)." *Mol. Cell. Biochem. 131*, 99–104.

171. Chmielewski, V., Drupt, F. and Morfin, R. (2000) "Dexamethasone-induced apoptosis of mouse thymocytes: prevention by native 7alpha-hydroxysteroids." *Immunol. Cell Biol. 78*, 238–246.

172. Loria, R.M. (1997) "Antiglucocorticoid function of androstenetriol." *Psychoneuroendocrinology 22*, Suppl 1, S103–S108.

173. Kimonides, V.G., Spillantini, M.G., Sofroniew, M.V., Fawcett, J.W. and Herbert, J. (1999) "Dehydroepiandrosterone antagonizes the neurotoxic effects of corticosterone and translocation of stress-activated protein kinase 3 in hippocampal primary cultures." *Neuroscience 89*, 429–436.

174. Strous, R.D., Golubchik, P., Maayan, R., Mozes, T., Tuati-Werner, D., Weizman, A. *et al.* (2005) "Lowered DHEA-S plasma levels in adult individuals with autistic disorder." *Eur. Neuropsychopharmacol. 15*, 305–309.

175. Insel, T.R. (1992) "Oxytocin – a neuropeptide for affiliation: evidence from behavioral, receptor autoradiographic, and comparative studies." *Psychoneuroendocrinology 17*, 3–35.

176. Insel, T.R., O'Brien, D.J. and Leckman, J.F. (1999) "Oxytocin, vasopressin, and autism: is there a connection?" *Biol. Psychiatry 45*, 145–157.

177. Neumann, I.D. (2002) "Involvement of the brain oxytocin system in stress coping: interactions with the hypothalamo-pituitary-adrenal axis." *Prog. Brain Res. 139*, 147–162.

178. Heinrichs, M., Baumgartner, T., Kirschbaum, C. and Ehlert, U. (2003) "Social support and oxytocin interact to suppress cortisol and subjective responses to psychosocial stress." *Biol. Psychiatry 54*, 1389–1398.

179. Modahl, C., Green, L., Fein, D., Morris, M., Waterhouse, L., Feinstein, C. *et al.* (1998) "Plasma oxytocin levels in autistic children." *Biol. Psychiatry 43*, 270–277.

180. Mueller-Heubach, E., Morris, M. and Rose, J.C. (1995) "Fetal oxytocin and its extended forms at term with and without labor." *Am. J. Obstet. Gynecol. 173*, 375–380.

181. Norenberg, U. and Richter, D. (1988) "Processing of the oxytocin precursor: isolation of an exopeptidase from neurosecretory granules of bovine pituitaries." *Biochem. Biophys. Res. Commun. 156*, 898–904.

182. Hollander, E., Novotny, S., Hanratty, M., Yaffe, R., DeCaria, C.M., Aronowitz, B.R. *et al.* (2003) "Oxytocin infusion reduces repetitive behaviors in adults with autistic and Asperger's disorders." *Neuropsychopharmacology 28*, 193–198.

183. Ludwig, M. (1998) "Dendritic release of vasopressin and oxytocin." *J. Neuroendocrinol. 10*, 881–895.

184. Ludwig, M., Sabatier, N., Bull, P.M., Landgraf, R., Dayanithi, G. and Leng, G. (2002) "Intracellular calcium stores regulate activity-dependent neuropeptide release from dendrites." *Nature 418*, 85–89.

185. Ferguson, J.N., Aldag, J.M., Insel, T.R. and Young, L.J. (2001) "Oxytocin in the medial amygdala is essential for social recognition in the mouse." *J. Neurosci. 21*, 8278–8285.

186. Amico, J.A., Mantella, R.C., Vollmer, R.R. and Li, X. (2004) "Anxiety and stress responses in female oxytocin deficient mice." *J. Neuroendocrinol. 16*, 319–324.

187. Winslow, J.T. and Insel, T.R. (2002) "The social deficits of the oxytocin knockout mouse." *Neuropeptides 36*, 221–229.

188. McGowan-Sass, B.K. and Timiras, P.S. (1975) "The hippocampus and hormonal cyclicity." In R.L. Isaacson and K.H. Pribram (eds) *The Hippocampus, Vol. 1. Structure and Development.* New York: Plenum; pp.355–391.

189. Geschwind, N. and Galaburda, A.M. (1985) "Cerebral lateralization. Biological mechanisms, associations and pathology: III. A hypothesis and a program for research." *Arch. Neurol. 42*, 634–654.

190. MacLusky, N.J. and Naftolin, F. (1981) "Sexual differentiation of the central nervous system." *Science 211*, 1294–1302.

191. McEwen, B.S. and Alves, S.E. (1999) "Estrogen actions in the central nervous system." *Endocr. Rev. 20*, 279–307.

192. Manning, J., Bundred, P. and Flanagan, B. (2002) "The ratio of 2nd to 4th digit length: a proxy for transactivation activity of the androgen receptor gene?" *Med. Hypotheses 59*, 334–336.

193. Okten, A., Kalyoncu, M. and Yaris, N. (2002) "The ratio of second- and fourth-digit lengths and congenital adrenal hyperplasia due to 21-hydroxylase deficiency." *Early Hum. Dev. 70*, 47–54.

194. Lutchmaya, S., Baron-Cohen, S., Raggatt, P., Knickmeyer, R. and Manning, J.T. (2004) "2nd to 4th digit ratios, fetal testosterone and estradiol." *Early Hum. Dev. 77*, 23–28.

195. Buck, J.J., Williams, R.M., Hughes, I.A. and Acerini, C.L. (2003) "In-utero androgen exposure and 2nd to 4th digit length ratio-comparisons between healthy controls and females with classical congenital adrenal hyperplasia." *Hum. Reprod. 18*, 976–979.

196. Manning, J.T., Baron-Cohen, S., Wheelwright, S. and Sanders, G. (2001) "The 2nd to 4th digit ratio and autism." *Dev. Med. Child Neurol. 43*, 160–164.

197. Williams, J.H., Greenhalgh, K.D. and Manning, J.T. (2003) "Second to fourth finger ratio and possible precursors of developmental psychopathology in preschool children." *Early Hum. Dev. 72*, 57–65.

198. Knickmeyer, R., Baron-Cohen, S., Raggatt, P. and Taylor, K. (2005) "Foetal testosterone, social relationships, and restricted interests in children." *J. Child Psychol. Psychiatry 46*, 198–210.

199. Ingudomnukul, E., Wheelwright, S., Baron-Cohen, S. and Knickmeyer, R. (2006) "Elevated rates of testosterone-related disorders in women with autism spectrum conditions." Submitted for publication.

200. Caviness, V.S., Jr., Kennedy, D.N., Richelme, C., Rademacher, J. and Filipek, P.A. (1996) "The human brain age 7–11 years: a volumetric analysis based on magnetic resonance images." *Cereb. Cortex 6,* 726–736.

201. Giedd, J.N., Castellanos, F.X., Rajapakse, J.C., Vaituzis, A.C. and Rapoport, J.L. (1997) "Sexual dimorphism of the developing human brain." *Prog. Neuropsychopharmacol. Biol. Psychiatry 21,* 1185–1201.

202. Filipek, P.A., Richelme, C., Kennedy, D.N. and Caviness, V.S., Jr. (1994) "The young adult human brain: an MRI-based morphometric analysis." *Cereb. Cortex 4,* 344–360.

203. Hines, M. (2003) "Sex steroids and human behavior: prenatal androgen exposure and sex-typical play behavior in children." *Ann. NY Acad. Sci. 1007,* 272–282.

204. Knickmeyer, R., Baron-Cohen, S., Fane, B.A., Wheelwright, S., Mathews, G.A., Conway, G.S. *et al.* (2005) "Androgens and autistic traits: a study of individuals with congenital adrenal hyperplasia (CAH)." In press.

205. Sloviter, R.S., Valiquette, G., Abrams, G.M., Ronk, E.C., Sollas, A.L., Paul, L.A. *et al.* (1989) "Selective loss of hippocampal granule cells in the mature rat brain after adrenalectomy." *Science 243,* 535–538.

206. Gould, E., Woolley, C.S. and McEwen, B.S. (1990) "Short-term glucocorticoid manipulations affect neuronal morphology and survival in the adult dentate gyrus." *Neuroscience 37,* 367–375.

207. Götz, F., Dörner, G., Malz, U., Rohde, W., Stahl, F., Poppe, I. *et al.* (1993) "Short- and long-term effects of perinatal interleukin-1 beta-application in rats." *Neuroendocrinology 58,* 344–351.

208. Dahlgren, J., Nilsson, C., Jennische, E., Ho, H.P., Eriksson, E., Niklasson, A. *et al.* (2001) "Prenatal cytokine exposure results in obesity and gender-specific programming." *Am. J. Physiol. Endocrinol. Metab. 281,* E326–E334.

209. Bowman, R.E., MacLusky, N.J., Sarmiento, Y., Frankfurt, M., Gordon, M. and Luine, V.N. (2004) "Sexually dimorphic effects of prenatal stress on cognition, hormonal responses, and central neurotransmitters." *Endocrinology 145,* 3778–3787.

210. Martin, M.B., Reiter, R., Pham, T., Avellanet, Y.R., Camara, J., Lahm, M. *et al.* (2003) "Estrogen-like activity of metals in MCF-7 breast cancer cells." *Endocrinology 144,* 2425–2436.

211. Johnson, M.D., Kenney, N., Stoica, A., Hilakivi-Clarke, L., Singh, B., Chepko, G. *et al.* (2003) "Cadmium mimics the in vivo effects of estrogen in the uterus and mammary gland." *Nat. Med. 9,* 1081–1084.

212. Martin, M.B., Voeller, H.J., Gelmann, E.P., Lu, J., Stoica, E.G., Hebert, E.J. *et al.* (2002) "Role of cadmium in the regulation of AR gene expression and activity." *Endocrinology 143,* 263–275.

213. Palnaes, H.C., Stadil, F. and Rehfeld, J.F. (2000) "Metabolism and acid secretory effect of sulfated and nonsulfated gastrin-6 in humans." *Am. J. Physiol. Gastrointest. Liver Physiol. 279,* G903–G909.

214. Gigoux, V., Escrieut, C., Silvente-Poirot, S., Maigret, B., Gouilleux, L., Fehrentz, J.A. *et al.* (1998) "Met-195 of the cholecystokinin-A receptor interacts with the sulfated tyrosine of cholecystokinin and is crucial for receptor transition to high affinity state." *J. Biol. Chem. 273,* 14380–14386.

215. Bateman, A., Solomon, S. and Bennett, H.P. (1990) "Post-translational modification of bovine pro-opiomelanocortin. Tyrosine sulfation and pyroglutamate formation, a mass spectrometric study." *J. Biol. Chem. 265,* 22130–22136.

216. Falany, J.L., Macrina, N. and Falany, C.N. (2002) "Regulation of MCF-7 breast cancer cell growth by beta-estradiol sulfation." *Breast Cancer Res. Treat. 74,* 167–176.

217. Park-Chung, M., Malayev, A., Purdy, R.H., Gibbs, T.T. and Farb, D.H. (1999) "Sulfated and unsulfated steroids modulate gamma-aminobutyric acidA receptor function through distinct sites." *Brain Res. 830,* 72–87.

218. Ferioli, A., Apostoli, P. and Romeo, L. (1989) "Alteration of steroid hormone sulfation and D-glucaric acid excretion in lead workers." *Biol. Trace Elem. Res. 21,* 289–294.

219. Visser, T.J. (1994) "Role of sulfation in thyroid hormone metabolism." *Chem. Biol. Interact. 92,* 293–303.

220. Cohen, D.J., Young, J.G., Lowe, T.L. and Harcherik, D. (1980) "Thyroid hormone in autistic children." *J. Autism Dev. Disord. 10,* 445–450.

221. Gillberg, I.C., Gillberg, C. and Kopp, S. (1992) "Hypothyroidism and autism spectrum disorders." *J. Child Psychol. Psychiatry 33,* 531–542.

222. Campbell, M., Small, A.M., Hollander, C.S., Korein, J., Cohen, I.L., Kalmijn, M. *et al.* (1978) "A controlled crossover study of triiodothyronine in autistic children." *J. Autism Child Schizophr. 8,* 371–381.

223. Haas, H.S. and Schauenstein, K. (1997) "Neuroimmunomodulation via limbic structures – the neuro-anatomy of psychoimmunology." *Prog. Neurobiol. 51,* 195–222.

224. Brooks, W.H., Cross, R.J., Roszman, T.L. and Markesbery, W.R. (1982) "Neuroimmunomodulation: neural anatomical basis for impairment and facilitation." *Ann. Neurol. 12*, 56–61.

225. Bratt, A.M., Kelley, S.P., Knowles, J.P., Barrett, J., Davis, K., Davis, M. *et al.* (2001) "Long term modulation of the HPA axis by the hippocampus. Behavioral, biochemical and immunological endpoints in rats exposed to chronic mild stress." *Psychoneuroendocrinology 26*, 121–145.

226. Devi, R.S., Sivaprakash, R.M. and Namasivayam, A. (2004) "Rat hippocampus and primary immune response." *Indian J. Physiol. Pharmacol. 48*, 329–336.

227. Marx, J. (1995) "How the glucocorticoids suppress immunity." *Science 270*, 232–233.

228. Mash, B., Bheekie, A. and Jones, P.W. (2001) "Inhaled vs oral steroids for adults with chronic asthma." *Cochrane Database Syst. Rev.*, CD002160.

229. Lionakis, M.S. and Kontoyiannis, D.P. (2003) "Glucocorticoids and invasive fungal infections." *Lancet 362*, 1828–1838.

230. Stubbs, E.G. and Crawford, M.L. (1977) "Depressed lymphocyte responsiveness in autistic children." *J. Autism Child Schizophr. 7*, 49–55.

231. Warren, R.P., Singh, V.K., Averett, R.E., Odell, J.D., Maciulis, A., Burger, R.A. *et al.* (1996) "Immunogenetic studies in autism and related disorders." *Mol. Chem. Neuropathol. 28*, 77–81.

232. Ferrante, P., Saresella, M., Guerini, F.R., Marzorati, M., Musetti, M.C. and Cazzullo, A.G. (2003) "Significant association of HLA A2-DR11 with CD4 naive decrease in autistic children." *Biomed. Pharmacother. 57*, 372–374.

233. Warren, R.P., Odell, J.D., Warren, W.L., Burger, R.A., Maciulis, A., Daniels, W.W. *et al.* (1997) "Brief report: immunoglobulin A deficiency in a subset of autistic subjects." *J. Autism Dev. Disord. 27*, 187–192.

234. Jyonouchi, H., Sun, S. and Le, H. (2001) "Proinflammatory and regulatory cytokine production associated with innate and adaptive immune responses in children with autism spectrum disorders and developmental regression." *J. Neuroimmunol. 120*, 170–179.

235. Webb, T., Meinzen-Derr, J., Wilson, S. and Wess, M. (2004) "Are children with autism more likely to have digestive, respiratory, or skin allergies compared with healthy controls?" *Proc. Ann. Conf. Pediatric Academic Societies*, San Francisco, May 1.

236. Comi, A.M., Zimmerman, A.W., Frye, V.H., Law, P.A. and Peeden, J.N. (1999) "Familial clustering of autoimmune disorders and evaluation of medical risk factors in autism." *J. Child Neurol. 14*, 388–394.

237. Croen, L.A., Grether, J.K., Yoshida, C.K., Odouli, R. and Van de, W.J. (2005) "Maternal autoimmune diseases, asthma and allergies, and childhood autism spectrum disorders: a case-control study." *Arch. Pediatr. Adolesc. Med. 159*, 151–157.

238. Sweeten, T.L., Posey, D.J. and McDougle, C.J. (2003) "High blood monocyte counts and neopterin levels in children with autistic disorder." *Am. J. Psychiatry 160*, 1691–1693.

239. Vargas, D.L., Nascimbene, C., Krishnan, C., Zimmerman, A.W. and Pardo, C.A. (2005) "Neuroglial activation and neuroinflammation in the brain of patients with autism." *Ann. Neurol. 57*, 67–81.

240. Rogers, T., Kalaydjieva, L., Hallmayer, J., Petersen, P.B., Nicholas, P., Pingree, C. *et al.* (1999) "Exclusion of linkage to the HLA region in ninety multiplex sibships with autism." *J. Autism Dev. Disord. 29*, 195–201.

241. Daniels, W.W., Warren, R.P., Odell, J.D., Maciulis, A., Burger, R.A., Warren, W.L. *et al.* (1995) "Increased frequency of the extended or ancestral haplotype B44-SC30-DR4 in autism." *Neuropsychobiology 32*, 120–123.

242. Warren, R.P., Odell, J.D., Warren, W.L., Burger, R.A., Maciulis, A., Daniels, W.W. *et al.* (1996) "Strong association of the third hypervariable region of HLA-DR beta 1 with autism." *J. Neuroimmunol. 67*, 97–102.

243. Torres, A.R., Maciulis, A., Stubbs, E.G., Cutler, A. and Odell, D. (2002) "The transmission disequilibrium test suggests that HLA-DR4 and DR13 are linked to autism spectrum disorder." *Hum. Immunol. 63*, 311–316.

244. Seto, K., Saito, H., Takeshima, Y., Kitaoka, K., Sasaki, Y., Kimura, F. *et al.* (1986) "Influence of microinjection of insulin into hippocampus on hepatic acetate metabolism in rabbits." *Exp. Clin. Endocrinol. 87*, 341–344.

245. Seto, K., Saito, H., Kaba, H., Ohri, A., Nojima, K., Takahashi, T. *et al.* (1988) "Influence of microinjection of corticosterone into hippocampus on hepatic acetate metabolism in rabbits." *Exp. Clin. Endocrinol. 91*, 123–126.

246. Saito, H., Kaba, H., Sato, T., Nojima, K., Li, C.S., Seto, K. *et al.* (1990) "Influence of dorsal hippocampal stimulation and dorsal fornix lesions on hepatic glucose metabolism in rabbits." *Exp. Clin. Endocrinol. 96,* 113–116.

247. Brewster, M.A. (1988) "Biomarkers of xenobiotic exposures." *Ann. Clin. Lab. Sci. 18,* 306–317.

248. Buchanan, N., Eyberg, C. and Davis, M.D. (1979) "Antipyrine pharmacokinetics and D-glucaric excretion in kwashiorkor." *Am. J. Clin. Nutr. 32,* 2439–2442.

249. Kato, N., Mochizuki, S., Kawai, K. and Yoshida, A. (1982) "Effect of dietary level of sulfur-containing amino acids on liver drug-metabolizing enzymes, serum cholesterol and urinary ascorbic acid in rats fed PCB." *J. Nutr. 112,* 848–854.

250. Labadarios, D., Dickerson, J.W., Parke, D.V., Lucas, E.G. and Obuwa, G.H. (1978) "The effects of chronic drug administration on hepatic enzyme induction and folate metabolism." *Br. J. Clin. Pharmacol. 5,* 167–173.

251. Kishi, T., Fujita, N., Eguchi, T. and Ueda, K. (1997) "Mechanism for reduction of serum folate by antiepileptic drugs during prolonged therapy." *J. Neurol. Sci. 145,* 109–112.

252. Billings, R.E. (1984) "Interactions between folate metabolism, phenytoin metabolism, and liver microsomal cytochrome P450." *Drug Nutr. Interact. 3,* 21–32.

253. Froscher, W., Maier, V., Laage, M., Wolfersdorf, M., Straub, R., Rothmeier, J. *et al.* (1995) "Folate deficiency, anticonvulsant drugs, and psychiatric morbidity." *Clin. Neuropharmacol. 18,* 165–182.

254. Schwaninger, M., Ringleb, P., Winter, R., Kohl, B., Fiehn, W., Rieser, P.A. *et al.* (1999) "Elevated plasma concentrations of homocysteine in antiepileptic drug treatment." *Epilepsia 40,* 345–350.

255. Nataf, R., Skorupka, C., Amet, L., Lam, A., Springbett, A. and Lathe, R. (2005) "Porphyrinuria in childhood autistic disorder." Submitted for publication.

256. Woods, J.S. (1996) "Altered porphyrin metabolism as a biomarker of mercury exposure and toxicity." *Can. J. Physiol. Pharmacol. 74,* 210–215.

257. Woods, J.S. and Miller, H.D. (1993) "Quantitative measurement of porphyrins in biological tissues and evaluation of tissue porphyrins during toxicant exposures." *Fundam. Appl. Toxicol. 21,* 291–297.

258. Bowers, M.A., Aicher, L.D., Davis, H.A. and Woods, J.S. (1992) "Quantitative determination of porphyrins in rat and human urine and evaluation of urinary porphyrin profiles during mercury and lead exposures." *J. Lab. Clin. Med. 120,* 272–281.

259. Woods, J.S. (1995) "Porphyrin metabolism as indicator of metal exposure and toxicity." In R.A. Goyer and M.G. Cherian (eds) *Handbook of Experimental Pharmacology, Vol. 115.* Berlin: Springer-Verlag; pp.19–52.

260. Woods, J.S., Echeverria, D., Heyer, N.J., Simmonds, P.L., Wilkerson, J. and Farin, F.M. (2005) "The association between genetic polymorphisms of coproporphyrinogen oxidase and an atypical porphyrinogenic response to mercury exposure in humans." *Toxicol. Appl. Pharmacol. 206,* 113–120.

261. Pingree, S.D., Simmonds, P.L., Rummel, K.T. and Woods, J.S. (2001) "Quantitative evaluation of urinary porphyrins as a measure of kidney mercury content and mercury body burden during prolonged methylmercury exposure in rats." *Toxicol. Sci. 61,* 234–240.

262. Gonzalez-Ramirez, D., Maiorino, R.M., Zuniga-Charles, M., Xu, Z., Hurlbut, K.M., Junco-Munoz, P. *et al.* (1995) "Sodium 2,3-dimercaptopropane-1-sulfonate challenge test for mercury in humans: II. Urinary mercury, porphyrins and neurobehavioral changes of dental workers in Monterrey, Mexico." *J. Pharmacol. Exp. Ther. 272,* 264–274.

263. Woods, J.S., Martin, M.D., Naleway, C.A. and Echeverria, D. (1993) "Urinary porphyrin profiles as a biomarker of mercury exposure: studies on dentists with occupational exposure to mercury vapor." *J. Toxicol. Environ. Health 40,* 235–246.

264. Rosen, J.F. and Markowitz, M.E. (1993) "Trends in the management of childhood lead poisonings." *Neurotoxicology 14,* 211–217.

265. Despaux, N., Bohuon, C., Comoy, E. and Boudene, C. (1977) "Postulated mode of action of metals on purified human ALA-dehydratase (EC 4-2-1-24)." *Biomedicine 27,* 358–361.

266. Woods, J.S., Kardish, R. and Fowler, B.A. (1981) "Studies on the action of porphyrinogenic trace metals on the activity of hepatic uroporphyrinogen decarboxylase." *Biochem. Biophys. Res. Commun. 103,* 264–271.

267. Woods, J.S., Eaton, D.L. and Lukens, C.B. (1984) "Studies on porphyrin metabolism in the kidney. Effects of trace metals and glutathione on renal uroporphyrinogen decarboxylase." *Mol. Pharmacol. 26,* 336–341.

268. Rossi, E., Attwood, P.V. and Garcia-Webb, P. (1992) "Inhibition of human lymphocyte coproporphyrinogen oxidase activity by metals, bilirubin and haemin." *Biochim. Biophys. Acta 1135*, 262–268.

269. Gaertner, R.R. and Hollebone, B.R. (1983) "The in vitro inhibition of hepatic ferrochelatase by divalent lead and other soft metal ions." *Can. J. Biochem. Cell Biol. 61*, 214–222.

270. Kappas, A. and Drummond, G.S. (1986) "Control of heme metabolism with synthetic metalloporphyrins." *J. Clin. Invest. 77*, 335–339.

271. Iesato, K., Wakashin, M., Wakashin, Y. and Tojo, S. (1977) "Renal tubular dysfunction in Minamata disease. Detection of renal tubular antigen and beta-2-microglobin in the urine." *Ann. Intern. Med. 86*, 731–737.

272. Fowler, B.A. (1993) "Mechanisms of kidney cell injury from metals." *Environ. Health Perspect. 100*, 57–63.

273. Zalups, R.K. (2000) "Molecular interactions with mercury in the kidney." *Pharmacol. Rev. 52*, 113–143.

274. Marks, G.S., Zelt, D.T. and Cole, S.P. (1982) "Alterations in the heme biosynthetic pathway as an index of exposure to toxins." *Can. J. Physiol. Pharmacol. 60*, 1017–1026.

275. Hill, R.H. (1985) "Effects of polyhalogenated aromatic compounds on porphyrin metabolism." *Environ. Health Perspect. 60*, 139–143.

276. Rumbeiha, W.K., Fitzgerald, S.D., Braselton, W.E., Roth, R.A., Pestka, J.J. and Kaneene, J.B. (2000) "Augmentation of mercury-induced nephrotoxicity by endotoxin in the mouse." *Toxicology 151*, 103–116.

Chapter 9 Body and Mind: Impact of Physiological Changes on Brain and Behavior in ASD

1. Shahar, E., Borenstein, A. and Filk, D. (2000) "Severe migraine associated with coarctation of aorta: complete recovery following balloon dilation." *J. Child Neurol. 15*, 826–827.

2. Pratesi, R., Modelli, I.C., Martins, R.C., Almeida, P.L. and Gandolfi, L. (2003) "Celiac disease and epilepsy: favorable outcome in a child with difficult to control seizures." *Acta Neurol. Scand. 108*, 290–293.

3. Dundar, B., Bober, E. and Buyukgebiz, A. (2003) "Successful therapy with L-T4 in a 5-year-old boy with generalized thyroid hormone resistance." *J. Pediatr. Endocrinol. Metab. 16*, 1051–1056.

4. Marion, R. (1995) "The girl who mewed: acute intermittent porphyria." *Discover 16*, 38–40.

5. Gorker, I. and Tuzun, U. (2005) "Autistic-like findings associated with a urea cycle disorder in a 4-year-old girl." *J. Psychiatry Neurosci. 30*, 133–135.

6. Kim, C., Choi, H., Kim, J.K., Kim, M.S. and Park, H.J. (1976) "Influence of hippocampectomy on gastric ulcer in rats." *Brain Res. 109*, 245–254.

7. Ben Menachem, E. (2002) "Vagus-nerve stimulation for the treatment of epilepsy." *Lancet Neurol. 1*, 477–482.

8. Olejniczak, P.W., Fisch, B.J., Carey, M., Butterbaugh, G., Happel, L. and Tardo, C. (2001) "The effect of vagus nerve stimulation on epileptiform activity recorded from hippocampal depth electrodes." *Epilepsia 42*, 423–429.

9. Druschky, A., Heckmann, J.G., Druschky, K., Huk, W.J., Erbguth, F. and Neundorfer, B. (2002) "Severe neurological complications of ulcerative colitis." *J. Clin. Neurosci. 9*, 84–86.

10. Wright, D.H. (1995) "The major complications of coeliac disease." *Baillieres Clin. Gastroenterol. 9*, 351–369.

11. Akhan, G., Andermann, F. and Gotman, M.J. (2002) "Ulcerative colitis, status epilepticus and intractable temporal seizures." *Epileptic. Disord. 4*, 135–137.

12. Bolte, E.R. (1998) "Autism and *Clostridium tetani*." *Med. Hypotheses 51*, 133–144.

13. Sandler, R.H., Finegold, S.M., Bolte, E.R., Buchanan, C.P., Maxwell, A.P., Vaisanen, M.L. *et al.* (2000) "Short-term benefit from oral vancomycin treatment of regressive-onset autism." *J. Child Neurol. 15*, 429–435.

14. Pangborn, J., Baker, S. and Rimland, B. (2005) *Autism: Effective Biomedical Treatments (The DAN Protocol)*. San Diego: Autism Research Institute.

15. Shaw, W. (2002) *Biological Treatments for Autism and PDD*. Lenexa, KS: Great Plains Laboratory.

16. Wakefield, A.J., Anthony, A., Murch, S.H., Thomson, M., Montgomery, S.M., Davies, S. *et al.* (2000) "Enterocolitis in children with developmental disorders." *Am. J. Gastroenterol. 95*, 2285–2295.

17. Brudnak, M.A., Rimland, B., Kerry, R.E., Dailey, M., Taylor, R., Stayton, B. *et al.* (2002) "Enzyme-based therapy for autism spectrum disorders – is it worth another look?" *Med. Hypotheses 58*, 422–428.

18. Lucarelli, S., Frediani, T., Zingoni, A.M., Ferruzzi, F., Giardini, O., Quintieri, F. *et al.* (1995) "Food allergy and infantile autism." *Panminerva Med. 37*, 137–141.

19. Knivsberg, A.M., Reichelt, K.L. and Nodland, M. (2001) "Reports on dietary intervention in autistic disorders." *Nutr. Neurosci. 4*, 25–37.

20. Knivsberg, A.M., Reichelt, K.L., Hoien, T. and Nodland, M. (2002) "A randomised, controlled study of dietary intervention in autistic syndromes." *Nutr. Neurosci. 5*, 251–261.

21. Jyonouchi, H., Sun, S. and Itokazu, N. (2002) "Innate immunity associated with inflammatory responses and cytokine production against common dietary proteins in patients with autism spectrum disorder." *Neuropsychobiology 46*, 76–84.

22. Jyonouchi, H., Geng, L., Ruby, A., Reddy, C. and Zimmerman-Bier, B. (2005) "Evaluation of an association between gastrointestinal symptoms and cytokine production against common dietary proteins in children with autism spectrum disorders." *J. Pediatr. 146*, 605–610.

23. Stark, H., Van Bree, J.B., de Boer, A.G., Jaehde, U. and Breimer, D.D. (1992) "In vitro penetration of des-tyrosine1-D-phenylalanine3-beta-casomorphin across the blood-brain barrier." *Peptides 13*, 47–51.

24. Nyberg, F., Lieberman, H., Lindstrom, L.H., Lyrenas, S., Koch, G. and Terenius, L. (1989) "Immuno-reactive beta-casomorphin-8 in cerebrospinal fluid from pregnant and lactating women: correlation with plasma levels." *J. Clin. Endocrinol. Metab. 68*, 283–289.

25. Pasi, A., Mahler, H., Lansel, N., Bernasconi, C. and Messiha, F.S. (1993) "Beta-casomorphin-immuno-reactivity in the brain stem of the human infant." *Res. Commun. Chem. Pathol. Pharmacol. 80*, 305–322.

26. Lindstrom, L.H., Nyberg, F., Terenius, L., Bauer, K., Besev, G., Gunne, L.M. *et al.* (1984) "CSF and plasma beta-casomorphin-like opioid peptides in postpartum psychosis." *Am. J. Psychiatry 141*, 1059–1066.

27. Dubynin, V.A., Malinovskaya, I.V., Ivleva, Y.A., Andreeva, L.A., Kamenskii, A.A. and Ashmarin, I.P. (2000) "Delayed behavioral effects of beta-casomorphin-7 depend on age and gender of albino rat pups." *Bull. Exp. Biol. Med. 130*, 1031–1034.

28. Sun, Z. and Cade, R. (2003) "Findings in normal rats following administration of gliadorphin-7 (GD-7)." *Peptides 24*, 321–323.

29. Reymann, K.G., Chepkova, A.N. and Matthies, H. (1983) "Effects of deprolorphin, a casomorphin analog, on hippocampal CA1 field potentials in vitro." *Peptides 4*, 283–286.

30. Reymann, K.G., Chepkova, A.N., Schulzeck, K. and Ott, T. (1985) "Effects of beta-casomorphin on dentate hippocampal field potentials in freely moving rats." *Biomed. Biochim. Acta 44*, 749–754.

31. Sahley, T.L. and Panksepp, J. (1987) "Brain opioids and autism: an updated analysis of possible linkages." *J. Autism Dev. Disord. 17*, 201–216.

32. Wakefield, A.J., Puleston, J.M., Montgomery, S.M., Anthony, A., O'Leary, J.J. and Murch, S.H. (2002) "Review article: the concept of entero-colonic encephalopathy, autism and opioid receptor ligands." *Aliment. Pharmacol. Ther. 16*, 663–674.

33. Trygstad, O.E., Reichelt, K.L., Foss, I., Edminson, P.D., Saelid, G., Bremer, J. *et al.* (1980) "Patterns of peptides and protein-associated-peptide complexes in psychiatric disorders." *Br. J. Psychiatry 136*, 59–72.

34. Reichelt, K.L., Hole, K., Hamberger, A., Saelid, G., Edminson, P.D., Braestrup, C.B. *et al.* (1981) "Biologically active peptide-containing fractions in schizophrenia and childhood autism." *Adv. Biochem. Psychopharmacol. 28*, 627–643.

35. Le Couteur, A., Trygstad, O., Evered, C., Gillberg, C. and Rutter, M. (1988) "Infantile autism and urinary excretion of peptides and protein-associated peptide complexes." *J. Autism Dev. Disord. 18*, 181–190.

36. Millward, C., Ferriter, M., Calver, S. and Connell-Jones, G. (2004) "Gluten- and casein-free diets for autistic spectrum disorder." *Cochrane Database Syst. Rev.*, CD003498.

37. Vargas, D.L., Nascimbene, C., Krishnan, C., Zimmerman, A.W. and Pardo, C.A. (2005) "Neuroglial activation and neuroinflammation in the brain of patients with autism." *Ann. Neurol. 57*, 67–81.

38. Zimmerman, A.W., Jyonouchi, H., Comi, A.M., Connors, S.L., Milstien, S., Varsou, A. *et al.* (2005) "Cerebrospinal fluid and serum markers of inflammation in autism." *Pediatr. Neurol. 33*, 195–201.

39. Feghali, C.A. and Wright, T.M. (1997) "Cytokines in acute and chronic inflammation." *Front Biosci. 2*, d12–d26.

40. Bilbo, S.D., Levkoff, L.H., Mahoney, J.H., Watkins, L.R., Rudy, J.W. and Maier, S.F. (2005) "Neonatal infection induces memory impairments following an immune challenge in adulthood." *Behav. Neurosci. 119,* 293–301.

41. Farrar, W.L., Kilian, P.L., Ruff, M.R., Hill, J.M. and Pert, C.B. (1987) "Visualization and characterization of interleukin 1 receptors in brain." *J. Immunol. 139,* 459–463.

42. Cunningham, E.T., Jr., Wada, E., Carter, D.B., Tracey, D.E., Battey, J.F. and De Souza, E.B. (1992) "In situ histochemical localization of type I interleukin-1 receptor messenger RNA in the central nervous system, pituitary, and adrenal gland of the mouse." *J. Neurosci. 12,* 1101–1114.

43. Takao, T., Culp, S.G., Newton, R.C. and De Souza, E.B. (1992) "Type 1 interleukin-1 receptors in the mouse brain-endocrine-immune axis labelled with (125I)recombinant human interleukin-1 receptor antagonist." *Neuroimmunology 41,* 51–60.

44. Ban, E.M.H. (1994) "Interleukin-1 receptors in the brain: characterization by quantitative in situ autoradiography." *Immunomethods 5,* 31–40.

45. Ericsson, A., Liu, C., Hart, R.P. and Sawchenko, P.E. (1995) "Type I interleukin-1 receptor in the rat brain: distribution, regulation, and relationship to sites of IL-1-induced cellular activation." *J. Comp. Neurol. 361,* 681–698.

46. Frost, P., Barrientos, R.M., Makino, S., Wong, M.L. and Sternberg, E.M. (2001) "IL-1 receptor type I gene expression in the amygdala of inflammatory susceptible Lewis and inflammatory resistant Fischer rats." *J. Neuroimmunol. 121,* 32–39.

47. Utsuyama, M. and Hirokawa, K. (2002) "Differential expression of various cytokine receptors in the brain after stimulation with LPS in young and old mice." *Exp. Gerontol. 37,* 411–420.

48. Wang, Y. and Zhou, C.F. (2005) "Involvement of interferon-gamma and its receptor in the activation of astrocytes in the mouse hippocampus following entorhinal deafferentation." *Glia 50,* 56–65.

49. Gadient, R.A. and Otten, U. (1994) "Identification of interleukin-6 (IL-6)-expressing neurons in the cerebellum and hippocampus of normal adult rats." *Neurosci. Lett. 182,* 243–246.

50. Schobitz, B., de Kloet, E.R., Sutanto, W. and Holsboer, F. (1993) "Cellular localization of interleukin 6 mRNA and interleukin 6 receptor mRNA in rat brain." *Eur. J. Neurosci. 5,* 1426–1435.

51. Rhodes, J.K., Andrews, P.J., Holmes, M.C. and Seckl, J.R. (2002) "Expression of interleukin-6 messenger RNA in a rat model of diffuse axonal injury." *Neurosci. Lett. 335,* 1–4.

52. Loscher, C.E., Donnelly, S., Lynch, M.A. and Mills, K.H. (2000) "Induction of inflammatory cytokines in the brain following respiratory infection with *Bordetella pertussis*." *J. Neuroimmunol. 102,* 172–181.

53. Nofech-Mozes, Y., Yuhas, Y., Kaminsky, E., Weizman, A. and Ashkenazi, S. (2000) "Induction of mRNA for tumor necrosis factor-alpha and interleukin-1 beta in mice brain, spleen and liver in an animal model of Shigella-related seizures." *Isr. Med. Assoc. J. 2,* 86–90.

54. Donnelly, S., Loscher, C.E., Lynch, M.A. and Mills, K.H. (2001) "Whole-cell but not acellular pertussis vaccines induce convulsive activity in mice: evidence of a role for toxin-induced interleukin-1beta in a new murine model for analysis of neuronal side effects of vaccination." *Infect. Immun. 69,* 4217–4223.

55. Laye, S., Bluthe, R.M., Kent, S., Combe, C., Medina, C., Parnet, P. *et al.* (1995) "Subdiaphragmatic vagotomy blocks induction of IL-1 beta mRNA in mice brain in response to peripheral LPS." *Am. J. Physiol. 268,* R1327–R1331.

56. Hansen, M.K., Taishi, P., Chen, Z. and Krueger, J.M. (1998) "Vagotomy blocks the induction of interleukin-1beta (IL-1beta) mRNA in the brain of rats in response to systemic IL-1beta." *J. Neurosci. 18,* 2247–2253.

57. Sapolsky, R.M. (2003) "Stress and plasticity in the limbic system." *Neurochem. Res. 28,* 1735–1742.

58. O'Connor, K.A., Johnson, J.D., Hansen, M.K., Wieseler Frank, J.L., Maksimova, E., Watkins, L.R. *et al.* (2003) "Peripheral and central proinflammatory cytokine response to a severe acute stressor." *Brain Res. 991,* 123–132.

59. Marquette, C., Linard, C., Galonnier, M., Van Uye, A., Mathieu, J., Gourmelon, P. *et al.* (2003) "IL-1beta, TNFalpha and IL-6 induction in the rat brain after partial-body irradiation: role of vagal afferents." *Int. J. Radiat. Biol. 79,* 777–785.

60. Bruccoleri, A., Brown, H. and Harry, G.J. (1998) "Cellular localization and temporal elevation of tumor necrosis factor-alpha, interleukin-1 alpha, and transforming growth factor-beta 1 mRNA in hippocampal injury response induced by trimethyltin." *J. Neurochem. 71,* 1577–1587.

61. Bruccoleri, A., Pennypacker, K.R. and Harry, G.J. (1999) "Effect of dexamethasone on elevated cytokine mRNA levels in chemical-induced hippocampal injury." *J. Neurosci. Res. 57*, 916–926.

62. Yabuuchi, K., Minami, M., Katsumata, S. and Satoh, M. (1993) "In situ hybridization study of interleukin-1 beta mRNA induced by kainic acid in the rat brain." *Brain Res. Mol. Brain Res. 20*, 153–161.

63. Eriksson, C., Tehranian, R., Iverfeldt, K., Winblad, B. and Schultzberg, M. (2000) "Increased expression of mRNA encoding interleukin-1beta and caspase-1, and the secreted isoform of interleukin-1 receptor antagonist in the rat brain following systemic kainic acid administration." *J. Neurosci. Res. 60*, 266–279.

64. Lehtimaki, K.A., Peltola, J., Koskikallio, E., Keranen, T. and Honkaniemi, J. (2003) "Expression of cytokines and cytokine receptors in the rat brain after kainic acid-induced seizures." *Brain Res. Mol. Brain Res. 110*, 253–260.

65. Bluthe, R.M., Michaud, B., Kelley, K.W. and Dantzer, R. (1996) "Vagotomy blocks behavioural effects of interleukin-1 injected via the intraperitoneal route but not via other systemic routes." *Neuroreport 7*, 2823–2827.

66. Konsman, J.P., Luheshi, G.N., Bluthe, R.M. and Dantzer, R. (2000) "The vagus nerve mediates behavioural depression, but not fever, in response to peripheral immune signals; a functional anatomical analysis." *Eur. J. Neurosci. 12*, 4434–4446.

67. Cartmell, T., Luheshi, G.N. and Rothwell, N.J. (1999) "Brain sites of action of endogenous interleukin-1 in the febrile response to localized inflammation in the rat." *J. Physiol. 518*, 585–594.

68. Palin, K., Bluthe, R.M., Verrier, D., Tridon, V., Dantzer, R. and Lestage, J. (2004) "Interleukin-1beta mediates the memory impairment associated with a delayed type hypersensitivity response to bacillus Calmette-Guerin in the rat hippocampus." *Brain Behav. Immun. 18*, 223–230.

69. Dantzer, R. (1994) "How do cytokines say hello to the brain? Neural versus humoral mediation." *Eur. Cytokine Netw. 5*, 271–273.

70. Hosoi, T., Okuma, Y. and Nomura, Y. (2000) "Electrical stimulation of afferent vagus nerve induces IL-1beta expression in the brain and activates HPA axis." *Am. J. Physiol. Regul. Integr. Comp. Physiol. 279*, R141–R147.

71. Strijbos, P.J. and Rothwell, N.J. (1995) "Interleukin-1 beta attenuates excitatory amino acid-induced neurodegeneration in vitro: involvement of nerve growth factor." *J. Neurosci. 15*, 3468–3474.

72. Wang, C.X. and Shuaib, A. (2002) "Involvement of inflammatory cytokines in central nervous system injury." *Prog. Neurobiol. 67*, 161–172.

73. Rothwell, N.J. and Luheshi, G.N. (2000) "Interleukin 1 in the brain: biology, pathology and therapeutic target." *Trends Neurosci. 23*, 618–625.

74. Li, Y., Liu, L., Barger, S.W. and Griffin, W.S. (2003) "Interleukin-1 mediates pathological effects of microglia on tau phosphorylation and on synaptophysin synthesis in cortical neurons through a p38-MAPK pathway." *J. Neurosci. 23*, 1605–1611.

75. Downen, M., Amaral, T.D., Hua, L.L., Zhao, M.L. and Lee, S.C. (1999) "Neuronal death in cytokine-activated primary human brain cell culture: role of tumor necrosis factor-alpha." *Glia 28*, 114–127.

76. Kanemoto, K., Kawasaki, J., Miyamoto, T., Obayashi, H. and Nishimura, M. (2000) "Interleukin (IL)1beta, IL-1alpha, and IL-1 receptor antagonist gene polymorphisms in patients with temporal lobe epilepsy." *Ann. Neurol. 47*, 571–574.

77. Kanemoto, K., Kawasaki, J., Yuasa, S., Kumaki, T., Tomohiro, O., Kaji, R. *et al.* (2003) "Increased frequency of interleukin-1beta-511T allele in patients with temporal lobe epilepsy, hippocampal sclerosis, and prolonged febrile convulsion." *Epilepsia 44*, 796–799.

78. Yang, L., Lindholm, K., Konishi, Y., Li, R. and Shen, Y. (2002) "Target depletion of distinct tumor necrosis factor receptor subtypes reveals hippocampal neuron death and survival through different signal transduction pathways." *J. Neurosci. 22*, 3025–3032.

79. Cacci, E., Claasen, J.H. and Kokaia, Z. (2005) "Microglia-derived tumor necrosis factor-alpha exaggerates death of newborn hippocampal progenitor cells in vitro." *J. Neurosci. Res. 80*, 789–797.

80. Smith, C.J., Emsley, H.C., Gavin, C.M., Georgiou, R.F., Vail, A., Barberan, E.M. *et al.* (2004) "Peak plasma interleukin-6 and other peripheral markers of inflammation in the first week of ischaemic stroke correlate with brain infarct volume, stroke severity and long-term outcome." *BMC Neurol. 4*, 2; http://www.biomedcentral.com/1471-2377/4/2

81. Rothwell, N.J., Busbridge, N.J., Lefeuvre, R.A., Hardwick, A.J., Gauldie, J. and Hopkins, S.J. (1991) "Interleukin-6 is a centrally acting endogenous pyrogen in the rat." *Can. J. Physiol. Pharmacol. 69*, 1465–1469.

82. Horrevoets, A.J., Fontijn, R.D., van Zonneveld, A.J., de Vries, C.J., ten Cate, J.W. and Pannekoek, H. (1999) "Vascular endothelial genes that are responsive to tumor necrosis factor-alpha in vitro are expressed in atherosclerotic lesions, including inhibitor of apoptosis protein-1, stannin, and two novel genes." *Blood 93*, 3418–3431.

83. Cuccaro, M.L., Wright, H.H., Abramson, R.K., Marsteller, F.A. and Valentine, J. (1993) "Whole-blood serotonin and cognitive functioning in autistic individuals and their first-degree relatives." *J. Neuropsychiatry Clin. Neurosci. 5*, 94–101.

84. Hanley, H.G., Stahl, S.M. and Freedman, D.X. (1977) "Hyperserotonemia and amine metabolites in autistic and retarded children." *Arch. Gen. Psychiatry 34*, 521–531.

85. Kuperman, S., Beeghly, J., Burns, T. and Tsai, L. (1987) "Association of serotonin concentration to behavior and IQ in autistic children." *J. Autism Dev. Disord. 17*, 133–140.

86. Franke, L., Schewe, H.J., Uebelhack, R., Berghofer, A. and Muller-Oerlinghausen, B. (2003) "Platelet-5HT uptake and gastrointestinal symptoms in patients suffering from major depression." *Life Sci. 74*, 521–531.

87. Yonan, A.L., Palmer, A.A., Smith, K.C., Feldman, I., Lee, H.K., Yonan, J.M. *et al.* (2003) "Bioinformatic analysis of autism positional candidate genes using biological databases and computational gene network prediction." *Genes Brain Behav. 2*, 303–320.

88. Jacoby, J.H. and Bryce, G.F. (1978) "The acute pharmacologic effects of serotonin on the release of insulin and glucagon in the intact rat." *Arch. Int. Pharmacodyn. Ther. 235*, 254–270.

89. Li, Y., Wu, X.Y., Zhu, J.X. and Owyang, C. (2001) "Intestinal serotonin acts as paracrine substance to mediate pancreatic secretion stimulated by luminal factors." *Am. J. Physiol. Gastrointest. Liver Physiol. 281*, G916–G923.

90. Niebergall-Roth, E. and Singer, M.V. (2001) "Central and peripheral neural control of pancreatic exocrine secretion." *J. Physiol. Pharmacol. 52*, 523–538.

91. Dabire, H., Cherqui, C., Safar, M. and Schmitt, H. (1990) "Haemodynamic aspects and serotonin." *Clin. Physiol. Biochem. 8*, Suppl 3, 56–63.

92. Zilbovicius, M., Boddaert, N., Belin, P., Poline, J.B., Remy, P., Mangin, J.F. *et al.* (2000) "Temporal lobe dysfunction in childhood autism: a PET study. Positron emission tomography." *Am. J. Psychiatry 157*, 1988–1993.

93. Boddaert, N. and Zilbovicius, M. (2002) "Functional neuroimaging and childhood autism." *Pediatr. Radiol. 32*, 1–7.

94. Boddaert, N., Chabane, N., Gervais, H., Good, C.D., Bourgeois, M., Plumet, M.H. *et al.* (2004) "Superior temporal sulcus anatomical abnormalities in childhood autism: a voxel-based morphometry MRI study." *Neuroimage 23*, 364–369.

95. Ito, H., Mori, K., Hashimoto, T., Miyazaki, M., Hori, A., Kagami, S. *et al.* (2005) "Findings of brain 99mTc-ECD SPECT in high-functioning autism – 3-dimensional stereotactic ROI template analysis of brain SPECT." *J. Med. Invest. 52*, 49–56.

96. Young, S.N., Smith, S.E., Pihl, R.O. and Ervin, F.R. (1985) "Tryptophan depletion causes a rapid lowering of mood in normal males." *Psychopharmacology (Berl.) 87*, 173–177.

97. Van der Does, A.J. (2001) "The effects of tryptophan depletion on mood and psychiatric symptoms." *J. Affect. Disord. 64*, 107–119.

98. Curzon, G. (1979) "Study of disturbed tryptophan metabolism in depressive illness." *Ann. Biol. Clin. (Paris) 37*, 27–33.

99. Young, S.N. and Leyton, M. (2002) "The role of serotonin in human mood and social interaction. Insight from altered tryptophan levels." *Pharmacol. Biochem. Behav. 71*, 857–865.

100. D'Eufemia, P., Finocchiaro, R., Celli, M., Viozzi, L., Monteleone, D. and Giardini, O. (1995) "Low serum tryptophan to large neutral amino acids ratio in idiopathic infantile autism." *Biomed. Pharmacother. 49*, 288–292.

101. Minderaa, R.B., Anderson, G.M., Volkmar, F.R., Harcherick, D., Akkerhuis, G.W. and Cohen, D.J. (1989) "Whole blood serotonin and tryptophan in autism: temporal stability and the effects of medication." *J. Autism Dev. Disord. 19*, 129–136.

102. Croonenberghs, J., Delmeire, L., Verkerk, R., Lin, A.H., Meskal, A., Neels, H. *et al.* (2000) "Peripheral markers of serotonergic and noradrenergic function in post-pubertal, caucasian males with autistic disorder." *Neuropsychopharmacology 22*, 275–283.

103. Arnold, G.L., Hyman, S.L., Mooney, R.A. and Kirby, R.S. (2003) "Plasma amino acids profiles in children with autism: potential risk of nutritional deficiencies." *J. Autism Dev. Disord. 33*, 449–454.

104. Schroecksnadel, K., Kaser, S., Ledochowski, M., Neurauter, G., Mur, E., Herold, M. *et al.* (2003) "Increased degradation of tryptophan in blood of patients with rheumatoid arthritis." *J. Rheumatol. 30*, 1935–1939.

105. McDougle, C.J., Naylor, S.T., Cohen, D.J., Aghajanian, G.K., Heninger, G.R. and Price, L.H. (1996) "Effects of tryptophan depletion in drug-free adults with autistic disorder." *Arch. Gen. Psychiatry 53*, 993–1000.

106. Kulman, G., Lissoni, P., Rovelli, F., Roselli, M.G., Brivio, F. and Sequeri, P. (2000) "Evidence of pineal endocrine hypofunction in autistic children." *Neuroendocrinol. Lett. 21*, 31–34.

107. Nir, I., Meir, D., Zilber, N., Knobler, H., Hadjez, J. and Lerner, Y. (1995) "Brief report: circadian melatonin, thyroid-stimulating hormone, prolactin, and cortisol levels in serum of young adults with autism." *J. Autism Dev. Disord. 25*, 641–654.

108. Ishizaki, A., Sugama, M. and Takeuchi, N. (1999) "Usefulness of melatonin for developmental sleep and emotional/behavior disorders – studies of melatonin trial on 50 patients with developmental disorders." *No To Hattatsu 31*, 428–437.

109. Lee, P.P. and Pang, S.F. (1993) "Melatonin and its receptors in the gastrointestinal tract." *Biol. Signals 2*, 181–193.

110. Stone, T.W. (2001) "Kynurenines in the CNS: from endogenous obscurity to therapeutic importance." *Prog. Neurobiol. 64*, 185–218.

111. Widner, B., Laich, A., Sperner-Unterweger, B., Ledochowski, M. and Fuchs, D. (2002) "Neopterin production, tryptophan degradation, and mental depression – what is the link?" *Brain Behav. Immun. 16*, 590–595.

112. Capuron, L., Neurauter, G., Musselman, D.L., Lawson, D.H., Nemeroff, C.B., Fuchs, D. *et al.* (2003) "Interferon-alpha-induced changes in tryptophan metabolism: relationship to depression and paroxetine treatment." *Biol. Psychiatry 54*, 906–914.

113. Hissong, B.D. and Carlin, J.M. (1997) "Potentiation of interferon-induced indoleamine 2,3-dioxygenase mRNA in human mononuclear phagocytes by lipopolysaccharide and interleukin-1." *J. Interferon Cytokine Res. 17*, 387–393.

114. Hu, B., Hissong, B.D. and Carlin, J.M. (1995) "Interleukin-1 enhances indoleamine 2,3-dioxygenase activity by increasing specific mRNA expression in human mononuclear phagocytes." *J. Interferon Cytokine Res. 15*, 617–624.

115. Southgate, G.S., Daya, S. and Potgieter, B. (1998) "Melatonin plays a protective role in quinolinic acid-induced neurotoxicity in the rat hippocampus." *J. Chem. Neuroanat. 14*, 151–156.

116. Southgate, G. and Daya, S. (1999) "Melatonin reduces quinolinic acid-induced lipid peroxidation in rat brain homogenate." *Metab. Brain Dis. 14*, 165–171.

117. Cabrera, J., Reiter, R.J., Tan, D.X., Qi, W., Sainz, R.M., Mayo, J.C. *et al.* (2000) "Melatonin reduces oxidative neurotoxicity due to quinolinic acid: in vitro and in vivo findings." *Neuropharmacology 39*, 507–514.

118. Calderon-Guzman, D., Hernandez-Islas, J.L., Espitia-Vazquez, I., Barragan-Mejia, G., Hernandez-Garcia, E., Santamaria-del Angel, D. *et al.* (2004) "Pyridoxine, regardless of serotonin levels, increases production of 5-hydroxytryptophan in rat brain." *Arch. Med. Res. 35*, 271–274.

119. Nye, C. and Brice, A. (2005) "Combined vitamin B6-magnesium treatment in autism spectrum disorder." *Cochrane Database Syst. Rev.*, CD003497.

120. James, S.J., Cutler, P., Melnyk, S., Jernigan, S., Janak, L., Gaylor, D.W. *et al.* (2004) "Metabolic biomarkers of increased oxidative stress and impaired methylation capacity in children with autism." *Am. J. Clin. Nutr. 80*, 1611–1617.

121. Tani, Y., Fernell, E., Watanabe, Y., Kanai, T. and Langstrom, B. (1994) "Decrease in 6R-5,6,7,8-tetrahydrobiopterin content in cerebrospinal fluid of autistic patients." *Neurosci. Lett. 181*, 169–172.

122. Gal, E.M. and Whitacre, D.H. (1981) "Biopterin. VII. Inhibition of synthesis of reduced biopterins and its bearing on the function of cerebral tryptophan-5-hydroxylase in vivo." *Neurochem. Res. 6*, 233–241.

123. Kobayashi, T., Hasegawa, H., Kaneko, E. and Ichiyama, A. (1991) "Gastrointestinal serotonin: depletion due to tetrahydrobiopterin deficiency induced by 2,4-diamino-6-hydroxypyrimidine administration." *J. Pharmacol. Exp. Ther. 256*, 773–779.

124. Miller, L., Insel, T., Scheinin, M., Aloi, J., Murphy, D.L., Linnoila, M. *et al.* (1986) "Tetrahydrobiopterin administration to rhesus macaques. Its appearance in CSF and effect on neurotransmitter synthesis." *Neurochem. Res. 11*, 291–298.

125. Fernell, E., Watanabe, Y., Adolfsson, I., Tani, Y., Bergstrom, M., Hartvig, P. *et al.* (1997) "Possible effects of tetrahydrobiopterin treatment in six children with autism – clinical and positron emission tomography data: a pilot study." *Dev. Med. Child Neurol. 39*, 313–318.

126. Baker, T.A., Milstien, S. and Katusic, Z.S. (2001) "Effect of vitamin C on the availability of tetrahydrobiopterin in human endothelial cells." *J. Cardiovasc. Pharmacol. 37*, 333–338.

127. Nakai, K., Urushihara, M., Kubota, Y. and Kosaka, H. (2003) "Ascorbate enhances iNOS activity by increasing tetrahydrobiopterin in RAW 264.7 cells." *Free Radic. Biol. Med. 35*, 929–937.

128. Rutter, M., Andersen-Wood, L., Beckett, C., Bredenkamp, D., Castle, J., Groothues, C. *et al.* (1999) "Quasi-autistic patterns following severe early global privation. English and Romanian Adoptees (ERA) Study Team." *J. Child Psychol. Psychiatry 40*, 537–549.

129. Gould, E., Cameron, H.A., Daniels, D.C., Woolley, C.S. and McEwen, B.S. (1992) "Adrenal hormones suppress cell division in the adult rat dentate gyrus." *J. Neurosci. 12*, 3642–3650.

130. Gould, E., Tanapat, P., McEwen, B.S., Flugge, G. and Fuchs, E. (1998) "Proliferation of granule cell precursors in the dentate gyrus of adult monkeys is diminished by stress." *Proc. Natl. Acad. Sci. USA 95*, 3168–3171.

131. Marx, J. (1995) "How the glucocorticoids suppress immunity." *Science 270*, 232–233.

132. Strous, R.D., Golubchik, P., Maayan, R., Mozes, T., Tuati-Werner, D., Weizman, A. *et al.* (2005) "Lowered DHEA-S plasma levels in adult individuals with autistic disorder." *Eur. Neuropsychopharmacol. 15*, 305–309.

133. Kalimi, M., Shafagoj, Y., Loria, R., Padgett, D. and Regelson, W. (1994) "Anti-glucocorticoid effects of dehydroepiandrosterone (DHEA)." *Mol. Cell. Biochem. 131*, 99–104.

134. Monks, D.A., Lonstein, J.S. and Breedlove, S.M. (2003) "Got milk? Oxytocin triggers hippocampal plasticity." *Nat. Neurosci. 6*, 327–328.

135. Petersson, M. and Uvnas-Moberg, K. (2003) "Systemic oxytocin treatment modulates glucocorticoid and mineralocorticoid receptor mRNA in the rat hippocampus." *Neurosci. Lett. 343*, 97–100.

136. Neumann, I.D. (2002) "Involvement of the brain oxytocin system in stress coping: interactions with the hypothalamo-pituitary-adrenal axis." *Prog. Brain Res. 139*, 147–162.

137. Yang, S.H., Perez, E., Cutright, J., Liu, R., He, Z., Day, A.L. *et al.* (2002) "Testosterone increases neurotoxicity of glutamate in vitro and ischemia-reperfusion injury in an animal model." *J. Appl. Physiol. 92*, 195–201.

138. Tordjman, S., Ferrari, P., Sulmont, V., Duyme, M. and Roubertoux, P. (1997) "Androgenic activity in autism." *Am. J. Psychiatry 154*, 1626–1627.

139. Gillberg, C. and Schaumann, H. (1981) "Infantile autism and puberty." *J. Autism Dev. Disord. 11*, 365–371.

140. Baron-Cohen, S. (2002) "The extreme male brain theory of autism." *Trends Cogn. Sci. 6*, 248–254.

141. Jaenisch, R. and Bird, A. (2003) "Epigenetic regulation of gene expression: how the genome integrates intrinsic and environmental signals." *Nat. Genet. 33*, Suppl, 245–254.

142. Meehan, R.R. (2003) "DNA methylation in animal development." *Semin. Cell Dev. Biol. 14*, 53–65.

143. Amir, R.E., Van de Veyver, Wan, M., Tran, C.Q., Francke, U. and Zoghbi, H.Y. (1999) "Rett syndrome is caused by mutations in X-linked MECP2, encoding methyl-CpG-binding protein 2." *Nat. Genet. 23*, 185–188.

144. Young, J.I., Hong, E.P., Castle, J.C., Crespo-Barreto, J., Bowman, A.B., Rose, M.F. *et al.* (2005) "Regulation of RNA splicing by the methylation-dependent transcriptional repressor methyl-CpG binding protein 2." *Proc. Natl. Acad. Sci. USA 102*, 17551–17558.

145. Bugl, H., Fauman, E.B., Staker, B.L., Zheng, F., Kushner, S.R., Saper, M.A. *et al.* (2000) "RNA methylation under heat shock control." *Mol. Cell 6*, 349–360.

146. Nataf, R., Skorupka, C., Amet, L., Lam, A., Springbett, A. and Lathe, R. (2005) "Porphyrinuria in childhood autistic disorder." Submitted for publication.

147. Costa, C.A., Trivelato, G.C., Pinto, A.M. and Bechara, E.J. (1997) "Correlation between plasma 5-aminolevulinic acid concentrations and indicators of oxidative stress in lead-exposed workers." *Clin. Chem. 43*, 1196–1202.

148. Gordon, N. (1999) "The acute porphyrias." *Brain Dev. 21*, 373–377.

149. Millward, L.M., Kelly, P., Deacon, A., Senior, V. and Peters, T.J. (2001) "Self-rated psychosocial consequences and quality of life in the acute porphyrias." *J. Inherit. Metab. Dis. 24*, 733–747.

150. Ruscito, B.J. and Harrison, N.L. (2003) "Hemoglobin metabolites mimic benzodiazepines and are possible mediators of hepatic encephalopathy." *Blood 102*, 1525–1528.

151. Mustajoki, P. (1980) "Variegate porphyria. Twelve years' experience in Finland. *Q. J. Med. 49*, 191–203.

152. Bonkowsky, H.L. and Schady, W. (1982) "Neurologic manifestations of acute porphyria." *Semin. Liver Dis. 2*, 108–124.

153. Lathe, R. and Seckl, J.R. (2002) "Neurosteroids and brain sterols." In J.I. Mason (ed) *Genetics of Steroid Biosynthesis and Function*. London: Taylor and Francis; pp.407–474.

154. Verma, A., Nye, J.S. and Snyder, S.H. (1987) "Porphyrins are endogenous ligands for the mitochondrial (peripheral-type) benzodiazepine receptor." *Proc. Natl. Acad. Sci. USA 84*, 2256–2260.

155. Wendler, G., Lindemann, P., Lacapere, J.J. and Papadopoulos, V. (2003) "Protoporphyrin IX binding and transport by recombinant mouse PBR." *Biochem. Biophys. Res. Commun. 311*, 847–852.

156. Nakayama, K., Takasawa, A., Terai, I., Okui, T., Ohyama, T. and Tamura, M. (2000) "Spontaneous porphyria of the Long-Evans cinnamon rat: an animal model of Wilson's disease." *Arch. Biochem. Biophys. 375*, 240–250.

157. Taketani, S., Kohno, H., Furukawa, T. and Tokunaga, R. (1995) "Involvement of peripheral-type benzodiazepine receptors in the intracellular transport of heme and porphyrins." *J. Biochem. (Tokyo) 117*, 875–880.

158. Opler, M.G., Brown, A.S., Graziano, J., Desai, M., Zheng, W., Schaefer, C. *et al.* (2004) "Prenatal lead exposure, delta-aminolevulinic acid, and schizophrenia." *Environ. Health Perspect. 112*, 548–552.

159. Brennan, M.J. and Cantrill, R.C. (1979) "The effect of delta-aminolaevulinic acid on the uptake and efflux of [3H]GABA in rat brain synaptosomes." *J. Neurochem. 32*, 1781–1786.

160. Muller, W.E. and Snyder, S.H. (1977) "Delta-aminolevulinic acid: influences on synaptic GABA receptor binding may explain CNS symptoms of porphyria." *Ann. Neurol. 2*, 340–342.

161. Emanuelli, T., Pagel, F.W., Alves, L.B., Regner, A. and Souza, D.O. (2001) "5-aminolevulinic acid inhibits [3H]muscimol binding to human and rat brain synaptic membranes." *Neurochem. Res. 26*, 101–105.

162. Murata, K., Sakai, T., Morita, Y., Iwata, T. and Dakeishi, M. (2003) "Critical dose of lead affecting delta-aminolevulinic acid levels." *J. Occup. Health 45*, 209–214.

163. Wehner, J.M. and Marley, R.J. (1986) "Genetic differences in the effects of delta-aminolevulinic acid on seizure latency in mice." *Exp. Neurol. 94*, 280–291.

164. Solinas, C. and Vajda, F.J. (2004) "Epilepsy and porphyria: new perspectives." *J. Clin. Neurosci. 11*, 356–361.

165. Stepien, H., Kunert-Radek, J., Stanisz, A., Zerek-Melen, G. and Pawlikowski, M. (1991) "Inhibitory effect of porphyrins on the proliferation of mouse spleen lymphocytes in vitro." *Biochem. Biophys. Res. Commun. 174*, 313–322.

166. Pastorino, J.G., Simbula, G., Gilfor, E., Hoek, J.B. and Farber, J.L. (1994) "Protoporphyrin IX, an endogenous ligand of the peripheral benzodiazepine receptor, potentiates induction of the mitochondrial permeability transition and the killing of cultured hepatocytes by rotenone." *J. Biol. Chem. 269*, 31041–31046.

167. Baldwin, D.R. and Marshall, W.J. (1999) "Heavy metal poisoning and its laboratory investigation." *Ann. Clin. Biochem. 36 (Pt 3)*, 267–300.

168. Vakharia, D.D., Liu, N., Pause, R., Fasco, M., Bessette, E., Zhang, Q.Y. *et al.* (2001) "Polycyclic aromatic hydrocarbon/metal mixtures: effect on PAH induction of CYP1A1 in human HEPG2 cells." *Drug Metab. Dispos. 29*, 999–1006.

169. Maines, M.D. and Trakshel, G.M. (1992) "Tin-protoporphyrin: a potent inhibitor of hemoprotein-dependent steroidogenesis in rat adrenals and testes." *J. Pharmacol. Exp. Ther. 260*, 909–916.

170. Lathe, R. (2002) "Steroid and sterol 7-hydroxylation: ancient pathways." *Steroids 67*, 967–977.

171. Rose, K., Allan, A., Gauldie, S., Stapleton, G., Dobbie, L., Dott, K. *et al.* (2001) "Neurosteroid hydroxylase CYP7B: vivid reporter activity in dentate gyrus of gene-targeted mice and abolition of a widespread pathway of steroid and oxysterol hydroxylation." *J. Biol. Chem. 276*, 23937–23944.

172. Weihua, Z., Lathe, R., Warner, M. and Gustafsson, J.-A. (2002) "A novel endocrine pathway in the prostate, ERbeta, AR, 5alpha-androstane-3beta,17beta-diol, and CYP7B, regulates prostate growth." *Proc. Natl. Acad. Sci. USA 99*, 13589–13594.

173. Edelson, S.B. and Cantor, D.S. (1998) "Autism: xenobiotic influences." *Toxicol. Ind. Health 14*, 553–563.

174. Sone, N., Larsstuvold, M.K. and Kagawa, Y. (1977) "Effect of methyl mercury on phosphorylation, transport, and oxidation in mammalian mitochondria." *J. Biochem. (Tokyo) 82*, 859–868.

175. Polster, B.M. and Fiskum, G. (2004) "Mitochondrial mechanisms of neural cell apoptosis." *J. Neurochem. 90*, 1281–1289.

176. Humphrey, M.L., Cole, M.P., Pendergrass, J.C. and Kiningham, K.K. (2005) "Mitochondrial mediated thimerosal-induced apoptosis in a human neuroblastoma cell line (SK-N-SH)." *Neurotoxicology 26*, 407–416.

177. Taoka, S., Lepore, B.W., Kabil, O., Ojha, S., Ringe, D. and Banerjee, R. (2002) "Human cystathionine beta-synthase is a heme sensor protein. Evidence that the redox sensor is heme and not the vicinal cysteines in the CXXC motif seen in the crystal structure of the truncated enzyme." *Biochemistry 41*, 10454–10461.

178. Taoka, S., Green, E.L., Loehr, T.M. and Banerjee, R. (2001) "Mercuric chloride-induced spin or ligation state changes in ferric or ferrous human cystathione beta-synthase inhibit enzyme activity." *J. Inorg. Biochem. 87*, 253–259.

179. Waly, M., Olteanu, H., Banerjee, R., Choi, S.W., Mason, J.B., Parker, B.S. *et al.* (2004) "Activation of methionine synthase by insulin-like growth factor-1 and dopamine: a target for neurodevelopmental toxins and thimerosal." *Mol. Psychiatry 9*, 358–370.

180. Kurth, C., Wegerer, V., Reulbach, U., Lewczuk, P., Kornhuber, J., Steinhoff, B.J. *et al.* (2004) "Analysis of hippocampal atrophy in alcoholic patients by a Kohonen feature map." *Neuroreport 15*, 367–371.

181. den Heijer, T., Vermeer, S.E., Clarke, R., Oudkerk, M., Koudstaal, P.J., Hofman, A. *et al.* (2003) "Homocysteine and brain atrophy on MRI of non-demented elderly." *Brain 126*, 170–175.

182. Shapre, L.G., Olney, J.W., Ohlendorf, C., Lyss, A., Zimmerman, M. and Gale, B. (1975) "Brain damage and associated behavioral deficits following the administration of L-cysteine to infant rats." *Pharmacol. Biochem. Behav. 3*, 291–298.

183. Streck, E.L., Bavaresco, C.S., Netto, C.A. and Wyse, A.T. (2004) "Chronic hyperhomocysteinemia provokes a memory deficit in rats in the Morris water maze task." *Behav. Brain Res. 153*, 377–381.

184. Alberti, A., Pirrone, P., Elia, M., Waring, R.H. and Romano, C. (1999) "Sulphation deficit in 'low-functioning' autistic children: a pilot study." *Biol. Psychiatry 46*, 420–424.

185. Pasca, S.P., Nemes, B., Vlase, L., Gagyi, C.E., Dronca, E., Miu, A.C. *et al.* (2006) "High levels of homocysteine and low serum paraoxonase 1 arylesterase activity in children with autism." *Life Sci.*, in press. Online at: http://www.sciencedirect.com/science/journal/00243205

186. Kang, S.S., Zhou, J., Wong, P.W., Kowalisyn, J. and Strokosch, G. (1988) "Intermediate homocysteinemia: a thermolabile variant of methylenetetrahydrofolate reductase." *Am. J. Hum. Genet. 43*, 414–421.

187. Frosst, P., Blom, H.J., Milos, R., Goyette, P., Sheppard, C.A., Matthews, R.G. *et al.* (1995) "A candidate genetic risk factor for vascular disease: a common mutation in methylenetetrahydrofolate reductase." *Nat. Genet. 10*, 111–113.

188. Rozen, R. (1996) "Molecular genetics of methylenetetrahydrofolate reductase deficiency." *J. Inherit. Metab. Dis. 19*, 589–594.

189. Perry, D.J. (1999) "Hyperhomocysteinaemia." *Baillieres Best Pract. Res. Clin. Haematol. 12*, 451–477.

190. Blom, H.J. (2000) "Genetic determinants of hyperhomocysteinaemia: the roles of cystathionine beta-synthase and 5,10-methylenetetrahydrofolate reductase." *Eur. J. Pediatr. 159*, Suppl 3, S208–S212.

191. Koch, H.G., Nabel, P., Junker, R., Auberger, K., Schobess, R., Homberger, A. *et al.* (1999) "The 677T genotype of the common MTHFR thermolabile variant and fasting homocysteine in childhood venous thrombosis." *Eur. J. Pediatr. 158*, Suppl 3, S113–S116.

192. James, S.J., Slikker, W., III, Melnyk, S., New, E., Pogribna, M. and Jernigan, S. (2005) "Thimerosal neurotoxicity is associated with glutathione depletion: protection with glutathione precursors." *Neurotoxicology 26*, 1–8.

193. Ren, S. and Correia, M.A. (2000) "Heme: a regulator of rat hepatic tryptophan 2,3-dioxygenase?" *Arch. Biochem. Biophys. 377*, 195–203.

194. Dick, R., Murray, B.P., Reid, M.J. and Correia, M.A. (2001) "Structure – function relationships of rat hepatic tryptophan 2,3-dioxygenase: identification of the putative heme-ligating histidine residues." *Arch. Biochem. Biophys. 392*, 71–78.

195. Littlejohn, T.K., Takikawa, O., Skylas, D., Jamie, J.F., Walker, M.J. and Truscott, R.J. (2000) "Expression and purification of recombinant human indoleamine 2,3-dioxygenase." *Protein Expr. Purif. 19*, 22–29.

196. Terentis, A.C., Thomas, S.R., Takikawa, O., Littlejohn, T.K., Truscott, R.J., Armstrong, R.S. *et al.* (2002) "The heme environment of recombinant human indoleamine 2,3-dioxygenase. Structural properties and substrate–ligand interactions." *J. Biol. Chem. 277*, 15788–15794.

197. Kaliman, P.A., Nikitchenko, I.V., Sokol, O.A. and Strel'chenko, E.V. (2001) "Regulation of heme oxygenase activity in rat liver during oxidative stress induced by cobalt chloride and mercury chloride." *Biochemistry (Mosc.) 66*, 77–82.

198. Sapolsky, R.M., Krey, L.C. and McEwen, B.S. (1986) "The neuroendocrinology of stress and aging: the glucocorticoid cascade hypothesis." *Endocr. Rev. 7*, 284–301.

199. Insausti, A.M., Gaztelu, J.M., Gonzalo, L.M., Romero-Vives, M., Barrenechea, C., Felipo, V. *et al.* (1997) "Diet induced hyperammonemia decreases neuronal nuclear size in rat entorhinal cortex." *Neurosci. Lett. 231*, 179–181.

200. Watanabe, A. (1998) "Cerebral changes in hepatic encephalopathy." *J. Gastroenterol. Hepatol. 13*, 752–760.

201. Messing, R.O. and Simon, R.P. (1986) "Seizures as a manifestation of systemic disease." *Neurol. Clin. 4*, 563–584.

Chapter 10 Biomedical Therapy: Typing and Correction

1. Eriksson, P.S., Perfilieva, E., Bjork-Eriksson, T., Alborn, A.M., Nordborg, C., Peterson, D.A. *et al.* (1998) "Neurogenesis in the adult human hippocampus." *Nat. Med. 4*, 1313–1317.

2. Kornack, D.R. and Rakic, P. (1999) "Continuation of neurogenesis in the hippocampus of the adult macaque monkey." *Proc. Natl. Acad. Sci. USA 96*, 5768–5773.

3. Gould, E., Reeves, A.J., Fallah, M., Tanapat, P., Gross, C.G. and Fuchs, E. (1999) "Hippocampal neurogenesis in adult Old World primates." *Proc. Natl. Acad. Sci. USA 96*, 5263–5267.

4. Gorker, I. and Tuzun, U. (2005) "Autistic-like findings associated with a urea cycle disorder in a 4-year-old girl." *J. Psychiatry Neurosci. 30*, 133–135.

5. Filipek, P.A., Accardo, P.J., Ashwal, S., Baranek, G.T., Cook, E.H., Jr., Dawson, G. *et al.* (2000) "Practice parameter: screening and diagnosis of autism: report of the Quality Standards Subcommittee of the American Academy of Neurology and the Child Neurology Society." *Neurology 55*, 468–479.

6. Rimland, B., Semon, B. and Kornblum, L. (1992) *Feast Without Yeast: 4 Stages to Better Health.* Wisconsin: Wisconsin Institute of Nutrition.

7. Shaw, W. (2002) *Biological Treatments for Autism and PDD.* Lenexa, KS: Great Plains Laboratory.

8. McCandless, J. (2003) *Children with Starving Brains: A Medical Treatment Guide for Autism Spectrum Disorder.* Putney, VT: Bramble Books.

9. Pangborn, J., Baker, S. and Rimland, B. (2005) *Autism: Effective Biomedical Treatments (The DAN Protocol).* San Diego: Autism Research Institute.

10. Amaral, D.G. (2003) "Report from the research director." *MIND Institute Newsletter 4*, 1, 1–2.

11. Powell, K. (2004) "Opening a window to the autistic brain." *PLOS Biol. 2*, 1054–1058.

12. Cuccaro, M.L., Shao, Y., Grubber, J., Slifer, M., Wolpert, C.M., Donnelly, S.L. *et al.* (2003) "Factor analysis of restricted and repetitive behaviors in autism using the Autism Diagnostic Interview-R." *Child Psychiatry Hum. Dev. 34*, 3–17.

13. Shao, Y., Cuccaro, M.L., Hauser, E.R., Raiford, K.L., Menold, M.M., Wolpert, C.M. *et al.* (2003) "Fine mapping of autistic disorder to chromosome 15q11–q13 by use of phenotypic subtypes." *Am. J. Hum. Genet. 72*, 539–548.

14. Brewster, M.A. (1988) "Biomarkers of xenobiotic exposures." *Ann. Clin. Lab Sci. 18*, 306–317.

15. Sakai, T. (2000) "Biomarkers of lead exposure." *Ind. Health 38*, 127–142.

16. Woods, J.S. (1996) "Altered porphyrin metabolism as a biomarker of mercury exposure and toxicity." *Can. J. Physiol. Pharmacol. 74*, 210–215.

17. Woods, J.S., Echeverria, D., Heyer, N.J., Simmonds, P.L., Wilkerson, J. and Farin, F.M. (2005) "The association between genetic polymorphisms of coproporphyrinogen oxidase and an atypical porphyrinogenic response to mercury exposure in humans." *Toxicol. Appl. Pharmacol. 206*, 113–120.

18. Cox, M.A., Lewis, K.O. and Cooper, B.T. (1999) "Measurement of small intestinal permeability markers, lactulose, and mannitol in serum: results in celiac disease." *Dig. Dis. Sci. 44*, 402–406.

19. Tibble, J.A. and Bjarnason, I. (2001) "Non-invasive investigation of inflammatory bowel disease." *World J. Gastroenterol. 7*, 460–465.

20. James, S.J., Cutler, P., Melnyk, S., Jernigan, S., Janak, L., Gaylor, D.W. *et al.* (2004) "Metabolic biomarkers of increased oxidative stress and impaired methylation capacity in children with autism." *Am. J. Clin. Nutr. 80*, 1611–1617.

21. Alberti, A., Pirrone, P., Elia, M., Waring, R.H. and Romano, C. (1999) "Sulphation deficit in 'low-functioning' autistic children: a pilot study." *Biol. Psychiatry 46*, 420–424.

22. Brouwer, O.F., Onkenhout, W., Edelbroek, P.M., de Kom, J.F., de Wolff, F.A. and Peters, A.C. (1992) "Increased neurotoxicity of arsenic in methylenetetrahydrofolate reductase deficiency." *Clin. Neurol. Neurosurg. 94*, 307–310.

23. Onalaja, A.O. and Claudio, L. (2000) "Genetic susceptibility to lead poisoning." *Environ. Health Perspect. 108*, Suppl 1, 23–28.

24. Frosst, P., Blom, H.J., Milos, R., Goyette, P., Sheppard, C.A., Matthews, R.G. *et al.* (1995) "A candidate genetic risk factor for vascular disease: a common mutation in methylenetetrahydrofolate reductase." *Nat. Genet. 10*, 111–113.

25. James, S.J., Melnyk, S. and Jernigan, S. (2005) "Low plasma methionine, cysteine, and glutathione levels are associated with increased frequency of common polymorphisms affecting methylation and glutathione pathways in children with autism." *Proc. XXXV Intl. Cong. Physiol. Sci., San Diego.* Online at: http://www.faseb.org/meetings/eb2005

26. Kelada, S.N., Shelton, E., Kaufmann, R.B. and Khoury, M.J. (2001) "Delta-aminolevulic acid dehydratase genotype and lead toxicity: a HuGE review." *Am.J. Epidemiol. 154*, 1–13.

27. Battistuzzi, G., Petrucci, R., Silvagni, L., Urbani, F.R. and Caiola, S. (1981) "Delta-aminolevulinate dehydrase: a new genetic polymorphism in man." *Ann. Hum. Genet. 45*, 223–229.

28. Ingelman-Sundberg, M. (2005) "Genetic polymorphisms of cytochrome P450 2D6 (CYP2D6): clinical consequences, evolutionary aspects and functional diversity." *Pharmacogenomics J. 5*, 6–13.

29. D'Amelio, M., Ricci, I., Sacco, R., Liu, X., D'Agruma, L., Muscarella, L.A. *et al.* (2005) "Paraoxonase gene variants are associated with autism in North America, but not in Italy: possible regional specificity in gene-environment interactions." *Mol. Psychiatry 10*, 1006–1016.

30. Aronson, S.M. (2005) "The dancing cats of Minamata Bay." *Med. Health RI 88*, 209.

31. Fonfria, E., Rodriguez-Farre, E. and Sunol, C. (2001) "Mercury interaction with the GABA(A) receptor modulates the benzodiazepine binding site in primary cultures of mouse cerebellar granule cells." *Neuropharmacology 41*, 819–833.

32. Jensen, M.L., Timmermann, D.B., Johansen, T.H., Schousboe, A., Varming, T. and Ahring, P.K. (2002) "The beta subunit determines the ion selectivity of the GABAA receptor." *J. Biol. Chem. 277*, 41438–41447.

33. Dunne, E.L., Hosie, A.M., Wooltorton, J.R., Duguid, I.C., Harvey, K., Moss, S.J. *et al.* (2002) "An N-terminal histidine regulates Zn(2+) inhibition on the murine GABA(A) receptor beta3 subunit." *Br. J. Pharmacol. 137*, 29–38.

34. Oliveira, G., Diogo, L., Grazina, M., Garcia, P., Ataide, A., Marques, C. *et al.* (2005) "Mitochondrial dysfunction in autism spectrum disorders: a population-based study." *Dev. Med. Child Neurol. 47*, 185–189.

35. Erlandson, A. and Hagberg, B. (2005) "MECP2 abnormality phenotypes: clinicopathologic area with broad variability." *J. Child Neurol. 20*, 727–732.

36. Nataf, R., Skorupka, C., Amet, L., Lam, A., Springbett, A. and Lathe, R. (2005) "Porphyrinuria in childhood autistic disorder." Submitted for publication.

37. Kaufman, B.N. (1995) *Son-Rise: The Miracle Continues.* Tiburon, CA: H.J. Kramer Press.

38. Scahill, L. and Koenig, K. (1999) "Pharmacotherapy in children and adolescents with pervasive developmental disorders." *J. Child Adolesc. Psychiatr. Nurs. 12*, 41–43.

39.   Hanft, A. and Hendren, R.L. (2004) "Pharmacotherapy of children and adolescents with pervasive developmental disorders." *Essent. Psychopharmacol. 6*, 12–24.

40.   Bostic, J.Q. and King, B.H. (2005) "Autism spectrum disorders: emerging pharmacotherapy." *Expert. Opin. Emerg. Drugs 10*, 521–536.

41.   Anderson, L.T., Campbell, M., Adams, P., Small, A.M., Perry, R. and Shell, J. (1989) "The effects of haloperidol on discrimination learning and behavioral symptoms in autistic children." *J. Autism Dev. Disord. 19*, 227–239.

42.   Remington, G., Sloman, L., Konstantareas, M., Parker, K. and Gow, R. (2001) "Clomipramine versus haloperidol in the treatment of autistic disorder: a double-blind, placebo-controlled, crossover study." *J. Clin. Psychopharmacol. 21*, 440–444.

43.   Malone, R.P., Cater, J., Sheikh, R.M., Choudhury, M.S. and Delaney, M.A. (2001) "Olanzapine versus haloperidol in children with autistic disorder: an open pilot study." *J. Am. Acad. Child Adolesc. Psychiatry 40*, 887–894.

44.   Lathe, R. and Seckl, J.R. (2002) "Neurosteroids and brain sterols." In J.I. Mason (ed) *Genetics of Steroid Biosynthesis and Function.* London: Taylor and Francis; pp.407–474.

45.   Ukai, W., Ozawa, H., Tateno, M., Hashimoto, E. and Saito, T. (2004) "Neurotoxic potential of haloperidol in comparison with risperidone: implication of Akt-mediated signal changes by haloperidol." *J. Neural. Transm. 111*, 667–681.

46.   Takahashi, S., Takagi, K. and Horikomi, K. (2001) "Effects of a novel, selective, sigma 1-ligand, MS-377, on phencyclidine-induced behaviour." *Naunyn Schmiedebergs Arch. Pharmacol. 364*, 81–86.

47.   Seeman, P. (1990) "Atypical neuroleptics: role of multiple receptors, endogenous dopamine, and receptor linkage." *Acta Psychiatr. Scand. Suppl. 358*, 14–20.

48.   McDougle, C.J., Scahill, L., Aman, M.G., McCracken, J.T., Tierney, E., Davies, M. *et al.* (2005) "Risperidone for the core symptom domains of autism: results from the study by the autism network of the research units on pediatric psychopharmacology." *Am. J. Psychiatry 162*, 1142–1148.

49.   Shea, S., Turgay, A., Carroll, A., Schulz, M., Orlik, H., Smith, I. *et al.* (2004) "Risperidone in the treatment of disruptive behavioral symptoms in children with autistic and other pervasive developmental disorders." *Pediatrics 114*, e634–e641.

50.   Di Martino, A., Melis, G., Cianchetti, C. and Zuddas, A. (2004) "Methylphenidate for pervasive developmental disorders: safety and efficacy of acute single dose test and ongoing therapy: an open-pilot study." *J. Child Adolesc. Psychopharmacol. 14*, 207–218.

51.   Handen, B.L., Johnson, C.R. and Lubetsky, M. (2000) "Efficacy of methylphenidate among children with autism and symptoms of attention-deficit hyperactivity disorder." *J. Autism Dev. Disord. 30*, 245–255.

52.   Gordon, C.T., State R.C., Nelson, J.E., Hamburger, S.D. and Rapoport, J.L. (1993) "A double-blind comparison of clomipramine, desipramine, and placebo in the treatment of autistic disorder." *Arch. Gen. Psychiatry 50*, 441–447.

53.   Moore, M.L., Eichner, S.F. and Jones, J.R. (2004) "Treating functional impairment of autism with selective serotonin-reuptake inhibitors." *Ann. Pharmacother. 38*, 1515–1519.

54.   Hollander, E., Phillips, A., Chaplin, W., Zagursky, K., Novotny, S., Wasserman, S. *et al.* (2005) "A placebo controlled crossover trial of liquid fluoxetine on repetitive behaviors in childhood and adolescent autism." *Neuropsychopharmacology 30*, 582–589.

55.   Figgitt, D.P. and McClellan, K.J. (2000) "Fluvoxamine. An updated review of its use in the management of adults with anxiety disorders." *Drugs 60*, 925–954.

56.   McDougle, C.J., Naylor, S.T., Cohen, D.J., Volkmar, F.R., Heninger, G.R. and Price, L.H. (1996) "A double-blind, placebo-controlled study of fluvoxamine in adults with autistic disorder." *Arch. Gen. Psychiatry 53*, 1001–1008.

57.   DeLong, G.R., Teague, L.A. and McSwain, K.M. (1998) "Effects of fluoxetine treatment in young children with idiopathic autism." *Dev. Med. Child Neurol. 40*, 551–562.

58.   Liston, H.L., DeVane, C.L., Boulton, D.W., Risch, S.C., Markowitz, J.S. and Goldman, J. (2002) "Differential time course of cytochrome P450 2D6 enzyme inhibition by fluoxetine, sertraline, and paroxetine in healthy volunteers." *J. Clin. Psychopharmacol. 22*, 169–173.

59.   Posey, D.J., Guenin, K.D., Kohn, A.E., Swiezy, N.B. and McDougle, C.J. (2001) "A naturalistic open-label study of mirtazapine in autistic and other pervasive developmental disorders." *J. Child Adolesc. Psychopharmacol. 11*, 267–277.

60. Kaduszkiewicz, H., Zimmermann, T., Beck-Bornholdt, H.P. and van den, B.H. (2005) "Cholinesterase inhibitors for patients with Alzheimer's disease: systematic review of randomised clinical trials." *BMJ 331,* 321–327.

61. Hardan, A.Y. and Handen, B.L. (2002) "A retrospective open trial of adjunctive donepezil in children and adolescents with autistic disorder." *J. Child Adolesc. Psychopharmacol. 12,* 237–241.

62. Chez, M.G., Aimonovitch, M., Buchanan, T., Mrazek, S. and Tremb, R.J. (2004) "Treating autistic spectrum disorders in children: utility of the cholinesterase inhibitor rivastigmine tartrate." *J. Child Neurol. 19,* 165–169.

63. Hertzman, M. (2003) "Galantamine in the treatment of adult autism: a report of three clinical cases." *Int. J. Psychiatry Med. 33,* 395–398.

64. Bratt, A.M., Kelley, S.P., Knowles, J.P., Barrett, J., Davis, K., Davis, M. *et al.* (2001) "Long term modulation of the HPA axis by the hippocampus. Behavioral, biochemical and immunological endpoints in rats exposed to chronic mild stress." *Psychoneuroendocrinology 26,* 121–145.

65. Campbell, M., Anderson, L.T., Small, A.M., Adams, P., Gonzalez, N.M. and Ernst, M. (1993) "Naltrexone in autistic children: behavioral symptoms and attentional learning." *J. Am. Acad. Child Adolesc. Psychiatry 32,* 1283–1291.

66. Willemsen-Swinkels, S.H., Buitelaar, J.K., Weijnen, F.G. and Van Engeland, H. (1995) "Placebo-controlled acute dosage naltrexone study in young autistic children." *Psychiatry Res. 58,* 203–215.

67. Kolmen, B.K., Feldman, H.M., Handen, B.L. and Janosky, J.E. (1995) "Naltrexone in young autistic children: a double-blind, placebo-controlled crossover study." *J. Am. Acad. Child Adolesc. Psychiatry 34,* 223–231.

68. Bouvard, M.P., Leboyer, M., Launay, J.M., Recasens, C., Plumet, M.H., Waller-Perotte, D. *et al.* (1995) "Low-dose naltrexone effects on plasma chemistries and clinical symptoms in autism: a double-blind, placebo-controlled study." *Psychiatry Res. 58,* 191–201.

69. Kolmen, B.K., Feldman, H.M., Handen, B.L. and Janosky, J.E. (1997) "Naltrexone in young autistic children: replication study and learning measures." *J. Am. Acad. Child Adolesc. Psychiatry 36,* 1570–1578.

70. Campbell, M., Anderson, L.T., Small, A.M., Locascio, J.J., Lynch, N.S. and Choroco, M.C. (1990) "Naltrexone in autistic children: a double-blind and placebo-controlled study." *Psychopharmacol. Bull. 26,* 130–135.

71. Willemsen-Swinkels, S.H., Buitelaar, J.K. and Van Engeland, H. (1996) "The effects of chronic naltrexone treatment in young autistic children: a double-blind placebo-controlled crossover study." *Biol. Psychiatry 39,* 1023–1031.

72. Knabe, R., Schulz, P. and Richard, J. (1990) "Initial aggravation of self-injurious behavior in autistic patients receiving naltrexone treatment." *J. Autism Dev. Disord. 20,* 591–593.

73. Benjamin, S., Seek, A., Tresise, L., Price, E. and Gagnon, M. (1995) "Case study: paradoxical response to naltrexone treatment of self-injurious behavior." *J. Am. Acad. Child Adolesc. Psychiatry 34,* 238–242.

74. Willemsen-Swinkels, S.H., Buitelaar, J.K., Nijhof, G.J. and Van Engeland, H. (1995) "Failure of naltrexone hydrochloride to reduce self-injurious and autistic behavior in mentally retarded adults. Double-blind placebo-controlled studies." *Arch. Gen. Psychiatry 52,* 766–773.

75. Symons, F.J., Thompson, A. and Rodriguez, M.C. (2004) "Self-injurious behavior and the efficacy of naltrexone treatment: a quantitative synthesis." *Ment. Retard. Dev. Disabil. Res. Rev. 10,* 193–200.

76. Fankhauser, M.P., Karumanchi, V.C., German, M.L., Yates, A. and Karumanchi, S.D. (1992) "A double-blind, placebo-controlled study of the efficacy of transdermal clonidine in autism." *J. Clin. Psychiatry 53,* 77–82.

77. Jaselskis, C.A., Cook, E.H., Jr., Fletcher, K.E. and Leventhal, B.L. (1992) "Clonidine treatment of hyperactive and impulsive children with autistic disorder." *J. Clin. Psychopharmacol. 12,* 322–327.

78. Tamura, T., Aiso, K., Johnston, K.E., Black, L. and Faught, E. (2000) "Homocysteine, folate, vitamin B-12 and vitamin B-6 in patients receiving antiepileptic drug monotherapy." *Epilepsy Res. 40,* 7–15.

79. Billings, R.E. (1984) "Interactions between folate metabolism, phenytoin metabolism, and liver microsomal cytochrome P450." *Drug Nutr. Interact. 3,* 21–32.

80. Kishi, T., Fujita, N., Eguchi, T. and Ueda, K. (1997) "Mechanism for reduction of serum folate by antiepileptic drugs during prolonged therapy." *J. Neurol. Sci. 145,* 109–112.

81. Yerby, M.S. (2003) "Management issues for women with epilepsy: neural tube defects and folic acid supplementation." *Neurology 61,* S23–S26.

82. Hancock, E., Osborne, J. and Milner, P. (2003) "Treatment of infantile spasms." *Cochrane Database Syst. Rev.*, CD001770.

83. Buitelaar, J.K., Dekker, M.E., Van Ree, J.M. and Van Engeland, H. (1996) "A controlled trial with ORG 2766, an ACTH-(4-9) analog, in 50 relatively able children with autism." *Eur. Neuropsychopharmacol. 6*, 13–19.

84. Freeman, J.M., Freeman, J.B. and Kelly, M.T. (2000) *The Ketogenic Diet*. New York: Demos Medical Publishing.

85. Vamecq, J., Vallee, L., Lesage, F., Gressens, P. and Stables, J.P. (2005) "Antiepileptic popular ketogenic diet: emerging twists in an ancient story." *Prog. Neurobiol. 75*, 1–28.

86. Glaze, D.G., Schultz, R.J. and Frost, J.D. (1998) "Rett syndrome: characterization of seizures versus non-seizures." *Electroencephalogr. Clin. Neurophysiol. 106*, 79–83.

87. Glaze, D.G. (2005) "Neurophysiology of Rett syndrome." *J. Child Neurol. 20*, 740–746.

88. Wada, J.A. (1985) "Differential diagnosis of epilepsy." *Electroencephalogr. Clin. Neurophysiol. Suppl. 37*, 285–311.

89. Kidd, P.M. (2002) "Autism, an extreme challenge to integrative medicine. Part 2: medical management." *Altern. Med. Rev. 7*, 472–499.

90. McFarland, L.V., Elmer, G.W. and Surawicz, C.M. (2002) "Breaking the cycle: treatment strategies for 163 cases of recurrent *Clostridium difficile* disease." *Am. J. Gastroenterol. 97*, 1769–1775.

91. Surawicz, C.M. (2004) "Treatment of recurrent *Clostridium difficile*-associated disease." *Nat. Clin. Pract. Gastroenterol. Hepatol. 1*, 32–38.

92. Sandler, R.H., Finegold, S.M., Bolte, E.R., Buchanan, C.P., Maxwell, A.P., Vaisanen, M.L. *et al.* (2000) "Short-term benefit from oral vancomycin treatment of regressive-onset autism." *J. Child Neurol. 15*, 429–435.

93. Posey, D.J., Kem, D.L., Swiezy, N.B., Sweeten, T.L., Wiegand, R.E. and McDougle, C.J. (2004) "A pilot study of D-cycloserine in subjects with autistic disorder." *Am. J. Psychiatry 161*, 2115–2117.

94. Seko, Y., Miura, T., Takahashi, M. and Koyama, T. (1981) "Methyl mercury decomposition in mice treated with antibiotics." *Acta Pharmacol. Toxicol. (Copenh.) 49*, 259–265.

95. Brudnak, M.A. (2002) "Probiotics as an adjuvant to detoxification protocols." *Med. Hypotheses 58*, 382–385.

96. Sartor, R.B. (2005) "Probiotic therapy of intestinal inflammation and infections." *Curr. Opin. Gastroenterol. 21*, 44–50.

97. Linday, L.A. (2001) "*Saccharomyces boulardii*: potential adjunctive treatment for children with autism and diarrhea." *J. Child Neurol. 16*, 387.

98. Dotan, I. and Rachmilewitz, D. (2005) "Probiotics in inflammatory bowel disease: possible mechanisms of action." *Curr. Opin. Gastroenterol. 21*, 426–430.

99. Groll, A.H., Just-Nuebling, G., Kurz, M., Mueller, C., Nowak-Goettl, U., Schwabe, D. *et al.* (1997) "Fluconazole versus nystatin in the prevention of candida infections in children and adolescents undergoing remission induction or consolidation chemotherapy for cancer." *J. Antimicrob. Chemother. 40*, 855–862.

100. Venkatakrishnan, K., von Moltke, L.L. and Greenblatt, D.J. (2000) "Effects of the antifungal agents on oxidative drug metabolism: clinical relevance." *Clin. Pharmacokinet. 38*, 111–180.

101. Edelson, S.B. and Cantor, D.S. (1998) "Autism: xenobiotic influences." *Toxicol. Ind. Health 14*, 553–563.

102. Lucarelli, S., Frediani, T., Zingoni, A.M., Ferruzzi, F., Giardini, O., Quintieri, F. *et al.* (1995) "Food allergy and infantile autism." *Panminerva Med. 37*, 137–141.

103. Knivsberg, A.M., Reichelt, K.L. and Nodland, M. (2001) "Reports on dietary intervention in autistic disorders." *Nutr. Neurosci. 4*, 25–37.

104. Knivsberg, A.M., Reichelt, K.L., Hoien, T. and Nodland, M. (2002) "A randomised, controlled study of dietary intervention in autistic syndromes." *Nutr. Neurosci. 5*, 251–261.

105. Millward, C., Ferriter, M., Calver, S. and Connell-Jones, G. (2004) "Gluten- and casein-free diets for autistic spectrum disorder." *Cochrane Database Syst. Rev.*, CD003498.

106. Adams, J.B. and Holloway, C. (2004) "Pilot study of a moderate dose multivitamin/mineral supplement for children with autistic spectrum disorder." *J. Altern. Complement. Med. 10*, 1033–1039.

107. Esch, B.E. and Carr, J.E. (2004) "Secretin as a treatment for autism: a review of the evidence." *J. Autism Dev. Disord. 34*, 543–556.

108. Sturmey, P. (2005) "Secretin is an ineffective treatment for pervasive developmental disabilities: a review of 15 double-blind randomized controlled trials." *Res. Dev. Disabil. 26*, 87–97.

109. Brudnak, M.A., Rimland, B., Kerry, R.E., Dailey, M., Taylor, R., Stayton, B. *et al.* (2002) "Enzyme-based therapy for autism spectrum disorders – is it worth another look?" *Med. Hypotheses 58*, 422–428.

110. Jaworek, J., Nawrot, K., Konturek, S.J., Leja-Szpak, A., Thor, P. and Pawlik, W.W. (2004) "Melatonin and its precursor, L-tryptophan: influence on pancreatic amylase secretion in vivo and in vitro." *J. Pineal Res. 36*, 155–164.

111. Malow, B.A. (2004) "Sleep disorders, epilepsy, and autism." *Ment. Retard. Dev. Disabil. Res. Rev. 10*, 122–125.

112. Vargas, D.L., Nascimbene, C., Krishnan, C., Zimmerman, A.W. and Pardo, C.A. (2005) "Neuroglial activation and neuroinflammation in the brain of patients with autism." *Ann. Neurol. 57*, 67–81.

113. Rothwell, N.J. and Luheshi, G.N. (2000) "Interleukin 1 in the brain: biology, pathology and therapeutic target." *Trends Neurosci. 23*, 618–625.

114. Kielar, M.L., Jeyarajah, D.R., Zhou, X.J. and Lu, C.Y. (2003) "Docosahexaenoic acid ameliorates murine ischemic acute renal failure and prevents increases in mRNA abundance for both TNF-alpha and inducible nitric oxide synthase." *J. Am. Soc. Nephrol. 14*, 389–396.

115. Verlengia, R., Gorjao, R., Kanunfre, C.C., Bordin, S., de Lima, T.M., Martins, E.F. *et al.* (2004) "Effects of EPA and DHA on proliferation, cytokine production, and gene expression in Raji cells." *Lipids 39*, 857–864.

116. Chen, W., Esselman, W.J., Jump, D.B. and Busik, J.V. (2005) "Anti-inflammatory effect of docosahexaenoic acid on cytokine-induced adhesion molecule expression in human retinal vascular endothelial cells." *Invest Ophthalmol. Vis. Sci. 46*, 4342–4347.

117. Young, G. and Conquer, J. (2005) "Omega-3 fatty acids and neuropsychiatric disorders." *Reprod. Nutr. Dev. 45*, 1–28.

118. Hallaway, N. and Strauts, Z. (1995) *Turning Lead into Gold: How Heavy Metal Poisoning Can Affect Your Child and How to Prevent and Treat It.* Vancouver: New Start.

119. Eppright, T.D., Sanfacon, J.A. and Horwitz, E.A. (1996) "Attention deficit hyperactivity disorder, infantile autism, and elevated blood-lead: a possible relationship." *Missouri Med. 93*, 136–138.

120. Lonsdale, D., Shamberger, R.J. and Audhya, T. (2002) "Treatment of autism spectrum children with thiamine tetrahydrofurfuryl disulfide: a pilot study." *Neuro. Endocrinol. Lett. 23*, 303–308.

121. Holmes, A.S. (2003) *Chelation of Mercury for the Treatment of Autism.* http://www.healing-arts.org /children/holmes.htm

122. Mercury Detoxification Consensus Group (2001) *Detoxification Position Paper.* San Diego, CA: Autism Research Institute.

123. Yates, J.C. (2005) "Autistic boy's death raises questions." Release by Associated Press. Online at: http://www.wjla.com/news/stories/0805/255037.html

124. Rogan, W.J., Dietrich, K.N., Ware, J.H., Dockery, D.W., Salganik, M., Radcliffe, J. *et al.* (2001) "The effect of chelation therapy with succimer on neuropsychological development in children exposed to lead." *N. Engl. J. Med. 344*, 1421–1426.

125. Liu, X., Dietrich, K.N., Radcliffe, J., Ragan, N.B., Rhoads, G.G. and Rogan, W.J. (2002) "Do children with falling blood lead levels have improved cognition?" *Pediatrics 110*, 787–791.

126. Marija, V., Piasek, M., Blanusa, M., Matek, S.M., Juresa, D. and Kostial, K. (2004) "Succimer treatment and calcium supplementation reduce tissue lead in suckling rats." *J. Appl. Toxicol. 24*, 123–128.

127. Markowitz, M.E. and Weinberger, H.L. (1990) "Immobilization-related lead toxicity in previously lead-poisoned children." *Pediatrics 86*, 455–457.

128. Walsh, W.J., Glab, L.B. and Haakenson, M.L. (2004) "Reduced violent behavior following biochemical therapy." *Physiol. Behav. 82*, 835–839.

129. Bradman, A., Eskenazi, B., Sutton, P., Athanasoulis, M. and Goldman, L.R. (2001) "Iron deficiency associated with higher blood lead in children living in contaminated environments." *Environ. Health Perspect. 109*, 1079–1084.

130. Flora, S.J., Pande, M., Kannan, G.M. and Mehta, A. (2004) "Lead induced oxidative stress and its recovery following co-administration of melatonin or N-acetylcysteine during chelation with succimer in male rats." *Cell Mol. Biol. (Noisy.-le-grand) 50*, Online Pub, OL543–OL551.

131. El Sokkary, G.H., Abdel-Rahman, G.H. and Kamel, E.S. (2005) "Melatonin protects against lead-induced hepatic and renal toxicity in male rats." *Toxicology 213*, 25–33.

132. Sivaprasad, R., Nagaraj, M. and Varalakshmi, P. (2004) "Combined efficacies of lipoic acid and 2,3-dimercaptosuccinic acid against lead-induced lipid peroxidation in rat liver." *J. Nutr. Biochem. 15*, 18–23.

133. Flora, S.J., Pande, M., Bhadauria, S. and Kannan, G.M. (2004) "Combined administration of taurine and meso 2,3-dimercaptosuccinic acid in the treatment of chronic lead intoxication in rats." *Hum. Exp. Toxicol. 23*, 157–166.

134. Flora, S.J., Pande, M. and Mehta, A. (2003) "Beneficial effect of combined administration of some naturally occurring antioxidants (vitamins) and thiol chelators in the treatment of chronic lead intoxication." *Chem. Biol. Interact. 145*, 267–280.

135. van Guldener, C. and Stehouwer, C.D. (2001) "Homocysteine-lowering treatment: an overview." *Expert. Opin. Pharmacother. 2*, 1449–1460.

136. Pasca, S.P., Nemes, B., Vlase, L., Gagyi, C.E., Dronca, E., Miu, A.C. *et al.* (2006) "High levels of homocysteine and low serum paraoxonase 1 arylesterase activity in children with autism." *Life Sci.* Online at: http://www.sciencedirect.com/science/journal/0024305

137. Rimland, B., Callaway, E. and Dreyfus, P. (1978) "The effect of high doses of vitamin B6 on autistic children: a double-blind crossover study." *Am. J. Psychiatry 135*, 472–475.

138. Nye, C. and Brice, A. (2005) "Combined vitamin B6-magnesium treatment in autism spectrum disorder." *Cochrane Database Syst. Rev.*, CD003497.

139. Fernell, E., Watanabe, Y., Adolfsson, I., Tani, Y., Bergstrom, M., Hartvig, P. *et al.* (1997) "Possible effects of tetrahydrobiopterin treatment in six children with autism – clinical and positron emission tomography data: a pilot study." *Dev. Med. Child Neurol. 39*, 313–318.

140. Baker, T.A., Milstien, S. and Katusic, Z.S. (2001) "Effect of vitamin C on the availability of tetrahydrobiopterin in human endothelial cells." *J. Cardiovasc. Pharmacol. 37*, 333–338.

141. Nakai, K., Urushihara, M., Kubota, Y. and Kosaka, H. (2003) "Ascorbate enhances iNOS activity by increasing tetrahydrobiopterin in RAW 264.7 cells." *Free Radic. Biol. Med. 35*, 929–937.

142. Dolske, M.C., Spollen, J., McKay, S., Lancashire, E. and Tolbert, L. (1993) "A preliminary trial of ascorbic acid as supplemental therapy for autism." *Prog. Neuropsychopharmacol. Biol. Psychiatry 17*, 765–774.

143. Dabbagh, O., Brismar, J., Gascon, G.G. and Ozand, P.T. (1994) "The clinical spectrum of biotin-treatable encephalopathies in Saudi Arabia." *Brain Dev. 16*, Suppl, 72–80.

144. Bressman, S., Fahn, S., Eisenberg, M., Brin, M. and Maltese, W. (1986) "Biotin-responsive encephalopathy with myoclonus, ataxia, and seizures." *Adv. Neurol. 43*, 119–125.

145. Valko, M., Morris, H. and Cronin, M.T. (2005) "Metals, toxicity and oxidative stress." *Curr. Med. Chem. 12*, 1161–1208.

146. Stites, T.E., Mitchell, A.E. and Rucker, R.B. (2000) "Physiological importance of quinoenzymes and the O-quinone family of cofactors." *J. Nutr. 130*, 719–727.

147. Steinberg, F., Stites, T.E., Anderson, P., Storms, D., Chan, I., Eghbali, S. *et al.* (2003) "Pyrroloquinoline quinone improves growth and reproductive performance in mice fed chemically defined diets." *Exp. Biol. Med. (Maywood) 228*, 160–166.

148. Strous, R.D., Golubchik, P., Maayan, R., Mozes, T., Tuati-Werner, D., Weizman, A. *et al.* (2005) "Lowered DHEA-S plasma levels in adult individuals with autistic disorder." *Eur. Neuropsychopharmacol. 15*, 305–309.

149. Kalimi, M., Shafagoj, Y., Loria, R., Padgett, D. and Regelson, W. (1994) "Anti-glucocorticoid effects of dehydroepiandrosterone (DHEA)." *Mol. Cell. Biochem. 131*, 99–104.

150. Lathe, R. (2002) "Steroid and sterol 7-hydroxylation: ancient pathways." *Steroids 67*, 967–977.

151. Maurice, C., Green, G. and Luce, S.C. (eds) (1996) *Behavioral Intervention for Young Children with Autism: A Manual for Parents and Professionals.* Austin, TX: Pro-Ed.

152. Harris, S.L. (1998) "Behavioural and educational approaches to the pervasive developmental disorders." In F. Volkmar and I.M. Goodyer (eds) *Autism and Pervasive Developmental Disorders.* Cambridge: Cambridge University Press; pp.195–208.

153. Mitchell, L.E., Adzick, N.S., Melchionne, J., Pasquariello, P.S., Sutton, L.N. and Whitehead, A.S. (2004) "Spina bifida." *Lancet 364*, 1885–1895.

154. Oblak, A., Cross, J.D. and Hollerman, J.R. (2005) "The effects of periconceptual supplementation of folic acid in an animal model of autism." *Proc. Soc. Neurosci. Congress Washington*. Online at: http://sfn .scholarone.com/itin2005/index.html, Abs. No. 448.7.

155. Hernandez-Avila, M., Gonzalez-Cossio, T., Hernandez-Avila, J.E., Romieu, I., Peterson, K.E., Aro, A. *et al*. (2003) "Dietary calcium supplements to lower blood lead levels in lactating women: a randomized placebo-controlled trial." *Epidemiology 14*, 206–212.

156. Food Standards Agency (2004) *Fish Consumption, Benefits and Risks, Part 3*. Online at: http://www.food .gov.uk/multimedia/pdfs/fishreport200403.pdf

157. Gesch, C.B., Hammond, S.M., Hampson, S.E., Eves, A. and Crowder, M.J. (2002) "Influence of supplementary vitamins, minerals and essential fatty acids on the antisocial behaviour of young adult prisoners. Randomised, placebo-controlled trial." *Br. J. Psychiatry 181*, 22–28.

Chapter 11 The Environmental Threat: From Autism and ADHD to Alzheimer's

1. Waddington, C.H. (1942) "Canalization of development and inheritance of acquired characters." *Nature 150*, 563.

2. Waddington, C.H. (1952) "Selection of the genetic basis for an acquired character." *Nature 169*, 625–626.

3. Waddington, C.H. (1961) "Genetic assimilation." *Adv. Genet. 10*, 257–293.

4. Waddington, C.H. (1959) "Canalization of development and genetic assimilation of acquired characters." *Nature 183*, 1654–1655.

5. McLaren, A. (1999) "Too late for the midwife toad: stress, variability and Hsp90." *Trends Genet. 15*, 169–171.

6. Rutherford, S.L. and Lindquist, S. (1998) "Hsp90 as a capacitor for morphological evolution." *Nature 396*, 336–342.

7. Wolpert, L. (1999) "Vertebrate limb development and malformations." *Pediatr. Res. 46*, 247–254.

8. Nau, H., Hauck, R.S. and Ehlers, K. (1991) "Valproic acid-induced neural tube defects in mouse and human: aspects of chirality, alternative drug development, pharmacokinetics and possible mechanisms." *Pharmacol. Toxicol. 69*, 310–321.

9. Mitchell, L.E., Adzick, N.S., Melchionne, J., Pasquariello, P.S., Sutton, L.N. and Whitehead, A.S. (2004) "Spina bifida." *Lancet 364*, 1885–1895.

10. Dorner, G., Geier, T., Ahrens, L., Krell, L., Munx, G., Sieler, H. *et al*. (1980) "Prenatal stress as possible aetiogenetic factor of homosexuality in human males." *Endokrinologie 75*, 365–368.

11. Susser, E.S. and Lin, S.P. (1992) "Schizophrenia after prenatal exposure to the Dutch Hunger Winter of 1944–1945." *Arch. Gen. Psychiatry 49*, 983–988.

12. Hoek, H.W., Susser, E., Buck, K.A., Lumey, L.H., Lin, S.P. and Gorman, J.M. (1996) "Schizoid personality disorder after prenatal exposure to famine." *Am. J. Psychiatry 153*, 1637–1639.

13. St. Clair, D., Xu, M., Wang, P., Yu, Y., Fang, Y., Zhang, F. *et al*. (2005) "Rates of adult schizophrenia following prenatal exposure to the Chinese famine of 1959–1961." *J. Am. Med. Assoc. 294*, 557–562.

14. Bauman, M.L. and Kemper, T.L. (2005) "Neuroanatomic observations of the brain in autism: a review and future directions." *Int. J. Dev. Neurosci. 23*, 183–187.

15. Juul-Dam, N., Townsend, J. and Courchesne, E. (2001) "Prenatal, perinatal, and neonatal factors in autism, pervasive developmental disorder – not otherwise specified, and the general population." *Pediatrics 107*, E63.

16. Rutter, M., Andersen-Wood, L., Beckett, C., Bredenkamp, D., Castle, J., Groothues, C. *et al*. (1999) "Quasi-autistic patterns following severe early global privation. English and Romanian Adoptees (ERA) Study Team." *J. Child Psychol. Psychiatry 40*, 537–549.

17. D'Amelio, M., Ricci, I., Sacco, R., Liu, X., D'Agruma, L., Muscarella, L.A. *et al*. (2005) "Paraoxonase gene variants are associated with autism in North America, but not in Italy: possible regional specificity in gene-environment interactions." *Mol. Psychiatry 10*, 1006–1016.

18. Nataf, R., Skorupka, C. and Lathe, R. (2005) Unpublished data.

19. Minder, B., Das-Smaal, E.A., Brand, E.F. and Orlebeke, J.F. (1994) "Exposure to lead and specific attentional problems in schoolchildren." *J. Learn. Disabil. 27*, 393–399.

20. Grandjean, P., Weihe, P., White, R.F., Debes, F., Araki, S., Yokoyama, K. *et al.* (1997) "Cognitive deficit in 7-year-old children with prenatal exposure to methylmercury." *Neurotoxicol. Teratol. 19*, 417–428.

21. Tuthill, R.W. (1996) "Hair lead levels related to children's classroom attention-deficit behavior." *Arch. Environ. Health 51*, 214–220.

22. Mendola, P., Selevan, S.G., Gutter, S. and Rice, D. (2002) "Environmental factors associated with a spectrum of neurodevelopmental deficits." *Ment. Retard. Dev. Disabil. Res. Rev. 8*, 188–197.

23. Capel, I.D., Pinnock, M.H., Dorrell, H.M., Williams, D.C. and Grant, E.C. (1981) "Comparison of concentrations of some trace, bulk, and toxic metals in the hair of normal and dyslexic children." *Clin. Chem. 27*, 879–881.

24. Marlowe, M., Cossairt, A., Moon, C., Errera, J., MacNeel, A., Peak, R. *et al.* (1985) "Main and interaction effects of metallic toxins on classroom behavior." *J. Abnorm. Child Psychol. 13*, 185–198.

25. Needleman, H.L., Riess, J.A., Tobin, M.J., Biesecker, G.E. and Greenhouse, J.B. (1996) "Bone lead levels and delinquent behavior." *J. Am. Med. Assoc. 275*, 363–369.

26. Dietrich, K.N., Ris, M.D., Succop, P.A., Berger, O.G. and Bornschein, R.L. (2001) "Early exposure to lead and juvenile delinquency." *Neurotoxicol. Teratol. 23*, 511–518.

27. Robertson, M., Evans, K., Robinson, A., Trimble, M. and Lascelles, P. (1987) "Abnormalities of copper in Gilles de la Tourette syndrome." *Biol. Psychiatry 22*, 968–978.

28. Bagedahl-Strindlund, M., Ilie, M., Furhoff, A.K., Tomson, Y., Larsson, K.S., Sandborgh-Englund, G. *et al.* (1997) "A multidisciplinary clinical study of patients suffering from illness associated with mercury release from dental restorations: psychiatric aspects." *Acta Psychiatr. Scand. 96*, 475–482.

29. Opler, M.G., Brown, A.S., Graziano, J., Desai, M., Zheng, W., Schaefer, C. *et al.* (2004) "Prenatal lead exposure, delta-aminolevulinic acid, and schizophrenia." *Environ. Health Perspect. 112*, 548–552.

30. Basun, H., Forssell, L.G., Wetterberg, L. and Winblad, B. (1991) "Metals and trace elements in plasma and cerebrospinal fluid in normal aging and Alzheimer's disease." *J. Neural Transm. Park Dis. Dement. Sect. 3*, 231–258.

31. Hock, C., Drasch, G., Golombowski, S., Muller-Spahn, F., Willershausen-Zonnchen, B., Schwarz, P. *et al.* (1998) "Increased blood mercury levels in patients with Alzheimer's disease." *J. Neural Transm. 105*, 59–68.

32. Farris, F.F., Dedrick, R.L., Allen, P.V. and Smith, J.C. (1993) "Physiological model for the pharmacokinetics of methyl mercury in the growing rat." *Toxicol. Appl. Pharmacol. 119*, 74–90.

33. Suzuki, T., Hongo, T., Yoshinaga, J., Imai, H., Nakazawa, M., Matsuo, N. *et al.* (1993) "The hair-organ relationship in mercury concentration in contemporary Japanese." *Arch. Environ. Health 48*, 221–229.

34. Holmes, A.S., Blaxill, M.F. and Haley, B.E. (2003) "Reduced levels of mercury in first baby haircuts of autistic children." *Int. J. Toxicol. 22*, 277–285.

35. Kobayashi, S., Fujiwara, S., Arimoto, S., Koide, H., Fukuda, J., Shimode, K. *et al.* (1989) "Hair aluminium in normal aged and senile dementia of Alzheimer type." *Prog. Clin. Biol. Res. 317*, 1095–1109.

36. Basha, M.R., Wei, W., Bakheet, S.A., Benitez, N., Siddiqi, H.K., Ge, Y.W. *et al.* (2005) "The fetal basis of amyloidogenesis: exposure to lead and latent overexpression of amyloid precursor protein and beta-amyloid in the aging brain." *J. Neurosci. 25*, 823–829.

37. Nakagawa, R. (1995) "Concentration of mercury in hair of diseased people in Japan." *Chemosphere 30*, 135–140.

38. Telisman, S., Cvitkovic, P., Jurasovic, J., Pizent, A., Gavella, M. and Rocic, B. (2000) "Semen quality and reproductive endocrine function in relation to biomarkers of lead, cadmium, zinc, and copper in men." *Environ. Health Perspect. 108*, 45–53.

39. Nemery, B. (1990) "Metal toxicity and the respiratory tract." *Eur. Respir. J. 3*, 202–219.

40. Chiappino, G. (1994) "Hard metal disease: clinical aspects." *Sci. Total Environ. 150*, 65–68.

41. Di Toro, R., Galdo, C.G., Gialanella, G., Miraglia, d.G., Moro, R. and Perrone, L. (1987) "Zinc and copper status of allergic children." *Acta Paediatr. Scand. 76*, 612–617.

42. Joseph, C.L., Havstad, S., Ownby, D.R., Peterson, E.L., Maliarik, M., McCabe, M.J., Jr. *et al.* (2005) "Blood lead level and risk of asthma." *Environ. Health Perspect. 113*, 900–904.

43. Croen, L.A., Grether, J.K., Yoshida, C.K., Odouli, R. and Van de, W.J. (2005) "Maternal autoimmune diseases, asthma and allergies, and childhood autism spectrum disorders: a case-control study." *Arch. Pediatr. Adolesc. Med. 159*, 151–157.

44. Woodruff, T.J., Axelrad, D.A., Kyle, A.D., Nweke, O., Miller, G.G. and Hurley, B.J. (2004) "Trends in environmentally related childhood illnesses." *Pediatrics 113*, 1133–1140.

45. Sverd, J. (2003) "Psychiatric disorders in individuals with pervasive developmental disorder." *J. Psychiatr. Pract. 9*, 111–127.

46. Stewart, P.W., Reihman, J., Lonky, E.I., Darvill, T.J. and Pagano, J. (2003) "Cognitive development in preschool children prenatally exposed to PCBs and MeHg." *Neurotoxicol. Teratol. 25*, 11–22.

47. Cohen, D.J., Paul, R., Anderson, G.M. and Harcherik, D.F. (1982) "Blood lead in autistic children." *Lancet 2*, 94–95.

48. Accardo, P., Whitman, B., Caul, J. and Rolfe, U. (1988) "Autism and plumbism. A possible association." *Clin. Pediatr. (Phila.) 27*, 41–44.

49. Shannon, M. and Graef, J.W. (1996) "Lead intoxication in children with pervasive developmental disorders." *J. Toxicol. Clin. Toxicol. 34*, 177–181.

50. Lidsky, T.I. and Schneider, J.S. (2005) "Autism and autistic symptoms associated with childhood lead poisoning." *J. Appl. Res. 5*, 80–87.

51. Edelson, S.B. and Cantor, D.S. (1998) "Autism: xenobiotic influences." *Toxicol. Ind. Health 14*, 553–563.

52. Wu, S., Jia, M., Ruan, Y., Liu, J., Guo, Y., Shuang, M. *et al.* (2005) "Positive association of the oxytocin receptor gene (OXTR) with autism in the Chinese Han population." *Biol. Psychiatry 58*, 74–77.

53. McEwen, B.S. (2003) "Mood disorders and allostatic load." *Biol. Psychiatry 54*, 200–207.

54. Lathe, R. (2004) "The individuality of mice." *Genes Brain Behav. 3*, 317–327.

55. Young, S.N. and Leyton, M. (2002) "The role of serotonin in human mood and social interaction. Insight from altered tryptophan levels." *Pharmacol. Biochem. Behav. 71*, 857–865.

56. Rosvold, H.E., Mirsky, A.F. and Pribram, K.H. (1954) "Influence of amygdalectomy on social behavior in monkeys." *J. Comp. Physiol. Psychol. 47*, 173–178.

57. Eriksson, P.S., Perfilieva, E., Bjork-Eriksson, T., Alborn, A.M., Nordborg, C., Peterson, D.A. *et al.* (1998) "Neurogenesis in the adult human hippocampus." *Nat. Med. 4*, 1313–1317.

58. Kornack, D.R. and Rakic, P. (1999) "Continuation of neurogenesis in the hippocampus of the adult macaque monkey." *Proc. Natl. Acad. Sci. USA 96*, 5768–5773.

59. Gould, E., Reeves, A.J., Fallah, M., Tanapat, P., Gross, C.G. and Fuchs, E. (1999) "Hippocampal neurogenesis in adult Old World primates." *Proc. Natl. Acad. Sci. USA 96*, 5263–5267.

60. Crowcroft, P. (1966) *Mice All Over*. London: G.T. Foulis & Co.

61. van Praag, H., Kempermann, G. and Gage, F.H. (1999) "Running increases cell proliferation and neurogenesis in the adult mouse dentate gyrus." *Nat. Neurosci. 2*, 266–270.

62. Kozorovitskiy, Y. and Gould, E. (2004) "Dominance hierarchy influences adult neurogenesis in the dentate gyrus." *J. Neurosci. 24*, 6755–6759.

63. Fiore, M., Amendola, T., Triaca, V., Tirassa, P., Alleva, E. and Aloe, L. (2003) "Agonistic encounters in aged male mouse potentiate the expression of endogenous brain NGF and BDNF: possible implication for brain progenitor cells' activation." *Eur. J. Neurosci. 17*, 1455–1464.

64. Palanza, P., Morellini, F., Parmigiani, S. and vom Saal, F.S. (1999) "Prenatal exposure to endocrine disrupting chemicals: effects on behavioral development." *Neurosci. Biobehav. Rev. 23*, 1011–1027.

65. Brown, J., Cooper-Kuhn, C.M., Kempermann, G., van Praag, H., Winkler, J., Gage, F.H. *et al.* (2003) "Enriched environment and physical activity stimulate hippocampal but not olfactory bulb neurogenesis." *Eur. J. Neurosci. 17*, 2042–2046.

66. Schneider, T., Turczak, J. and Przewlocki, R. (2006) "Environmental enrichment reverses behavioral alterations in rats prenatally exposed to valproic acid: issues for a therapeutic approach in autism." *Neuropsychopharmacology 31*, 36–46.

67. Santarelli, L., Saxe, M., Gross, C., Surget, A., Battaglia, F., Dulawa, S. *et al.* (2003) "Requirement of hippocampal neurogenesis for the behavioral effects of antidepressants." *Science 301*, 805–809.

68. Kaufman, B.N. (1995) *Son-Rise: The Miracle Continues*. Tiburon, CA: H.J. Kramer Press.

69. Oskarsson, A., Palminger, H. and Sundberg, J. (1995) "Exposure to toxic elements via breast milk." *Analyst 120*, 765–770.

70. Oskarsson, A., Schultz, A., Skerfving, S., Hallen, I.P., Ohlin, B. and Lagerkvist, B.J. (1996) "Total and inorganic mercury in breast milk in relation to fish consumption and amalgam in lactating women." *Arch. Environ. Health 51*, 234–241.

71. Palmer, R.F., Blanchard, S., Stein, Z., Mandell, D. and Miller, C. (2006) "Environmental mercury release, special education rates, and autism disorder: an ecological study of Texas." *Health and Place 12*, 203–209.

72. Walkowiak, J., Wiener, J.A., Fastabend, A., Heinzow, B., Kramer, U., Schmidt, E. *et al.* (2001) "Environmental exposure to polychlorinated biphenyls and quality of the home environment: effects on psychodevelopment in early childhood." *Lancet 358*, 1602–1607.

73. Koopmann-Esseboom, C., Huisman, M. and Weisglas-Kuperus, N. (1994) "PCB and dioxin levels in plasma and human milk of 418 Dutch women and their infants: predictive value of PCB congener level in maternal plasma for feta and infant exposure to PCBs and dioxins." *Chemosphere 28*, 1721–1732.

74. Wingspread Conference (1991) "The Wingspread consensus statement." In S.F. Gilbert (ed) *DevBio; A Companion to Developmental Biology.* http://www.devbio.com/article.php?ch=22&id=217

75. Daston, G.P., Cook, J.C. and Kavlock, R.J. (2003) "Uncertainties for endocrine disrupters: our view on progress." *Toxicol. Sci. 74*, 245–252.

76. Hong, S., Candelone, J.P., Patterson, C.C. and Boutron, C.F. (1994) "Greenland ice evidence of hemispheric lead pollution two millennia ago by Greek and Roman civilizations." *Science 265*, 1841–1843.

77. Le Couteur, A., Bailey, A., Goode, S., Pickles, A., Robertson, S., Gottesman, I. *et al.* (1996) "A broader phenotype of autism: the clinical spectrum in twins." *J. Child Psychol. Psychiatry 37*, 785–801.

78. Bailey, A., Palferman, S., Heavey, L. and Le Couteur, A. (1998) "Autism: the phenotype in relatives." *J. Autism Dev. Disord. 28*, 369–392.

79. Gilfillan, S.C. (1965) "Roman culture and dysgenic lead poisoning." *The Mankind Quarterly (Edinburgh) 5*, 131–148.

Abbreviations and Glossary

ABA applied behavioral analysis

ACTH adrenocorticotrophic hormone; a pituitary hormone that acts on the adrenal to stimulate hormone release

ADD attention deficit disorder

ADHD attention deficit hyperactivity disorder

ADI-R autism diagnostic interview – revised

ADOS-G autism diagnostic observation schedule – generic

AGRE Autism Genetic Resource Exchange

ALAD δ-ALA dehydratase; enzyme of the heme synthesis pathway

allele a functional gene variant, ascribed to one or more mutations

Ammon's horn alternative name for the hippocampus

amygdala nut-shaped extension of the hippocampus (Latin, almond), regarded as a separate organ within the limbic system but with overlapping functionality

androgen a steroid hormone with masculinizing effects; includes testosterone and related hormones

antigen a novel structure or molecule that is recognized by the immune system

AR androgen receptor; responds to androgens including the sex steroid testosterone

ASD autism (or autistic) spectrum disorder; generally equates to the group of pervasive developmental disorders as defined by international criteria; these include autistic disorder, PDD – not otherwise specified, childhood disintegrative disorder, Asperger disorder, and Rett disorder

Asperger disorder/syndrome a type of high-functioning autism where speech and intelligence are preserved but other social deficits may be apparent

autism spectrum see ASD

autistic disorder autism proper; a subcategory of the pervasive developmental disorders (PDD) or autism spectrum disorders (ASD)

axon the long communicating fiber (or fibers) of a neuron

B12 vitamin B12, cyanocobalamin; cofactor in several enzyme reactions

β-E beta-endorphin; one of the endogenous opioids produced by the pituitary

benzodiazepine one of a group of structurally related drugs, including diazepam, with anxiolytic, sedative, and anticonvulsant activity

BH4 tetrahydrobiopterin; a cofactor in several enzyme reactions

bisphenol A an estrogenic endocrine disruptor; 4,4'-dihydroxy-2,2-diphenylpropane

brainstem the lower part of the brain extending toward the spinal cord

broader phenotype refers to the extended, often milder, phenotype sometimes seen in close relatives of subjects with autism spectrum disorders

CA regions subregions of the cornu ammonis (Ammon's horn), the hippocampus; as in CA1, CA2, CA3

CARS Childhood Autism Rating Scale

catecholamines the group of neurotransmitters including adrenalin (epinephrine), nor-adrenalin (nor-epinephrine), and dopamine

CBS cystathionine beta-synthase; key enzyme degrading homocysteine

CDD childhood disintegrative disorder; a subcategory of PDD

cerebellum at the lower rear of the brain (the "little brain"); involved in posture and locomotion

CHAT Checklist for Autism in Toddlers

chelating agent a chemical compound that binds particular heavy metals and may mobilize them for export

COMT catecholamine-O-methyltransferase; an enzyme degrading catecholamines

concordance the extent to which twins share the same defined behavior or disorder, usually expressed as a percentage

cornu ammonis see CA regions

corpus callosum major neuronal connecting tract between the two halves of the brain

cortex major (upper and outer) part of the brain, the cerebrum

CPOX coproporphyrinogen oxidase, a key enzyme in the heme synthesis pathway

CRF corticotropin-releasing factor, a hypothalamic hormone that acts on the pituitary

CSF cerebrospinal fluid; the fluid output of the brain that irrigates the cavities of the brain (ventricles) and the spinal cord

CYP cytochrome P450 hemoprotein (haemoprotein) involved in oxidative reactions; contains a tightly bound heme molecule

cytochrome literally a cellular pigment; most usually one of a group of proteins that form tight complexes with heme

cytokine protein signaling molecule produced by one cell to act on an adjacent cell; prominent regulator of immunity and inflammation

δALA δ-aminolevulinic acid; precursor to heme synthesis

DDT dichloro-diphenyl-trichloroethane; an insecticide and environmental pollutant

dendrite a short thin filament that allows neurons to communicate with adjacent cells including other neurons in the same tissue

DG dentate gyrus; subregion of the hippocampus so-named because of its tooth-like appearance

DHA docosahexaenoic acid; natural anti-inflammatory found in fish oils

DHEA dehydroepiandrosterone; steroid with androgenic properties, reputed to be an "anti-ageing" hormone

diazepam better known as Valium (7-chloro-1,3-dihydro-1-methyl-5-phenyl-2H-1,4-benzodiazepin-2-one), a member of the benzodiazepine group of drugs

DMPS dimercapto-propanesulfonic acid; metal-chelating agent

DMSA dimercapto-succinic acid, also known as succimer; metal-chelating agent

Down (Down's) syndrome a childhood disorder associated with an extra copy of chromosome 21 (or part of this chromosome); often associated with mental retardation

DSM (-III, -IIIR, -IV) Diagnostic and Statistical Manual of Mental Disorders, issued by the American Psychiatric Association (versions III, III-revised, IV)

DZ dizygotic, from two independent eggs, as in non-identical twins

ED endocrine disruptor; agent that causes long-lasting changes in reproductive and developmental status by mimicking natural sex hormones

EDTA ethylenediamine tetraacetic acid; metal-chelating agent

EEG electroencephalogram; a recording of brainwave activity from the scalp

endocrine pertaining to hormone secretion and action

entorhinal cortex cortical region immediately adjacent to the hippocampus

epigenetic refers to the acquired (*non-genetic*) characteristics of a cell that are passed on through division and often through generations; associated with changes in the methylation pattern of specific chromosomal DNA sequences

ER (ERα, ERβ) estrogen (oestrogen) receptor, the receptor responding to estrogens including estradiol; ERalpha, ERbeta are two non-identical subtypes

ErCx entorhinal cortex

erythroid relating to the blood, and more specifically to red blood cells

FMR-1 gene at the Fragile-X locus (for Fragile-X mental retardation)

fMRI functional magnetic resonance imaging

folic acid also known as vitamin B9; folic acid (folate) and its metabolites are required for several enzyme reactions

folinic acid 5-formyl-derivative of tetrahydrofolic acid, natural form of folic acid, readily converted to other reduced folic acid derivatives including tetrahydrofolate

Fragile X X chromosome anomaly often associated with mental retardation and autism

GABA gamma-amino butyric acid, a major inhibitory neurotransmitter

GI gastrointestinal; pertaining to the digestive system

Gilles de la Tourette syndrome Also known as Tourette's, a disorder often commencing in childhood; characterized by tics or repetitive involuntary movements or vocalizations

glucocorticoid a group of structurally related steroids produced by the adrenal gland with immunosuppressive, anti-inflammatory, and salt-regulatory properties

GnRH gonadotrophin-releasing hormone, formerly called LHRH (luteinizing hormone-releasing hormone); released from the hypothalamus to stimulate luteinizing hormone release from the pituitary

GPX glutathione peroxidase; a selenium-containing enzyme that uses

glutathione to remove peroxides and prevent oxidative damage

gray matter areas of the brain, seen in cross-section, that are dark colored because the structural cell bodies containing nuclei are enriched in these layers

GST glutathione S-transferase; one of several detoxification enzymes that link glutathione to metabolites and xenobiotics, so facilitating degradation and excretion

haplotype the collective genotype of a group of genetic markers, usually located on the same chromosome; also used to refer to an individual's overall collection of genetic markers

heme, haem the iron-containing pigment contained in hemoglobin (haemoglobin) and other proteins involved in oxygen transfer including cytochromes

heritability a mathematical calculation of the degree to which a disorder is dependent on genes

5HIAA (5-HIAA) indole acetic acid; degradation product of serotonin

hippocampus central region of the limbic brain, named from its shape (*hippocampus*, sea-horse); included in the medial temporal lobe

histocompatibility literally tissue compatibility; the major determinants of acceptance or rejection during transplant procedures from one individual to another; the chromosome region(s) determining histocompatibility encompass the HLA locus genes in humans and the H-2 locus genes in mice

histology the study of tissue (*histos*, Greek), usually involving microscope analysis of thin sections

HLA human leukocyte antigen; major antigens determining histocompatibility

HM initials of a renowned amnesic patient with bilateral hippocampal lesions

homocysteine a neurotoxic derivative of the essential amino acid cysteine

HPA axis hypothalamus–pituitary–adrenal axis; a sequential activation pathway of the three organs that more properly includes other target organs including the thyroid gland, GI tract, and gonads

HSP90 heat-shock protein-90k, a cellular stress-response protein

5HT (5-HT) serotonin, also known as 5-hydroxytryptamine; a major neurotransmitter in the brain

hypothalamus a structure of the lower brain; produces hormone-releasing factors that prominently control the activity of the pituitary

hypoxia reduced oxygen supply generally due to respiratory problems; usually pathologic in its consequences

IBS irritable bowel syndrome

ICD (-9, -10) International Classification of Diseases, issued by the World Health Organization; versions 9, 10

IDO indoleamine 2,3 di-oxygenase, an enzyme degrading tryptophan

IFN interferon, as in IFN-γ; a cytokine of the immune system

Ig immunoglobulin (antibody), as in IgG, IgA

IGF-1 insulin-like growth factor type-1

IL (IL-1, IL-6) interleukin (types -1 and -6)

IL1-RA interleukin-1 receptor antagonist; blocks IL-1 action

interleukin one of a group of cytokines, often associated with the immune system

ischemia (ischaemia) localized deficiency of oxygen in a tissue, notably in the brain, due to obstruction of a blood vessel; often pathologic in effect

karyotype the chromosome complement of a cell (or individual) determined by microscope analysis; shows the number, type, and size of each chromosome type

Klüver-Bucy syndrome (KBS) disorder produced by bilateral temporal lobe lesion including hippocampus and amygdala; named after the first physicians to report this condition

LH luteinizing hormone; a pituitary hormone that acts to stimulate gonadal activity and sex steroid production in both genders

LHRH luteinizing hormone-releasing hormone; see GnRH

limbic system region involved in emotion and memory; includes the hippocampus and amygdala (from *limbus*, fringe), between the cortex and the brainstem

LNH lymphoid nodular hyperplasia, swollen lymph nodes, often in the GI tract

LOD score log of the odds, a measure of statistical probability of gene association

LPS lipopolysaccharide, the inflammatory component of bacterial cell walls

M-CHAT Modified Checklist for Autism in Toddlers

MeCP2 methyl-cytosine binding protein type 2; function of the gene encoding MeCP2 is reduced in Rett syndrome

medial temporal lobe the brain lobe overlying and encompassing the hippocampus and amygdala

MET methionine, an essential amino acid

Me-THF methylene tetrahydrofolate, a cofactor in several enzyme reactions notably in methionine synthesis; produced from folic acid

methylmercury an organic form of mercury and the major metabolite of metallic mercury

MMR measles-mumps-rubella (as in MMR vaccine)

monocyte a large white cell of the blood; destroys invading bacteria or other cells, involved in inflammatory reactions (in tissues, monocytes are termed phagocytes)

MRI magnetic resonance imaging

MS methionine synthase, the major enzyme synthesizing methionine

MTF-1 metal regulatory transcription factor-1

MTHFR methylene tetrahydrofolate reductase; an enzyme involved in the regeneration of folic acid-derived cofactors

MZ monozygotic, from a single egg; as with identical twins

NAAR National Alliance for Autism Research

neuroleptic one of a diverse group of drugs used to treat psychoses and mood disorders; their mechanism of action is generally unknown

neuron the major information-carrying cell type of the brain

neurotransmitter a low molecular weight substance released in fast pulses by one neuron to impinge upon another neuron to stimulate (or inhibit) its activity; mediate information transfer in the brain

OT oxytocin; a polypeptide hormone involved in aspects of social behavior

OT-X oxytocin extended form; an abnormal (possibly juvenile) form of oxytocin

P450 properly termed cytochrome P450 enzymes (often contracted to CYP) in virtue of their characteristic color (peak wavelength of absorption in nanometers) after complexing with carbon monoxide, a molecule with high affinity for heme; involved in oxidative metabolism and detoxification

PAPS phosphoadenosine-5'-phosphosulfate; a major sulfate donor in enzyme reactions

PBR peripheral benzodiazepine receptor; an atypical receptor responding to benzodiazepines such as diazepam

PCB polychlorinated biphenyl, one of a group of related biphenyl molecules with one or more chlorine substituents; environmental pollutant deriving from industrial processes notably involving electrical equipment

PDD pervasive developmental disorder; see ASD

PDD-NOS pervasive developmental disorder – not otherwise specified; see ASD

PET positron-emission tomography

phenotype the appearance and manifestation of the combined effects of an individual's genetic complement (genotype) and the environment

pituitary a gland at the base of the brain that secretes hormones controlling growth and fertility; regulated by the hypothalamus

polymorphism any DNA sequence difference between two genes (or chromosomes); the majority of polymorphisms are thought to be silent in that they do not affect the function of nearby genes

POMC pro-opiomelanocortin, the pituitary precursor polypeptide to ACTH, beta-endorphin, and certain other small peptide hormones

PP pyridoxal phosphate, from pyridoxine (vitamin B6); cofactor in several enzyme reactions

ppm parts per million (micrograms per gram, or $\mu g/g$)

PQQ pyrroloquinoline quinine, a new vitamin presumed to be an enzyme cofactor

pro-inflammatory cytokine one of a group of cytokines that are released on inflammation and themselves can cause inflammation; includes interleukins, interferons, and tumor necrosis factor

Proto IX protoporphyrin IX, the last metabolite before heme (haem) during biosynthesis

p value probability value; a statistical measure of the likelihood that a difference between two groups of values might occur purely by chance. A value less than 0.05 reflects a greater than 95% chance that the difference is meaningful (not by chance) and is generally accepted as the cut-off point for statistical significance; a p value under 0.01 reflects a 99% chance that the difference is meaningful and is considered to be highly significant. In graphs and charts, p values are conventionally represented by stars or asterisks as follows: $\star$ = p<0.05; $\star\star$ = p<0.01; $\star\star\star$ = p<0.001; $(\star)$ = marginal significance, p<0.1

QUIN quinolinic acid; neurotoxic metabolite of tryptophan

Rett a syndrome (disorder) in the group of pervasive developmental disorders (autism spectrum disorders) most commonly associated with deficiency in MeCP2

Reye (syndrome or disorder) a rapid-onset debilitating childhood disorder attributed to combined viral infection and adverse response to medication; characterized by gastrointestinal involvement and brain effects including lethargy, confusion, and convulsions

rhinencephalon from Greek *rhis* (nose), *enkephalos* (brain); historical term for the part of the brain responsible for chemical sensing; includes the olfactory system and parts of the limbic brain including the hippocampus

Rho(D) rhesus immunoglobulin; given to mothers during pregnancy who are rhesus incompatible with their child

SAHH S-adenosyl homocysteine hydrolase

SAM S-adenosyl methionine; an essential cofactor derived from methionine and involved in methylation and methyl transfer reactions

serotonin a major neurotransmitter in the brain and gut, structurally known as 5-hydroxytryptamine (5HT)

SPECT single positron emission computed tomography

SSPE subacute sclerosing panencephalitis; a rare disease attributed to measles virus infection in the first two years of life and characterized by progressive, often fatal, brain inflammation

SSRI selective serotonin reuptake inhibitor; one of a group of antidepressants that increase serotonin action in the brain by inhibiting removal

statistical significance see p value

subiculum cortical region adjacent to the entorhinal cortex and hippocampus

T3 triiodothyronine; a thyroid hormone

T4 thyroxine or tetraiodothyronine; a thyroid hormone

TBT tributyltin

TCDD 2,3,7,8-tetrachlorodibenzo-p-dioxin; the most toxic of a group of related polychlorinated aromatic hydrocarbons, produced by incineration of industrial and domestic waste

TCII transcobalamin II synthase reductase; an enzyme involved in recycling vitamin B12

TDO tryptophan dioxygenase; enzyme involved in the degradation of tryptophan

temporal lobe the brain lobes underlying the temples

TET triethyltin

thalidomide 2-(2,6-dioxo-3-piperidinyl)-1H-isoindole-1,3(2H)-dione; drug formerly given during pregnancy to alleviate morning sickness and later found responsible for producing birth defects

THF tetrahydrofolate; intermediate form of folic acid (vitamin B9) regeneration

thimerosal, thiomersal a mercury-containing preservative (tradename Merthiolate), ethylmercurithiosalicylic acid sodium salt; breaks down to release ethylmercury in the body

TMT trimethyltin

TNF tumor necrosis factor, as in TNF-α; a cytokine of the immune system

Tourette's see Gilles de la Tourette syndrome

triad of impairments the three central impairments associated with autism and related spectrum disorders language and communication, social interaction, and behavioral repertoire

TRP tryptophan, an essential amino acid

TSC1, TSC2 genes involved in tuberous sclerosis

TTFD thiamine tetrahydrofurfuryl disulfide; a metal-chelating agent

TTQ tryptophan tryptophylquinone; a new vitamin and presumed enzyme cofactor

TUNEL terminal transferase dUTP-fluorescein nick end-labeling; a detection method for DNA fragmentation produced by programmed cell death

white matter layers of brain tissue particularly depleted in dark-colored neuronal cell bodies; primarily contains axonal projections linking neurons

Further Reading

Note: this bibliography is restricted to published books; where possible the reader is encouraged to consult original reviews published as journal articles, many of which are available on the internet. The selection is a personal choice.

Ader, R., Felten, D.L. and Cohen, N. (1991) *Psychoneuroimmunology, Second Edition*. San Diego: Academic Press.
This remarkable and pioneering work describes at length, with many illustrative case studies, how brain perception can have immediate and long-lasting effects on the immune system. The treatment is scholarly and comprehensive but the book is very readable.

Bauman, M. and Kemper, T.L. (eds) (1994) *The Neurobiology of Autism*. Baltimore: Johns Hopkins University Press.
A compendium of academic articles on diverse aspects of autism, from psychology to genetics. A second edition has been published in 2005.

Benton, A. (2000) *Exploring the History of Neuropsychology*. Oxford: Oxford University Press.
A masterly and unusual collection of key papers reflecting on the history and development of the field of neuropsychology; emphasizes unusual aspects of speech disorders and memory. Much of this material is accessible to the interested general reader.

Clarkson, T.W., Friberg, L., Nordberg, G.F. and Sager, P.R. (eds) (1986) *Biological Monitoring of Toxic Metals*. New York: Plenum.
A scientific treatise covering all aspects of tissue sampling and analysis for heavy metal contamination; for professionals.

Cohen, N.J. and Eichenbaum, H. (1993) *Memory, Amnesia and the Hippocampal System*. Cambridge, MA: MIT.
An introduction to the key issues surrounding the understanding of the limbic brain and its relationship to memory; aimed at graduate students and scientists but accessible to the informed reader.

Coleman, M. (ed) (2005) *The Neurology of Autism*. Oxford: Oxford University Press.
A scientific compilation of articles covering brain anatomic features in autism, reversibility of the condition, and outlines of therapeutic approaches.

Crowcroft, P. (1966) *Mice All Over*. London: G.T. Foulis & Co.
A brilliant anecdotal account of the complexities of rodent society. A must for students of all aspects of sociobiology but eminently accessible and informative for the general reader.

Delacour, J. (ed) (1994) *The Memory System of the Brain*. Singapore: World Scientific.
A scholarly compendium of articles on aspects of memory; the approach is philosophical and many of the articles have stood the test of time. For the student of memory function.

Denton, D. (1982) *The Hunger for Salt*. Berlin: Springer.
An extraordinary and outstanding treatise on all aspects of salt, from history to sociology to physiology. The central conjecture is that there is a specific motivation or hunger for salt consumption

that is unleashed on salt deprivation; Denton provides a clear exposition of the subservience of the mind to physiological stimuli. For the scientist and philosopher, with many sections being accessible to the general reader.

Diamond, A. (ed) (1991) *Developmental and Neural Basis of Higher Cognitive Function.* New York: New York Academy of Sciences.
This collection of scientific papers is published as a special issue of the Annals of the New York Academy of Sciences. While researchers for the most part dwell on brain function in the adult, the collection emphasizes aspects of cognition and memory in young children. For specialists.

Freeman, J.M., Freeman, J.B. and Kelly, M.T. (2000) *The Ketogenic Diet.* New York: Demos Medical Publishing.
A practical guide to implementing the ketogenic diet as a therapy for epilepsy. For families and practitioners. A new version of this book will become available in late 2006.

Frith, U.T. (ed) (1992) *Autism and Asperger Syndrome.* Cambridge: Cambridge University Press.
A compendium of articles dealing primarily with Asperger syndrome and overlaps with autism proper. A must for students with Asperger.

Gillberg, C. and Coleman, M. (2000) *The Biology of the Autistic Syndromes.* Cambridge: MacKeith–Cambridge University Press.
This book covers all aspects of autism and related developmental disorders. It is an authoritative and informative academic work, and required reading for the student and professional. Some sections may not be entirely accessible to the non-specialist, but overall the book is outstanding.

Grandin, T. (1995) *Thinking in Pictures.* New York: Doubleday.
An unusual first-hand account of what it means to be a scientist with an autism spectrum disorder; provides a fascinating insight into how perception of the everyday world is subtly skewed in autism, and how some simple behavioral remedies can reattune the affected individual. Recommended reading for both professional and the general reader.

Gray, J.A. (1982) *The Neuropsychology of Anxiety: An Enquiry into the Function of the Septo-Hippocampal System.* Oxford: Oxford University Press.
Gray, J.A. and McNaughton, N. (2000) *The Neuropsychology of Anxiety: An Enquiry into the Functions of the Septo-Hippocampal System.* Oxford: Oxford University Press.
In two editions, this highly technical work covers the structure and function of the limbic brain. The central thesis is that anxiety is determined by the hippocampus and conjoined brain regions. Required reading for the student of the limbic brain.

Hallaway, N. and Strauts, Z. (1995) *Turning Lead into Gold: How Heavy Metal Poisoning Can Affect Your Child and How to Prevent and Treat It.* Vancouver: New Start.
A first-hand anecdotal account written by a parent of a child on the autistic spectrum and her practitioner. Very readable with many insights, a useful and informative introduction to the problems of detecting and treating heavy metal toxicity. For the interested reader.

Isaacson, R.L. and Pribram, K.H. (eds) (1975) *The Hippocampus, Vol. 1. Structure and Development;* and *Vol. 2, Neurophysiology and Behavior.* New York: Plenum.
Although now somewhat dated, this excellent compendium of scientific articles addresses many aspects of hippocampal function that are sometimes forgotten. The treatment is academic, but essential reading for the keen student of brain function.

Kandel, E., Schwartz, J.H. and Jessel, T.M. (eds) (2000) *Principles of Neural Science.* New York: McGraw-Hill.

The classic student textbook of brain science. Comprehensively explains all aspects of the brain, from molecules to psychiatry. Although written for students and academics, it is very well presented and many topics are accessible to the non-specialist.

Kaufman, B.N. (1995) *Son-Rise: The Miracle Continues.* Tiburon, CA: H.J. Kramer Press.

A first-hand account of the evolution of a seriously affected child with autism into an adult with few if any traces of the disorder. Kaufman provides a detailed history of this transition and many pointers to the unusual features of autism. For the general reader, but as a case-study merits consideration by professionals.

McCandless, J. (2003) *Children with Starving Brains: A Medical Treatment Guide for Autism Spectrum Disorder.* Putney, VT: Bramble Books.

A guide to medical intervention in autism and related disorders, covering the field from gastrointestinal involvement to heavy metal detoxification. Written by a medical practitioner, the book avoids technical discussion and is designed for families and physicians.

Maurice, C., Green, G. and Luce, S.C. (eds) (1996) *Behavioral Intervention for Young Children with Autism: A Manual for Parents and Professionals.* Austin, TX: Pro-Ed.

An excellent and fairly comprehensive guide to behavioral therapy in autism, presented in a way that is easily assimilated by both families and professionals.

Pangborn, J., Baker, S. and Rimland, B. (2005) *Autism: Effective Biomedical Treatments (The DAN Protocol).* San Diego: Autism Research Institute.

This 2005 guide is the most up-to-date biomedical treatment manual for autism and related disorders, and contains many details of nutritional aspects written in a style open to the general reader. For families and physicians.

Rimland, B., Sermon, B. and Kornblum, L. (1992) *Feast Without Yeast: 4 Stages to Better Health.* Wisconsin: Wisconsin Institute of Nutrition.

A practical guide to avoiding yeast overgrowth, including gluten-free and casein-free diets. For families.

Shaw, W. (2002) *Biological Treatments for Autism and PDD.* Lenexa, KS: Great Plains Laboratory.

A useful and fairly comprehensive manual for families and practitioners, providing accessible scientific explanations of treatments and therapies.

Volkmar, F. (ed) (1998) *Autism and Pervasive Developmental Disorders.* Cambridge: Cambridge University Press.

A compendium of scientific articles on autism prevalence, diagnosis, and therapy. For the specialist and academic.

Williams, D. (1996) *Autism: An Inside Out Approach.* London: Jessica Kingsley Publishers.

Complementary to Grandin's book, this work gives a highly readable first-hand account of what it means to live with autism, and provides many insights into the condition and practical recommendations for how to work with individuals on the autism spectrum. For families and practitioners.

Index

The following abbreviations are used: DSM-IV for *Diagnostic and Statistical Manual of Mental Disorders, 4th edition*, ICD-10 for *International Classification of Diseases, issue 10*. Figures and tables are denoted by italic page numbers.